Neurocircuitry and Neuroautonomic Disorders

Neurocircuitry and Neuroautonomic Disorders

Reviews and Therapeutic Strategies

Fuad Lechin Caracas
Bertha van der Dijs Caracas
Marcel E. Lechin College Station, Tex.

72 figures, 28 in color, 12 tables, 2002

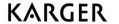 **KARGER**   Basel · Freiburg · Paris · London · New York ·
New Delhi · Bangkok · Singapore · Tokyo · Sydney

Dr. Fuad Lechin

Instituto de Medicina Experimental
Facultad de Medicina
Universidad Central de Venezuela
Caracas (Venezuela)
Fax +58 212 575 3161
E-Mail flechin@telcel.net.ve

Dr. Bertha van der Dijs

Instituto de Medicina Experimental
Facultad de Medicina
Universidad Central de Venezuela
Caracas (Venezuela)

Dr. Marcel E. Lechin

School of Medicine at Texas
A&M University College Station
1605 Rock Prairie Road
College Station, TX 77845 (USA)

Library of Congress Cataloging-in-Publication Data

Bibliographic Indices. This publication is listed in bibliographic services, including Current Contents:®

Drug Dosage. The authors and the publisher have exerted every effort to ensure that drug selection and dosage set forth in this text are in accord with current recommendations and practice at the time of publication. However, in view of ongoing research, changes in government regulations, and the constant flow of information relating to drug therapy and drug reactions, the reader is urged to check the package insert for each drug for any change in indications and dosage and for added warnings and precautions. This is particularly important when the recommended agent is a new and/or infrequently employed drug.

© Copyright 2002 by S. Karger AG,
P.O. Box, CH–4009 Basel (Switzerland)
Printed in Switzerland on acid-free paper by
Reinhardt Druck, Basel
www.karger.com
ISBN 3–8055–7413–4

Contents

Contents

Preface

Upon receiving my MD from the Central University of Venezuela, I entered directly into postdoctoral studies and earned degrees in Internal Medicine and Gastroenterology, followed by special training at the Hopital Saint Antoine in Paris and the Philadelphia Postgraduate Hospital. For several years afterward, while practicing medicine in Caracas, I underwent psychoanalysis five times a week (11 years) under the direction of senior psychoanalysts of the International Association of Psychoanalysis. This training encouraged me to use psychoanalysis in the study of many of my patients diagnosed as having duodenal ulcer, ulcerative colitis, irritable bowel syndrome, headache and other ailments.

At the same time, I began a rigorous study of the basic sciences including physiology, pharmacology, biochemistry, immunology, mathematics and statistics. I won a departmental staff position in physiology at the School of Medicine of the Central University of Venezuela where my group began experimental research with mammals. My group published their work on gastric, pancreatic, hepatic, metabolic and physiological studies in basic science journals. I brought my knowledge of the sciences of physiology, pharmacology and psychology into my clinical practice.

My research on the physiology and physiopathology of gastrointestinal motility began in the 1960s. I studied the effects of emotions (principally anger, fear and happiness) and of drugs affecting the brain on gastrointestinal motility in humans and dogs. I learned that strong emotion, like the central-acting drugs (lacking peripheral action), can significantly affect gastrointestinal motility that is the tone or contraction of intestinal muscles. I published

these findings, leading me to the major concept of 'brain-gut axis', in journals of pharmacology, physiology, gastroenterology and psychiatry. The discovery by Dr. Michael Gershon that myenteric plexa neurons (nerve cells located between the intestinal muscle layers) of the gastrointestinal tract form part of the central nervous system enabled me to understand that intestinal physiological disorders (malfunctioning) are also related to the brain. A blood-intestinal barrier similar to the blood-brain barrier that isolates the central nervous system from the peripheral circulation protects the nerve cells of the intestinal wall. These neurons do not make contact with blood. Step by step, I finally concluded that the brain is involved in the cause, or etiology, of all disease.

Since the late 1960s, my group has been immersed in the systematic study of the physiology (functioning), chemistry and central or brain circuitry of neurons, and the mechanisms of their physiological interactions. Finally, I turned to the study of the complex role of neuropharmacological drugs, i.e. those that act on brain neurons. From these studies I have published two books and numerous papers correlating my research findings with data gained from reading and rereading thousands of articles published in scientific journals. This dynamic process gradually reshaped my diagnostic and therapeutic procedures. The growing success of my treatment of patients who had formerly failed to respond encouraged me to keep working.

The functioning of the autonomic nervous system (ANS) reflects the activity of monoamines in the brain (noradrenaline = NA, adrenaline = Ad, dopamine = DA, serotonin = 5HT, acetylcholine = ACh, etc.). These neurotransmitters do not cross the blood-brain barrier. However, the assessment in plasma of NA, Ad, DA, 5HT and their metabolites reveals information about their central activity. In addition, the administration of low doses of central acting drugs, oral glucose or different types of stress challenges (orthostasis, exercise) triggers plasma neurotransmitter changes, which afford information about neurochemical changes in the CNS circuitry. To this end, my group installed a plasma neurotransmitters laboratory (the only in the world at the hospital level) where all brain monoamines may be routinely investi-

gated during both health and nonhealth situations. This valuable tool gave us the opportunity to assess the CNS neurochemical state. Up to the present, we have investigated some 25,000 normal and diseased subjects throughout the last 30 years. Endocrine and immunological investigations have also been included systematically throughout the last 25 years.

Finally, a sleep research lab was installed 2 years ago in order to assess plasma neurotransmitters throughout the different sleep stages (SWS 1, 2, 3, 4 and REM).

Fuad Lechin

Overview

The first part of this book is devoted to the outlining of neurocircuitry throughout the wake-sleep cycle in normal subjects. These postulations are made on the bases of findings of hundreds of experiments carried out on mammals. Thus, active waking, quiet waking (drowsiness), SWS and REM sleep are depicted. Other proposals are made dealing with endogenous depression (ED), dysthymic depression (DD), uncoping stress (US) situation, psychotics, bipolar disorder and panic attacks. These oversimplified models do not include all the neuronal connections involved in them, but highlight the most relevant disorders dealing with them. We hope that these schematic models will help doctors understand the neurophysiological and neurochemical disorders underlying those syndromes and thus help them prescribe more accurate and scientific therapeutic approaches. We ourselves have outlined successful therapeutic approaches for thousands of patients. Many of our double-blind crossover trials have been published in scientific journals.

We developed the only clinical neurochemistry lab in which plasma neurotransmitters are routinely investigated in both normal and diseased subjects. Circulating neurotransmitters include NA, Ad, DA, f5HT and p5HT. Plasma TRP is also assessed routinely. All these parameters are dosified during supine resting condition and after several types of stress challenge (orthostasis, moderate exercise, oral glucose) as well as after administration of several central-acting drugs (buspirone, clonidine, tianeptine, etc.).

Results obtained in normal as well as in psychiatric or somatic diseased subjects led us to postulate the existence of at least 3 well-defined types of profile: (a) ED; (b) DD, and (c) US. In accordance with this paradigm, ED = increased NA/Ad ratio (>5) + low TRP plasma level; DD = low NA + raised TRP, and US = low NA/Ad ratio (<2) + high f5HT. Increased platelet aggregability was found routinely in US patients. According to the above, we propose the paradigm ED vs. US. Higher than normal central NA activity + lower than normal central 5HT activity (low plasmaTRP) is registered in ED patients. Conversely, exhausted central NA activity + increased adrenomedullary (compensatory) sympathetic activity is registered in US patients. Therefore, patients showing those opposite neurochemical + neurophysiological disorders should receive distinct neuropharmacological therapies. This hypothesis has been supported by successful treatments in some 25,000 psychiatric and somatic patients.

Furthermore, our research work showed that those autoimmune diseases labeled Th-1 type (increased cellular immunity) always present with an ED neurochemical profile. Conversely, those autoimmune diseases associated with a Th-2 profile always present with a US neurochemical profile. These findings led us to design successful neuropharmacological therapies for many types of autoimmune disease. Special mention should be made of successful treatment in some 800 myasthenia gravis patients and some 16,000 asthmatic subjects.

The book gives illustrations of some successfully treated patients who were affected by cancer, Crohn's disease, psoriasis, pemphigus, atopic dermatitis or Sjögren disease.

Fuad Lechin
Bertha van der Dijs
Marcel E. Lechin

Introduction

The scientific tools necessary to provide the best therapeutic approaches are available but underutilized by physicians. Instead, physicians often 'cure' diseases by using treatments that address only symptoms or peripheral disturbances. These disturbances are the last link in a long chain of complex events. True diagnoses and successful treatments can only be achieved when physicians use scientific information to follow the physiological chain of events underlying the disease.

The practice of medicine is divided into two camps of doctors engaged in combating disease: scientists and clinicians. The former acquires knowledge about physiology, pathophysiology, pharmacology, neurochemistry, neuroendocrinology, immunology, genetics, biochemistry, and many other disciplines. Unfortunately, these scientific doctors do not practice medicine.

Conversely, many physicians or clinical practitioners possess only superficial knowledge of the above disciplines and so are limited to rudimentary and simplistic diagnostic and therapeutic procedures for suppressing symptoms. They do their best, although sadly it is seldom enough. Furthermore, such doctors spend most of their working life acquiring skills and perfecting techniques and so are unable to keep abreast with the scientific advances which could generate novel treatment strategies. For example, elderly people often have debilitating diseases such as diabetes, hypertension, cardiac arrest and strokes. Physicians usually prescribe for elderly patients symptomatic treatment, such as antihypertensive, antidiabetic, and vascular antispasmodic drugs, which leaves intact the physiologic disorders that trigger the illness. Another example is the standard therapy for duodenal ulcers, omeprazole, which is used to reduce HCl levels by blocking the sodium pump. Physicians are attempting to heal the mucosal damage while creating a physiological disorder. They prescribe antibiotics to kill *Helicobacter pylori*, but leave unchanged the abnormal underlying immunological disorder that allowed the bacteria to damage the mucosa.

In most sleep disorders some phases of slow wave sleep (SWS) disappear. Growth hormone (GH), which is normally produced and released during SWS, is severely suppressed under these circumstances. Considering that GH is one of the most important immunoactivating and restorative agents, it is easy to understand the association between sleep disorders and immunodeficiency, sleep disorders and osteoporosis, etc. However, doctors routinely prescribe benzodiazepines (BDZ) to treat sleep disorders, unaware that these drugs suppress phases 3 and 4 of SWS as well as REM sleep, which is responsible for the recovery of intellectual functions.

In late 1996, one of us (Dr. F. Lechin) suddenly developed myasthenia gravis during a period of excessive stress. Although neurologists prescribed pyridostigmine (Mestinon), steroids, and other immunosuppressant drugs, he refused this potentially deleterious regimen and conducted a neurochemical and immunological analysis. This revealed that he had a neurochemical and neuroimmune uncoping-stress profile in addition to acetylcholine-receptor autoantibodies in his blood. His adrenaline and free serotonin plasma levels were high; his noradrenaline levels were low, and platelet aggregability was increased. In addition, he had increased numbers of CD5+ B autoreactive lymphocytes and NK cells, high levels of IgM and

IL-6, and decreased NK cell cytotoxicity against K562 target cells. Because of these findings, he began a neuro-pharmacological antistress treatment addressed to reversing his neurochemical disorders. His regimen comprised doxepin (10 mg), phenylalanine (a NA precursor, 50 mg), buspirone (5 mg) (before breakfast) and 5-OH-tryptophan (25 mg before supper). All symptoms disappeared after 3 weeks of treatment. Normalization of the neurochemical disorder paralleled clinical improvement. Acetylcholine autoantibodies disappeared progressively over the next 6 months. His immunological status returned to normal by 3 months. Currently, Dr. Lechin does not take any drugs and he continues to walk 5 km daily.

Dr. F. Lechin's research group has treated (free of charge) about 800 patients with myasthenia gravis from various countries. We published 2 papers on our preliminary findings. Although all MG patients benefit significantly from our treatment, thymectomized MG patients (but not non-thymectomized patients) do not recover totally. Neurologists and other physicians cannot prescribe this type of neuropharmacological and neuroimmunological therapy because of a lack of training in the necessary scientific disciplines.

As a member of the American Physiological Society, Dr. F. Lechin published a letter to the editor in the journal *The Physiologist*. He argued vehemently for an increase in the number of courses in physiology and other basic sciences in the curriculum of medical schools. He believes that a stronger basic sciences curriculum in training clinicians will benefit society by improving clinical care.

The final chapters of this book refer to various neuro-pharmacological therapeutic approaches which are able to cure or improve many types of disease including cancer, multiple sclerosis, Crohn's enteritis, RCU, pancreatitis, biliary dyskinesia, IBS, Sjögren's disease, psoriasis, pemphigus, rheumatoid arthritis, dermatomyositis, uveitis, pulmonary fibrosis, Takayashu's disease, and others.

Our research work on the physiology and pathophysiology of gastrointestinal motility began in the 1960s. We studied and learned that emotions as well as central-acting drugs (lacking peripheral action) can significantly affect gastrointestinal motility. We published many research papers dealing with this issue, which allowed us to establish the brain-gut axis. This bulk of research was useful to the better understanding of gastrointestinal disorders but, at the same time, allowed us to demonstrate that

psychiatric disturbances and illness reflect on gastrointestinal motility and other visceral areas. We showed that schizophrenic patients present a typical distal colon motility profile that was normalized with clonidine. This 'antihypertensive' drug was able to suppress acute psychotic episodes. Further, we demonstrated that psychotic patients present a plasma neurotransmitter disorder characterized by excessive adrenaline (Ad), low noradrenaline (NA), high platelet serotonin (p5HT) and high free serotonin (f5HT). These findings allowed us to understand the physiological and physiopathological integration of the human being. The fact that both uncoping stressed and schizophrenic patients share similar distal colon motility plus plasma neurotransmitters and immunological profiles supports the postulation that neuroautonomic, neurochemical and immune systems are closely interrelated and maintain a permanent dialogue. The finding that clonidine [an α_2-agonist drug which bridles the C1-Ad medullary and/or the A6-LC-NA (pontine nuclei)] is able to reduce colonic motility, suppress pancreatic inflammation, suppress acute psychotic episodes, increase growth hormone release and lower BP demonstrates that central-acting drugs should no longer be labeled as 'antipsychotics', 'antidiarrheics', 'antihypertensives', 'antidepressants', etc. Science should make incursion into the practice of medicine. Science means physiology, physiopathology, pharmacology, immunology, neurochemistry, etc. While doctors are still trained as technicians but not scientists, the pharmaceutical industry but not doctors prescribe treatments to patients.

Here are some examples of the above statements. In 1994, our group reported that free serotonin (f5HT) in the plasma increased during asthma attacks. In 1996, we published another paper ratifying the above findings, and in 1998, published two research papers showing that tianeptine (a drug which reduces f5HT plasma levels) provokes a dramatic and sudden decrease of both clinical rating and f5HT, at the same time normalizing pulmonary function. Despite these impressive results doctors who treat asthmatic patients have been not able to assimilate its significance. They have inadequate information about plasma serotonin, platelet uptake of serotonin, pulmonary functioning and serotonin, etc. They only know that tianeptine is an 'antidepressant'. In the meanwhile, 600 million people are waiting for an appropriate therapy which will be able to save them from suffocation.

Chapter 1

....

Central Neurocircuitry Functioning during the Wake-Sleep Cycle

The wake-sleep cycle includes: (1) active waking; (2) drowsiness; (3) slow wave sleep (SWS), and (4) rapid eye movement (REM) sleep; SWS includes four stages or phases: 1, 2, 3 and 4.

Active Waking

Noradrenergic Nucleus

The locus coeruleus (LC) or A6 noradrenergic (NA) pontine cell group (blue nucleus in the figures) displays maximal activity (4 rings) during this period (fig. 1.1). Excitatory inputs: glutamic, corticotropin-releasing factor or hormone (CRF), ACh (nicotinic) and β-adrenergic predominate over inhibitory inputs: GABA, $5HT_2$, α_2, imidazole and opiates. NA is released at brain cortex and at all subcortical, pontine, medullary and spinal areas receiving NA-LC axons. Serotonergic (5HT), dopaminergic (DA), CRF, acetylcholinergic (ACh) and Ad neurons receive excitatory and/or inhibitory (monosynaptic or polysynaptic) influences from the LC (fig. 1.5, 1.6).

Serotonergic Nuclei

The dorsal raphe (DR), median raphe (MR) and the periaqueductal gray (PAG) serotonergic pontine nuclei receive LC-NA axons. Noradrenaline released from NA axons exerts excitatory influences on 5HT neurons by acting at the postsynaptic α_1-receptors. Physiological studies have demonstrated that NA-DR innervation plays an important role in maintaining the tonic firing activity of 5HT neurons. There is strong evidence suggesting that the NA input to DR-5HT neurons may exert its α_1-excitatory effect through an interposed GABA neuron. In addition, experimental evidence demonstrates that NA input inhib-

its DR-5HT neurons through α_2-adrenoceptors. Despite this inhibitory effect, NA facilitation of DR-5HT activity is well established. Although recent pharmacological evidence demonstrates that LC-NA axons trigger MR-5HT neuron excitation through α_1-postsynaptic receptors located at this level, this effect requires maximal doses of microinjected α_1-agonists.

DR- and MR-5HT nuclei send inhibitory axons to LC-NA neurons. This effect is mediated through $5HT_2$ postsynaptic receptors. In addition, both DR-5HT and MR-5HT nuclei interchange inhibitory axons. Serotonergic receptors involved in this inhibitory interchange include $5HT_{1A}$ and $5HT_{1b}$ receptors located at the soma-dendritic areas. According to the above, both LC-NA and DR-5HT + MR-5HT neurons display maximal activity during active waking periods. Therefore, NA and 5HT are released in all brain areas innervated by these nuclei.

The DR-5HT nucleus sends projections to the brain cortex, mainly in the temporoparietal and frontal areas, as well as to the striatum, amygdala, nucleus accumbens, lateral septum and hypothalamus (ventromedial mainly). The median eminence, outside the blood-brain barrier (BBB), is also innervated by DR axons. Some DR axons project to the dorsal hippocampus and brain stem reticular formation, and pedunculo-pontine nucleus (PPN).

The MR-5HT nucleus projects into the brain cortex, mainly the prefrontal, temporal, and parietal, hippocampus, septum, and other mesolimbic structures. The anterior preoptic hypothalamic area is selectively innervated by MR-5HT axons. Further, MR innervates brain stem reticular formation, also.

Raphe magnus (RM) and raphe pallidus (RP) medullary serotonergic nuclei display maximal activity during active waking periods. On the contrary, activity of the

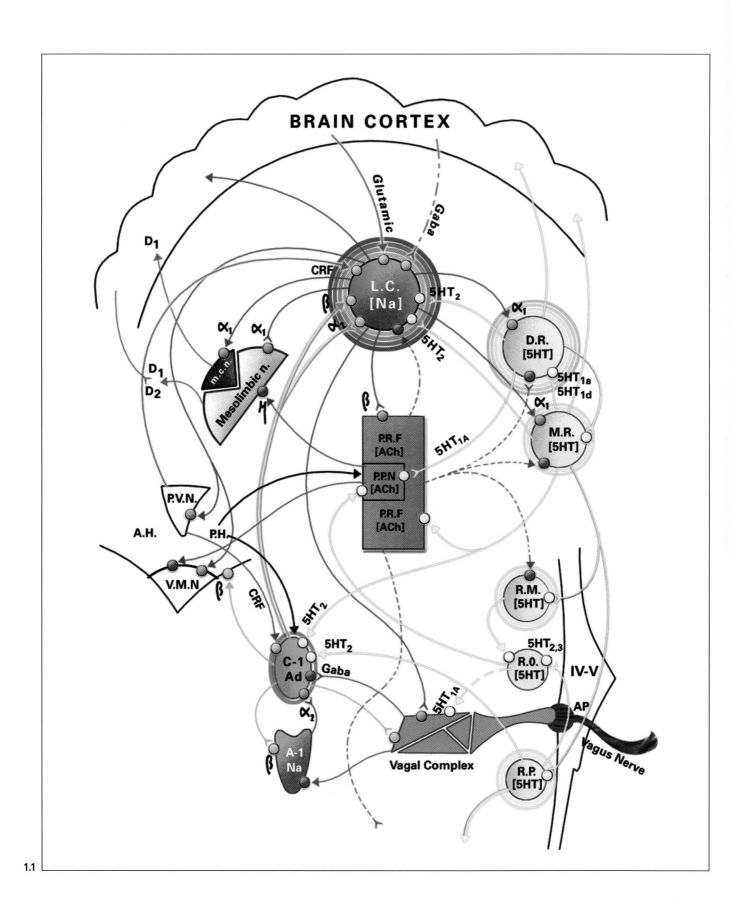

Central Neurocircuitry Functioning during
the Wake-Sleep Cycle

1.1

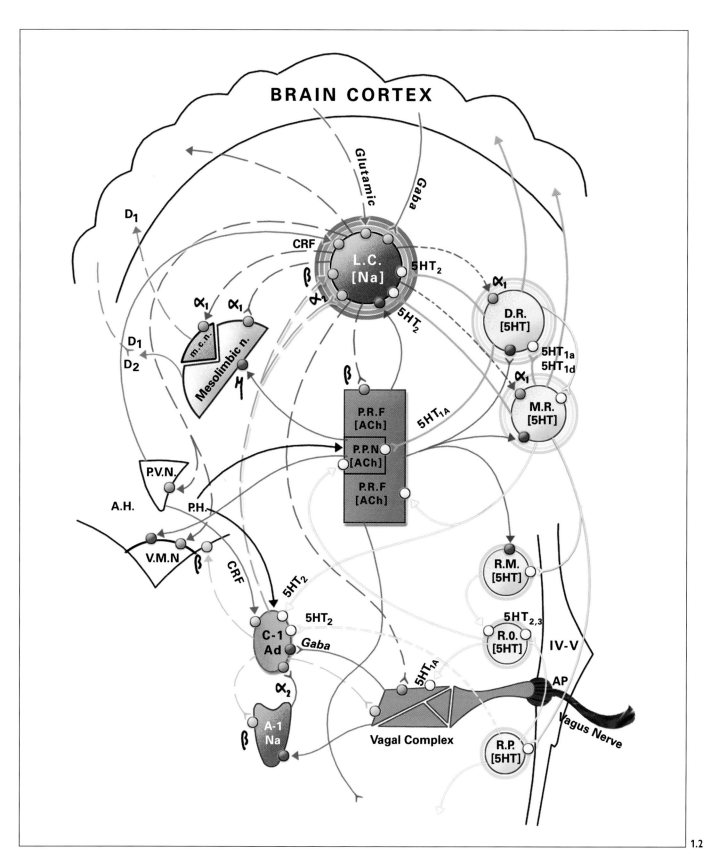

raphe obscurus (RO) nuclei correlates positively with parasympathetic activity periods (postprandial, drowsiness and sleep). These statements are consistent with findings that whereas RM and RP serotonergic nuclei send excitatory axons to the C1-Ad neurons and to the spinal preganglionic sympathetic neurons, the RO-5HT nucleus sends excitatory axons to vagal motoneurons.

Dopaminergic Nuclei

The LC-NA nucleus sends excitatory and inhibitory axons to the mesocortical and mesolimbic DA neurons, respectively. Both mesocortical and mesolimbic DA neurons integrate the ventral tegmental area (VTA = A10) neuronal group. According to this, DA is released at cortical level during waking periods (only at deep layers of the cortex: 5 and 6 layers). On the other hand, mesolimbic DA neurons receive excitatory signals from the pedunculo-pontine nucleus (PPN) (glutamic) and inhibitory signals from the LC-NA nucleus (α_1-receptor mediated). DR-5HT and MR-5HT axons reach the A10-DA and ACh (muscarinic) neurons, respectively, and display excitatory effects at these levels.

However, serotonin released from the DR axons at the mesocortical and mesolimbic areas inhibits the dopamine released from DA axons by acting at the $5HT_2$ receptors located at the DA terminals. Maximal release of cortical DA occurs during active waking periods. This cortical DA activity exerts an inhibitory control over subcortical DA release (mesolimbic and mesostriate areas).

Paraventricular Nucleus

LC-NA axons innervate the paraventricular nucleus (PVN) and excite CRF neurons. CRF axons innervate and stimulate LC-NA neurons. Thus, a positive feedback exists between these two nuclei. In addition, although LC-NA axons do not reach Ad neurons of the C1 medullary nucleus, NA-activated CRF axons stimulate the C1 nucleus. Thus, a polysynaptic excitatory circuit exists between the LC-NA and the C1-Ad nuclei. The latter sends axons to the LC-NA nucleus. These Ad axons reaching the LC-NA exert stimulatory and inhibitory effects through, respectively, the β- and α_2-postsynaptic receptors located at the LC-NA neurons. Considering that the C1-Ad nucleus is responsible for adrenal gland secretion, the neuronal circuitry LC-PVN-C1 governs the sympathetic activity associated with active waking periods. Finally, both LC-NA and C1-Ad nuclei send inhibitory axons to the vagal complex, whose activity is reduced during active waking periods.

Drowsiness

Fading of LC-NA and C1-Ad activities governs the main neurophysiological changes registered during this period. Reduction of dopamine (DA) mesocortical activity results from minimization of the NA excitatory influence. The vagal complex is disinhibited from the LC + C1 inhibitory influences, thus parasympathetic activity is increased (fig. 1.2, 1.5, 1.6).

Slow Wave Sleep

Although SWS includes four progressive stages (1, 2, 3 and 4) we depict here the two deepest stages (3 and 4) only. LC-NA, DR-5HT and MR-5HT nuclei show progressive reduction of their firing activities (fig. 1.3, 1.5,

Fig. 1.1. Active waking. LC = Locus coeruleus; DR = dorsal raphe; MR = median raphe; RM = raphe magnus; RO = raphe obscurus; RP = raphe pallidus; mcn = mesocortical nucleus; PVN = paraventricular nucleus; AH = anterior hypothalamus; PH = posterior hypothalamus; VMN = ventromedial nucleus; PRF = pontoreticular formation; PPN = pedunculopontine nucleus; CRF = corticotrophin-releasing factor; AP = area postrema; Na = noradrenaline; Ad = adrenaline; ACh = acetylcholine; 5HT = serotonin. → Excitation; ─< inhibition. Concentric circles, bright and faded colors indicate neuronal activity; dashed lines indicate reduced output.

Fig. 1.2. Drowsiness. LC = Locus coeruleus; DR = dorsal raphe; MR = median raphe; RM = raphe magnus; RO = raphe obscurus; RP = raphe pallidus; mcn = mesocortical nucleus; PVN = paraventricular nucleus; AH = anterior hypothalamus; PH = posterior hypothalamus; VMN = ventromedial nucleus; PRF = pontoreticular formation; PPN = pedunculo pontine nucleus; CRF = corticotrophin-releasing factor; AP = area postrema; Na = noradrenaline; Ad = adrenaline; ACh = acetylcholine; 5HT = serotonin. → Excitation; ─< inhibition. Concentric circles, bright and faded colors indicate neuronal activity. Dashed lines indicate reduced output.

Fig. 1.3. Slow wave sleep. LC = Locus coeruleus; DR = dorsal raphe; MR = median raphe; RM = raphe magnus; RO = raphe obscurus; RP = raphe pallidus; mcn = mesocortical nucleus; PVN = paraventricular nucleus; AH = anterior hypothalamus; PH = posterior hypothalamus; VMN = ventromedial nucleus; PRF = pontoreticular formation; PPN = pedunculopontine nucleus; CRF = corticotrophin-releasing factor; AP = area postrema; Na = noradrenaline; Ad = adrenaline; ACh = acetylcholine; 5HT = serotonin. → Excitation; ─< inhibition. Concentric circles, bright and faded colors indicate neuronal activity. Dashed lines indicate reduced output.

Central Neurocircuitry Functioning during the Wake-Sleep Cycle

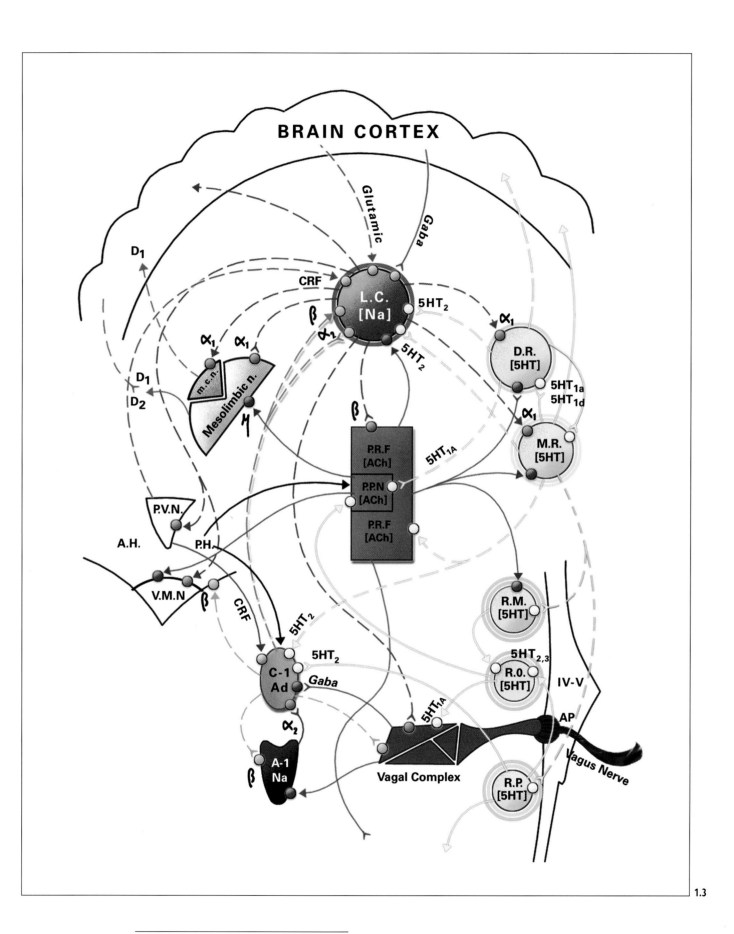

1.6). Although MR-5HT nucleus also shows progressive inhibition, this serotonergic nucleus does not fall to zero firing activity during SWS. MR activity cooperates with RO-serotonergic nucleus in the facilitation of vagal complex activity, which is progressively disinhibited from the LC-NA axons. All this results in a predominance of vagal complex activity over the C1-Ad medullary nucleus activity responsible for peripheral adrenal gland secretion. With respect to this, we found that whereas NA + Ad plasma levels fall during SWS, platelet serotonin (p5HT) shows raised blood levels. Additionally, plasma levels of free serotonin (f5HT) increase during SWS. Conversely, tryptophan plasma levels decrease during SWS. Accordingly, whereas p5HT correlates positively with RO-5HT and parasympathetic nuclei, plasma tryptophan levels correlate positively with the pontine serotonergic nuclei (DR and MR). Therefore, whereas tryptophan plasma levels correlates positively with blood pressure and heart rate (both decrease during SWS), p5HT correlates negatively with these two parameters. Central dopaminergic activity remains constant throughout SWS. Acetylcholinergic (ACh) neurons from the midbrain and medullary reticular formation (red color) become disinhibited from the LC-NA axons during SWS and show increased activity. These midbrain and medullary ACh neurons send motor inhibitory axons to the spinal anterior horns. This inhibitory influence is antagonized by serotonergic axons arising from the RP medullary serotonergic nucleus. This explains why muscular atonia is not registered during SWS. However, muscular atonia will occur during REM sleep when the RP-5HT nucleus is totally inhibited.

Rapid Eye Movement Sleep

LC-NA, DR-5HT, MR-5HT nuclei display zero activity during this period, whereas midbrain and medullary ACh neurons show maximal activity (figs. 1.4–1.6). Dopaminergic activity is constantly present throughout REM sleep. ACh released from ACh axons at the spinal motor neuron level triggers muscular atonia because RP-5HT axons do not release serotonin at this level during REM sleep. Maximal vagal complex activity is registered during REM sleep. Acetylcholine released from ACh axons reaching the LC-NA neurons will stimulate NA neurons and REM sleep will end (± 10 min). Several mechanisms underlie this phenomenon. Although both DR-5HT and MR-5HT nuclei receive excitatory influences from the LC-NA axons, the α_1-DR receptors show higher responsiveness than the α_1-MR receptors. On the other

hand, although both DR and MR nuclei interchange inhibitory axons, the DR-5HT neurons are provided with more $5HT_{1A}$ +$5HT_{1D}$ inhibitory autoreceptors than are the MR neurons. Finally, ACh neurons of the midbrain reticular formation send inhibitory axons to the DR-5HT but not the MR-5HT neurons. These ACh neurons become disinhibited from the bridle of LC-NA axons during both the SWS and the REM sleep periods. According to the above, although both DR-5HT and MR-5HT neurons show progressive reduction of their firing activity throughout SWS and REM sleep, only DR but not MR neurons became completely silent.

Periaqueductal gray-5HT and raphe magnus-5HT neurons become disinhibited from the DR-5HT neurons bridle during SWS sleep and REM sleep. Other medullary serotonergic nuclei (raphe obscurus and raphe pallidus) remain active during SWS; the former is responsible for the excitation of the vagal complex (including nucleus tractus solitarius (NTS) and nucleus ambiguus). The raphe pallidus nucleus is responsible for maintenance of muscle tone during SWS, an effect exerted through release of 5HT at the spinal motoneurons located at the anterior horns. However, this effect disappears during REM sleep. ACh axons arising from midbrain and medullary neurons override release of 5HT at those levels and trigger total muscle atonia during REM sleep.

Circulating Neurotransmitter Profiles throughout the Normal Wake-Sleep Cycle

Circulating parameters: NA, Ad, DA, f5HT, plasma TRP and p5HT have been routinely investigated by us during the last 22 years in some 25,000 normal and diseased subjects. These parameters were assessed during supine resting, orthostasis and moderate exercise conditions. In addition, we also tested the effects of oral glucose, as well as of many central-acting drugs such as cloni-

Fig. 1.4. REM sleep. LC = Locus coeruleus; DR = dorsal raphe; MR = median raphe; RM = raphe magnus; RO = raphe obscurus; RP = raphe pallidus; mcn = mesocortical nucleus; PVN = paraventricular nucleus; AH = anterior hypothalamus; PH = posterior hypothalamus; VMN = ventromedial nucleus; PRF = pontoreticular formation; PPN = pedunculo pontine nucleus; CRF = corticotrophin-releasing factor; AP = area postrema; Na = noradrenaline; Ad = adrenaline; ACh = acetylcholine; 5HT = serotonin. → Excitation; ⊸ inhibition. Concentric circles, bright and faded colors indicate neuronal activity. Dashed lines indicate reduced output.

Central Neurocircuitry Functioning during the Wake-Sleep Cycle

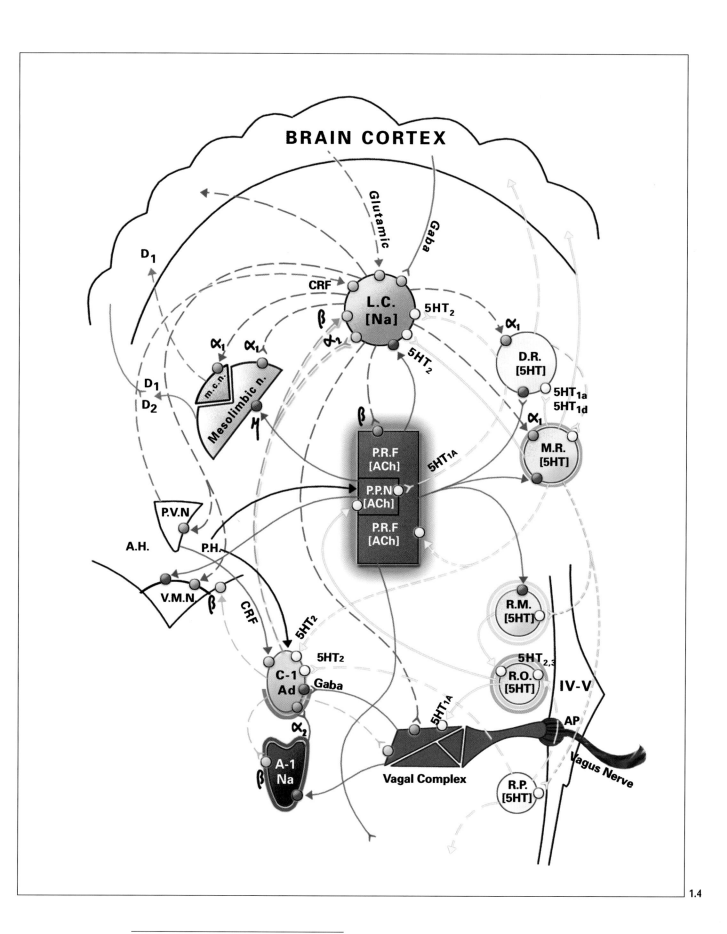

Circulating Neurotransmitter Profiles
throughout the Normal Wake-Sleep Cycle

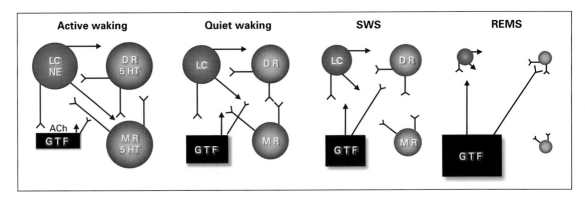

Fig. 1.5. Sleep-wake cycle. Sequence of monoaminergic and cholinergic nuclei predominances. LC-NE axons activates DR-5HT and MR-5HT neurons and in addition, inhibit ACh-giganto tegmental field neurons. Fading of LC-NE neurons disinhibit ACh-GTF neurons, which show maximal activity during REM sleep period. ACh released from GTF axons triggers activation of LC-NE neurons, which recover activity. At this time, NE is released at both DR and MR neurons. The latter is responsible for the end of REM sleep and re-starting of SWS. → Activates; –< inhibits [Lechin and van der Dijs, Res Commun Psychiatr Behav 1984;9:227–262].

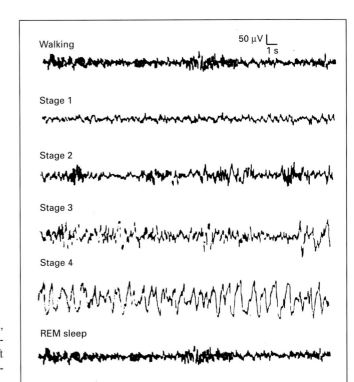

Fig. 1.6. The EEG of sleep in a human adult, shown for each stage of sleep in a single-channel, monopolar recording from the left parietal area, with the ears as a neutral reference point.

dine, atropine, and buspirone [Lechin et al., 1994a, b; Lechin, 2000; Lechin and van der Dijs, 1984; Lechin et al., 1979a–c, 1985a, b, 1987, 1989–1998, 2001]. From the above, we learned that neither absolute nor isolated values of the resulting parameters afford valuable information about the central and/or peripheral neuroautonomic

activities. Conversely, a global profile including all parameters as well as their responsiveness to physiological and pharmacological stimuli provided us with a valuable approach to understanding the above target.

Although absolute NA and Ad plasma values oscillate on a wide range, we found that the normal NA/Ad ratio is

Central Neurocircuitry Functioning during
the Wake-Sleep Cycle

3 to 5. This NA/Ad ratio rises during orthostasis and moderate exercise (5 min walking). Our investigations showed that oral glucose ingestion (75–100 g) and oral buspirone (20 mg) trigger an NA/Ad ratio rise similar to that provoked by orthostasis and/or moderate exercise stress tests. Plasma DA levels do not show a predictable profile of response to these stress tests.

However, circulating indolamines (f5HT and p5HT) show significant increases after oral glucose but not after orthostasis or moderate exercise. Plasma tryptophan levels, which are positively correlated with central serotonergic activity, do not show acute oscillation in these stress tests.

We have also routinely investigated heart rate and blood pressure changes in response to the above-mentioned physiological and pharmacological stimuli.

In view of these findings from tests performed during waking periods, before and after physiological and pharmacological stimuli, we were led to investigate these circulating parameter profiles during drowsiness and the different phases of sleep: SWS and REM sleep. The fact that it has been fully investigated the activities of central NA, 5HT, DA and ACh transmitters in the different sleep stages in experimental mammals allowed us to attempt in this research work the establishment of a possible parallelism between central and peripheral activities.

The results of neurotransmitter parameters registered in the wake period of the wake-sleep cycle showed that NA but not Ad or DA increased in the plasma during short-lasting (1 min) orthostasis (fig. 1.7). Furthermore, an additional rise of NA during moderate exercise (5 min walking) was paralleled by Ad increase. DA showed no significant change at any period. The NA rise during exercise was significantly greater than that of Ad, seen in additional increase of the NA/Ad ratio over that registered at orthostasis. The NA/DA ratio but not the Ad/DA ratio showed significant increase during exercise period (fig. 1.8). The foregoing results are consistent with the postulation that the two sources of plasma catecholamines, the adrenal glands and sympathetic nerves, can function either associatedly or dissociatedly. They are associated during exercise and dissociated at orthostasis. On the other hand, the significant rise of NA/DA ratio during exercise is consistent with the postulation that sympathetic nerves do not release DA at this period. Although tryptophane (TRP) plasma levels did not show significant oscillation throughout the test, TRP values showed negative correlations vs. both Ad and NA, as well as positive correlations with DA. Analysis of these correlations supports the postulation that adrenal rather than

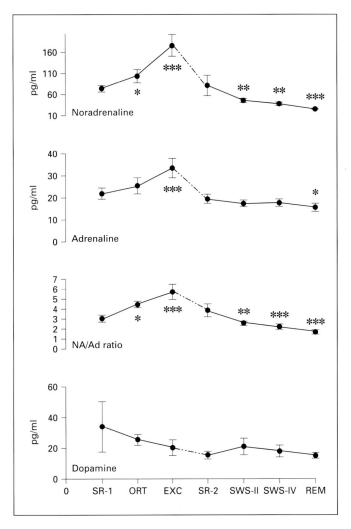

Fig. 1.7. NA, Ad, DA, and NA/Ad plasma values (mean ± SE) obtained from 13 normal subjects throughout supine-resting (SR-1)/orthostasis (ORT)/exercise (EXC) morning test and supine-resting (SR-2)/slow wave sleep-II (SWS-II)/slow wave sleep-IV (SWS-IV)/REM sleep nocturnal test. Both tests were performed on the same day. *, **, *** Levels of significance vs. SR-1 and SR-2, respectively.

neural sympathetic activity is involved in this peripheral indole vs. catechole antagonism. The analysis of correlations is also consistent with the hypothesis that the pool of DA located at the sympathetic nerves plays an inhibitory role in neural sympathetic activity.

While neither plasma f5HT nor p5HT showed significant changes throughout the test, the f5HT/p5HT ratio showed a significant drop at orthostasis when NA, NA/Ad and NA/DA peaks were registered (fig. 1.9).

Analysis of correlations between f5HT vs. TRP allowed us to postulate that these parameters are positively

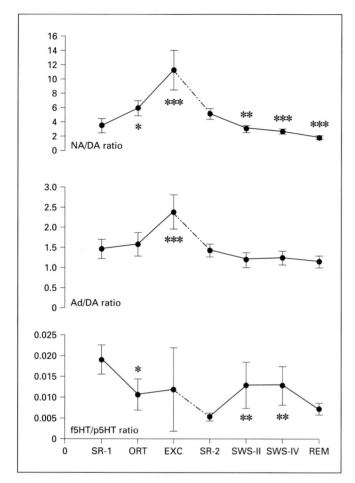

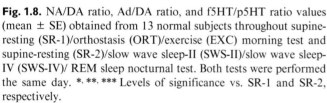

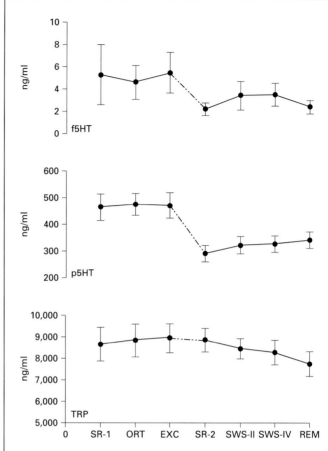

Fig. 1.8. NA/DA ratio, Ad/DA ratio, and f5HT/p5HT ratio values (mean ± SE) obtained from 13 normal subjects throughout supine-resting (SR-1)/orthostasis (ORT)/exercise (EXC) morning test and supine-resting (SR-2)/slow wave sleep-II (SWS-II)/slow wave sleep-IV (SWS-IV)/ REM sleep nocturnal test. Both tests were performed the same day. *, **, *** Levels of significance vs. SR-1 and SR-2, respectively.

Fig. 1.9. f5HT, p5HT and TRP plasma values (mean ± SE) obtained from 13 normal subjects throughout supine-resting (SR-1)/orthostasis (ORT)/exercise (EXC) morning test and supine-resting (SR-2)/ slow wave sleep-II (SWS-II)/slow wave sleep-IV (SWS-IV/REM sleep nocturnal test. Both tests were performed the same day.

associated with parasympathetic activity during the supine resting state. Moreover, it was also shown that p5HT is positively associated with neural sympathetic activity and negatively associated with adrenal sympathetic activity. In addition, analysis of correlations as well as the f5HT/p5HT vs. NA antagonism registered during orthostasis support the postulation that the f5HT/p5HT ratio is an accurate index of parasympathetic activity. Finally, we discuss the possible involvement of two central circuits: the locus coeruleus-NA vs. dorsal raphe + median raphe-5HT pontine nuclei as well as the medullary circuit integrated by the C1-Ad vs. the serotonergic nuclei raphe obscurus and raphe pallidus + the vagal complex.

The results emerging from the study of sleep period of the sleep wake cycle demonstrated that Ad but not NA plasma levels showed significant reduction at the nocturnal supine resting period (SR-2). Although dopamine (DA) plasma values tend to be lower during SR-2 and higher throughout SWS, these oscillations were not significant. NA, NA/Ad and NA/DA values were significantly lower during sleep periods than at the SR-2 period. f5HT and p5HT were found significantly lower throughout the nocturnal than during the diurnal test; however, both parameters showed a progressive rise throughout the SWS and REM periods. Nevertheless, although the mean ± SE values of both parameters were significantly greater than

Central Neurocircuitry Functioning during
the Wake-Sleep Cycle

those registered at the SR-2 period, both remained significantly lower than the SR-1 $\pm$ SE mean values. The f5HT/p5HT ratio level showed significantly lower mean $\pm$ SE values at SR-2 and REM periods, when compared with the SR-1 and SWS periods. TRP plasma levels showed a slow and progressive but not significant decrease throughout the nocturnal periods. Our findings are consistent with the postulation that the two branches of the sympathetic system (adrenal and neural) function in association during SWS-IV and REM sleep but are dissociated during SR-2 and SWS-II. In addition, it is reasonable to assume that nocturnal DA plasma values arise from the sympathetic nerves, mainly, and that the decrease of the NA/DA ratio registered throughout sleep reflects the inhibitory role exerted by the DA pool on NA release from the sympathetic nerves. The positive correlations registered in this study allow us to postulate that both neural and adrenal sympathetic activities tend to increase platelet serotonin stores; however, these positive correlations disappear during exercise, at which period excessive Ad is released to the plasma. In addition, the global analysis of correlations allows us to postulate that tryptophan plasma levels are positively associated with parasympathetic activity (f5HT/p5HT ratio). This association is disrupted during exercise, a period when parasympathetic activity is null. Finally, it was postulated that a close parallelism exists between the peripheral neuroautonomic profile and the central NA, Ad, DA, 5HT and ACh circuitry.

Chapter 2

....

Some Neuroautonomic and Neuroendocrine Changes Registered during the Wake and Sleep Periods

Active Waking Period

During this period, autonomic activity is reflected in the rise of blood pressure and heart rate. This is secondary to increased neural (LC-NA) sympathetic activity + adrenal gland sympathetic activity. CRF + ACTH + cortisol (CRT) + somatostatin are secreted from the hypothalamus, hypophysis and adrenal glands (cortex and medulla), respectively. This neuroendocrine activation results in minimization of parasympathetic tone as well as reduction of growth hormone (GH), GHRH, and gonadotropin secretion.

Prolongation and/or exacerbation of active waking activity may lead to exhaustion of LC-NA activity and depletion of brain NA stores (uncoping stress situation). During these circumstances, all sympathetic activity depends on adrenal gland secretion. At this time, release of NA by sympathetic nerves is reduced to a minimum. The CRF-ACTH-CRT axis predominates over the GHRH-GH and gonadotropins-ovarian axis.

Slow Wave Sleep Period

Autonomic activity is verted to parasympathetic predominance. This is reflected in the reduction of heart rate and blood pressure. LC-NA activity is decreased. The GHRH-GH and gonadotropins ovarian cascades are increased. Adrenomedullary secretions (adrenaline + cortisol) shrink to a minimum. Restorative processes occur. The immunological profile is also reverted to an antistress situation.

Rapid Eye Movement Sleep Period

Maximal parasympathetic activity occurs during this period. Consolidation of memory occurs during REM sleep.

Summarizing, whereas active waking periods travel towards stress, SWS and REM periods take an antistress direction.

Postprandial and Sleep Periods (Antistress Mechanisms)

In addition to sedation and sleep, postprandial and reward periods constitute physiological conditions during which antistress mechanisms are kindled. Parasympathetic hyperactivity is present during these periods (fig. 2.1, 2.2). The vagus nerve provokes serotonin release from the enterochromaffin cells located at the small intestine mucosa. A part of this serotonin (5HT) is verted to the intestinal lumen to facilitate peristalsis; another fraction is verted to the bloodstream. About 70% of circulating serotonin is taken up by the liver, 20% by the lungs and the remaining 10% by platelets. As little as 2% of platelet serotonin (p5HT) is released and circulates free in the plasma (f5HT). Although free serotonin does not cross the BBB, it is able to reach and excite the area postrema (outside the BBB) at the medullary IVth ventricle area. The area postrema constitutes an important sensory structure of the vagal complex. It is crowded with serotonin receptors ($5HT_3$ type) which are excited by free serotonin (f5HT) circulating in the plasma. Free serotonin is greatly increased during postprandial periods because of

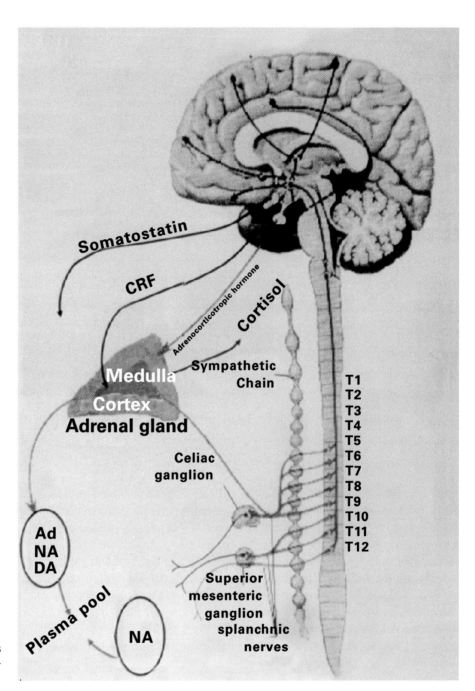

Fig. 2.1. Emotional tension, anxiety states and other mental stresses induce hypothalamic stimulation of CRF and somatostatin.

raised serotonin release at intestinal level and, in addition, because during parasympathetic predominance (postprandial, sedation, sleep) the short-lived circulating ACh interferes with platelet 5HT uptake. Excitatory drive from the sensory area postrema to motor nuclei of the vagus (dorsal and ambiguus) generates a positive feedback which increases and prolongs 5HT release from the small intestine. At the medullary level, excitation of the vagal complex bridles activity of the adrenergic rostral ventral lateral area (C1-Ad nuclei). This nucleus is one of the most important medullary nuclei for the secretion of adrenaline (Ad) by adrenal glands. Injections of retrovirus tracer at the adrenal glands level show that they go directly to the C1-Ad medullary nuclei. The C1-Ad nuclei send axons to the LC-NA nucleus where they are able to trigger excitation of NA neurons (β-receptors) or their inhibition

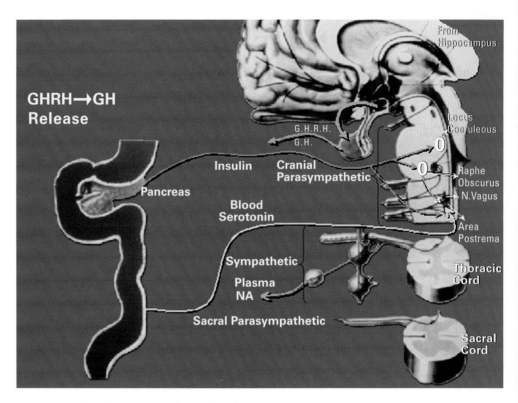

Fig. 2.2. Postprandial state as antistress situation.

(α_2-receptors). Conversely, the LC-NA nucleus does not send monosynaptic innervation to the C1-Ad medullary nuclei. The LC-NA is able to drive C1-Ad activity through polysynaptic mechanisms to the nucleus paraventricularis of the hypothalamus, posterior hypothalamic area and the vagal complex. In light of the above, it may be understood how it is possible for central (neural) sympathetic and peripheral (adrenal glands) sympathetic activity to function in associative or dissociative ways. For these reasons, it is no longer appropriate to refer to hypersympathetic activity in simplistic terms. It becomes necessary to describe precisely the particular participation of the sympathetic system components as either noradrenergic (LC) or adrenergic (C1). The only approach to this target is through the measurement of NA/Ad plasma ratios during both supine-resting and activated situations (both physiological and pharmacological).

We have tested the effects of orthostasis, moderate exercise, oral glucose, emotions, and intellectual activities, as well as many central-acting drugs (clonidine, buspirone, yohimbine, aminoacids, β-blockers, etc.). We have investigated not only NA, Ad and DA, but also indolamines (p5HT and f5HT), amino acids such as TRP,

and metabolites of catecholamines (MHPG, MOPEG, VMA) and of indolamines (5-HIAA). We have also assessed most of these parameters throughout the different sleep stages in normal sleepers and also in sleep-disordered subjects. As an outcome of our experience, we have learned to distrust all papers reporting only partial plasma neurotransmitter results. Such papers have fostered great confusion and misunderstanding.

Summarizing, we found the existence of 3 types of central sympathetic activities: LC-NA, C1-Ad and LC + C1. The only possibility for obtaining objective information regarding their roles is by means of the NA/Ad plasma ratio (normally = 3–5) both during basal and stimulated situations. The greater the NA/Ad ratio, the greater the LC-NA activity and conversely. Coping stress situation and major (endogenous) depression showed the greatest values of NA/Ad ratio (usually more than 7). Uncoping stress situations showed the lowest values (usually less than 1). Some intermediate values (1–3) obtained during basal periods are easily seen clarified throughout the different types of stress tests (orthostasis, moderate exercise, oral glucose, buspirone, etc.), when NA/Ad values fall to one or less. When this happens, patients may suffer many

Some Neuroautonomic and
Neuroendocrine Changes Registered during
the Wake and Sleep Periods

undesirable side effects (anxiety, dizziness, headache, tachycardia, abdominal pain, nausea, chest pain, etc.). On the other hand, no side effects are registered during NA/Ad increment periods.

Increases in f5HT plasma levels parallel Ad plasma peaks, according to our results. At the same time, we routinely registered platelet aggregation increases. No platelet aggregability is registered in normals or patients with elevated NA/Ad plasma levels. Headache and asthma attacks occur frequently in subjects showing low NA/Ad plasma levels plus increased platelet aggregability. The fact that such side effects are easily suppressed by the oral administration of 12.5 mg of tianeptine (a drug that increases the uptake of serotonin by platelets) has been reported in many published papers. These and other findings clearly demonstrate that it is not possible to accurately interpret the significance of isolated, basal plasma neurotransmitter values.

Chapter 3

....

Stress

Uncoping (Uncontrollable) Stress Situation

During an acute stress situation, all NA, DA and 5HT monoaminergic circuits are activated. The C1 adrenaline nucleus is also stimulated (fig. 3.1). All except for the DR and RO serotonergic nuclei show an increased firing rate. Activation of the PVN is responsible for the enhanced release of CRF, vasopressin and oxytocin hormones. Noradrenergic, serotonergic and CRF mechanisms converge to trigger the ACTH → cortisol cascade. On the contrary, the GHRH → GH cascade is inhibited at the hypothalamic-hypophysis level whereas somatostatin secretion is increased. Gonadotropin secretion is inhibited whereas prolactin secretion is enhanced.

Both neural (sympathetic nerves) and adrenomedullary glands are active. A rise of NA, DA, and Ad plasma levels is registered. Increased Ad plasma levels are responsible for platelet aggregation and the rise of f5HT in the plasma. Circulating serotonin is normally shared by platelets (98–99%) = p5HT and plasma (1–2%) = f5HT.

Neural sympathetic nerves release NA (90%) + DA (10%) which are verted to the bloodstream. These NA nerves are postsynaptic axons arising from sympathetic ganglia. At this level, preganglionic ACh axons establish synaptic contact with NA postsynaptic neurons. Preganglionic ACh axons have their cell bodies at the intermediolateral spinal column. These preganglionic spinal sympathetic cells receive polysynaptic activation from the LC-NA nucleus, in such a way that stimulation of this NA nucleus provokes neural sympathetic activation and a rise of NA plasma level. Other preganglionic sympathetic neurons located at the thoracic segment of the intermediolateral spinal column receive excitatory axons from the C1-medullary Ad nucleus. These preganglionic sympathetic neurons send axons to the adrenomedullary glands where they trigger catecholamine secretion: Ad 80% + NA 10% + DA 10%.

According to the above, the NA/Ad plasma ratio reflects the participation of neural/adrenomedullary sympathetic activity. In normal subjects during supine-resting conditions, the NA/Ad ratio = 3 to 5. This ratio will increase when LC-NA activity predominates over C1-Ad activity (fig. 3.2). Conversely, the NA/Ad ratio will decrease in the opposite situation. Normally, several physiologic stimuli such as orthostasis, moderate exercise, and glucose ingestion raise the NA/Ad ratio. This response is also registered after administration of various central acting drugs, for instance buspirone.

p5HT, which shows no change during short-lived acute stress situations, falls during prolonged acute stress. At this time, parasympathetic activity is lowered and both the f5HT/p5HT ratio and tryptophan are positively correlated with this activity. Blood serotonin arises from the small bowel enterochromaffin cells, which release serotonin when stimulated by vagal nerve endings.

Prolongation and/or repetition of acute stress situation can lead to adaptation (coping) or maladaptation (uncoping) stress. During coping stress, an increase of the NA/Ad ratio + a reduction of cortisol values are registered. Conversely, reduction of the NA/Ad ratio is observed during prolonged acute and chronic uncoping stress situations. The therapeutic approach employed for treating uncop-

Fig. 3.1. Uncoping stress. LC = Locus coeruleus; DR = dorsal raphe; MR = median raphe; RM = raphe magnus; RO = raphe obscurus; RP = raphe pallidus; mcn = mesocortical nucleus; PVN = paraventricular nucleus; AH = anterior hypothalamus; PH = posterior hypothalamus; VMN = ventromedial nucleus; PRF = pontoreticular formation; PPN = pedunculopontine nucleus; CRF = corticotrophin-releasing factor; AP = area postrema; Na = noradrenaline; Ad = adrenaline; ACh = acetylcholine; 5HT = serotonin. → Excitation; ─< inhibition. Concentric circles, bright and faded colors indicate neuronal activity. Dashed lines indicate reduced output.

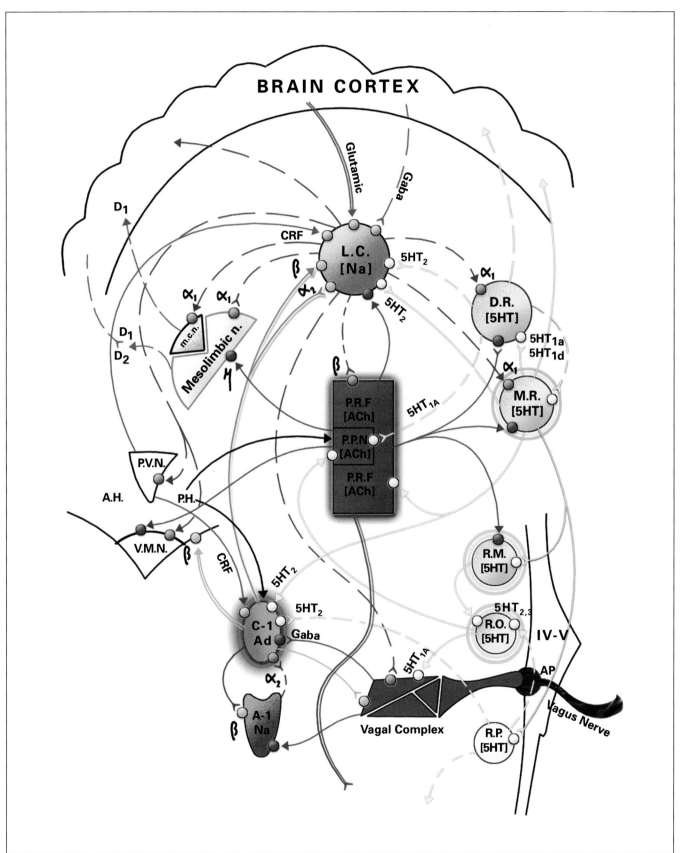

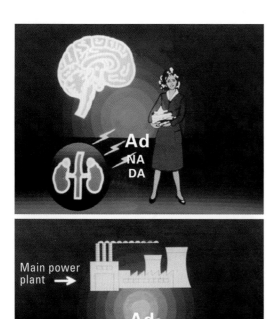

Fig. 3.2. Uncoping stress.

ing-stressed patients is consistent with small doses (25 mg) of NA-uptake inhibitors (desipramine, maprotyline, doxepin, etc.) + small doses of NA precursors (phenylalanine 50 mg or *L*-tyrosine 50 mg). At times we add small doses of an NA-releasing agent such as yohimbine (2.5–5 mg). All these drugs are taken before breakfast in order to preserve the normal wake-sleep cycle. This cycle requires greater diurnal than nocturnal NA activity and greater nocturnal than diurnal 5HT activity. 20 mg of propranolol after breakfast was added for patients showing tachycardia as a result of yohimbine. Such patients release more Ad than NA when taking yohimbine.

Central neuronal circuitry during uncoping stress would include the following changes (fig. 3.1): (a) exhaustion of NA stores = LC-NA reduction (zero rings) (blue); (b) maximal activity of the C1-Ad medullary nuclei (green), and (c) reduction of mesocortical DA activity (lilac).

Reduction of serotonergic activity of those 5HT nuclei which receive tonic excitatory stimulation from the LC-NA nucleus (DR and MR- yellow). Other 5HT nuclei which receive inhibitory innervation from the LC-DR-MR nuclei become disinhibited. The RM and the RO

now have facilitated potency for stimulating vagal activity (vagal complex). The RM-facilitated activity is responsible for 'stress-induced analgesia'. The periaqueductal gray nucleus (not shown in the figure) is also disinhibited from the LC-DR bridle. Activation of the PAG serotonergic system is involved in the mechanisms underlying the panic syndrome. Stimulation of the PAG-amygdala serotonergic axons triggers panic attacks and is involved in the aversive (anxiety) syndrome, a behavior pattern commonly observed in uncoping stressed mammals.

The C1-Ad and vagal complex medullary nuclei (red) become free from the inhibitory LC-NA+DR-5HT influence (fig. 3.1). Then adrenal-sympathetic ↔ parasympathetic oscillations are produced because the LC-NA modulatory influence is lacking. Cardiovascular, gastrointestinal, metabolic, endocrine, and immunological disorders are routinely registered during uncoping stress situation (fig. 3.2). We observed sleep disorders in these patients, always.

Coping Stress Situation

Mammals submitted to experimental uncoping (uncontrollable, inescapable) stress situation, also known as 'behavioral despair', show maximal exhaustion of CNS NA stores. On the contrary, increased NA stores are found in those mammals which have been able to cope with stress (fig. 3.3, 3.4). During experimental situations, 'coping stressed' mammals show peaks of NA but not Ad when they are submitted to stressors; neither do they register any increase of plasma cortisol. However, augmentation as well as excessive prolongation of stressor application may lead to a reversion of coping to uncoping stress situation. When this happens, central NA depletion is produced. Such mammals show Ad and cortisol plasma peaks when submitted to the impact of stressors.

Fig. 3.3. Coping stress. LC = Locus coeruleus; DR = dorsal raphe; MR = median raphe; RM = raphe magnus; RO = raphe obscurus; RP = raphe pallidus; mcn = mesocortical nucleus; PVN = paraventricular nucleus; AH = anterior hypothalamus; PH = posterior hypothalamus; VMN = ventromedial nucleus; PRF = pontoreticular formation; PPN = pedunculopontine nucleus; CRF = corticotrophin-releasing factor; AP = area postrema; Na = noradrenaline; Ad = adrenaline; ACh = acetylcholine; 5HT = serotonin. → Excitation; ⊸ inhibition. Concentric circles, bright and faded colors indicate neuronal activity. Dashed lines indicate reduced output.

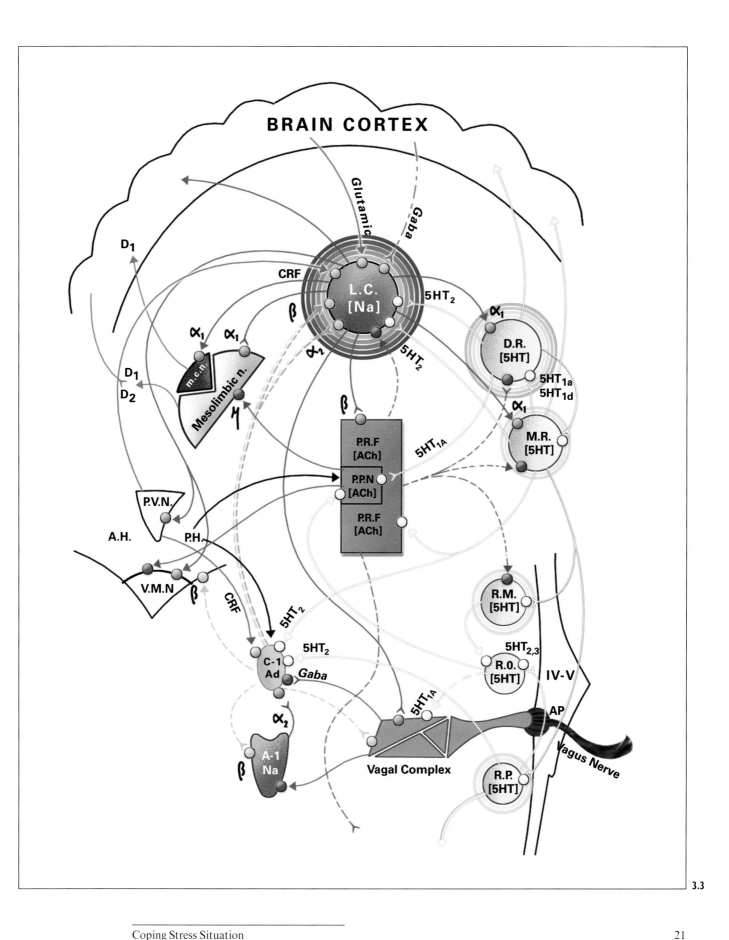

3.3

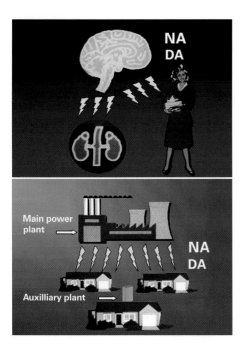

Fig. 3.4. Coping stress.

Normal humans show rises of NA, but not Ad, when submitted to orthostasis (1 min), moderate exercise, glucose, and buspirone challenges. We have shown this in tests on some 15,000 subjects. Conversely, diseased patients suffering infections, cancer, etc., and anxious people, show an uncoping stress profile when they are submitted to orthostasis, moderate exercise, glucose, and buspirone stress tests. We have tested some 25,000 patients over the last 24 years. These patients showed normal responses once their symptoms were normalized, either spontaneously or through neuropharmacological treatment to increase CNS NA activity. Wrongly treated patients did not show either clinical or plasma neurotransmitter profile normalization.

The diagram of CNS circuitry for coping stress shows a profile similar to the scheme presented for the active waking period (fig. 1.1), with the addition of one more blue ring to the LC-NA nucleus, and a smaller disk (green) for the C1-Ad nucleus (fig. 3.3).

Chapter 4

Depression

Major (Endogenous) Depression

In 1995, we published two research papers in *Biological Psychiatry* dealing with plasma neurotransmitter profiles in two types of depressed patients: major (endogenous) and dysthymic. These two types of depression show opposite profiles. Whereas the former presents increased noradrenergic activity + reduced serotonergic activity, the latter shows a low NA + high 5HT profile. Similar results were reported by us in other papers appearing in *Clinical Science* [1991], *Clinical Experimental Hypertension* [1993], *Psychotherapy and Psychosomatics* [1996], and in several scientific meetings. We established that the two types of depression, although apparently opposite, have a common factor: low levels of plasma Ad. Furthermore, Ad levels did not rise when patients were submitted to the usual stress challenges routinely employed in our institute: oral glucose, orthostasis, moderate exercise, and buspirone. According to the above, we were able to differentiate, from a neurochemical and neuropharmacological viewpoint, that the two types of depression share a poor adrenomedullary responsiveness, as distinct to an uncoping stress profile which is characterized by a high adrenomedullary responsiveness. These findings allowed us to design well-defined neuropharmacological therapies addressed to normalizing these pathophysiological profiles. Under this approach, therapeutic success was routinely obtained in 100% of the cases (endogenous and dysthymic depression as well as uncoping stress). This therapeutic success was obtained with consistently low doses of psychoactive drugs which, moreover, were reduced progressively until totally suppressed (2–3 months). This allowed administration of the drugs to be restarted when necessary.

The major depression diagram is characterized by a large blue LC-NA disk + a small (exhausted) yellow DR-5HT disk. The lilac mesocortical DA nucleus is depicted in brighter tone because NA axons excite it, intensely (fig. 4.1). Conversely, LC-NA axons trigger inhibition of mesolimbic DA activity. Excessive NA stimulation of the PVN hypothalamic nucleus is responsible for the excessive CRF → ACTH → cortisol cascade activation. Predominance of the A1-NA medullary nuclei reduces the activity of C1-Ad medullary nuclei. Inhibition of the C1-Ad activity favors disinhibition of the vagal complex. These mechanisms would be enough to explain the increased parasympathetic activity registered in major depressed patients. The MR-5HT would show predominance over DR-5HT activity. This MR-5HT predominance is compatible with a suicidal tendency often observed in such patients. In effect, MR-5HT activity is usually experimentally associated with aggressive and 'killing' behavior in mammals.

The very low levels of plasma tryptophan always registered in patients with major depression are consistent with the low DR-5HT activity postulated in them. Although consensus exists regarding the association of low tryptophan plasma levels with a reduction of central serotonergic activity, we think that the latter should not include the medullary serotonergic nuclei. High level (pontine) and low level (medullary) serotonergic nuclei usually present different and frequently opposing profiles of activity. For instance, the PAG serotonergic nucleus receives inhibitory axons from the DR-5HT nucleus. The RM and the RO serotonergic nuclei receive excitatory and inhibitory input from the PAG-5HT and MR-5HT nuclei, respectively, which in turn are positively associated with the vagal complex activity. On the contrary, the

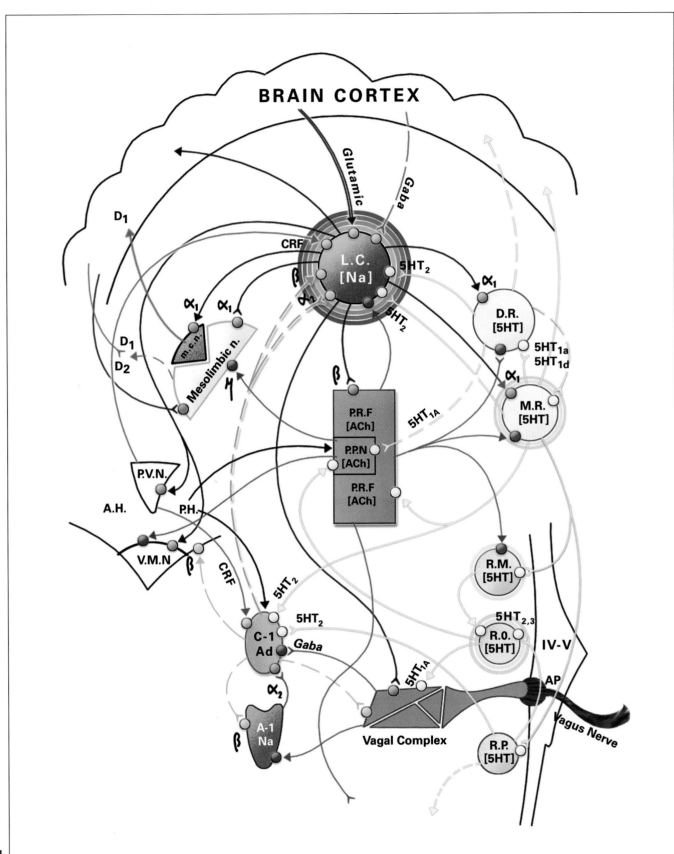

RP medullary nucleus antagonizes both the RM-5HT + RO-5HT nuclei and vagal complex activity. The RP sends excitatory axons to C1-Ad medullary nuclei as well as to presynaptic sympathetic spinal neurons (fig. 4.1).

The profile of major depression that we depict is consistent with the short REM latency usually registered in these patients. In effect, activity of LC-NA and DR-5HT neurons is reduced to zero during REM sleep. Normally, the LC-NA fall occurs slowly and progressively (60–90 min). This LC-NA landing is possible when the DR-5HT + MR-5HT bridle is working. However, poor activity of the former, postulated in patients with major depression, facilitates the 'crash-landing' of LC-NA activity registered in them.

Patients with major depression are treated routinely (in our institute) with low doses of 5-OH-tryptophan (25–50 mg) + low doses of an inhibitor of serotonin uptake: sertraline (25–50 mg) or paroxetine (20 mg) or clomipramine (25–50 mg). Normalization of the clinical and neurochemical profiles occurs in almost 100% of cases within 3–4 weeks of therapy. After this period, we usually reduce the antidepressant doses but not the serotonin precursor dose. We found no failures in several hundred patients. We add small doses of pindolol (2.5 mg) in some refractory patients. This $5HT_{1A}$ antagonist favors the release of serotonin from DR-5HT neurons, mainly. These DR-5HT neurons have the highest population of $5HT_{1A}$ inhibiting autoreceptors. The foregoing therapeutic approach is opposite to that employed for treating uncoping-stressed patients, who receive small doses of NA uptake inhibitors (desipramine, maprotyline, doxepin, etc.) + small doses of NA precursors (phenylalanine 50 mg or *L*-tyrosine 50 mg). At times, we add small doses of an NA-releasing agent such as yohimbine (2.5–5 mg). All these drugs are taken before breakfast by uncoping stressed patients. The normal wake-sleep cycle requires greater diurnal than nocturnal NA activity and greater

nocturnal than diurnal 5HT activity. 20 mg of propranolol after breakfast was added for patients showing tachycardia as a result of yohimbine. Such patients release more Ad than NA when taking yohimbine.

We call this kind of treatment physiological therapy. Physiological treatments do not require great doses of drugs. Massive doses are prescribed by those doctors who ignore what is wrong and what is happening to the patient. We believe that physiology implies God, and that we must seek God. God (physiology) is the boss; we always endeavor to act with, and not against, Him. We realize that the pharmaceutical industry recommends high doses of the so-called antidepressants, but we never needed to use large doses. Our patients never needed them.

Many papers appearing in psychiatric journals support the use of NA uptake inhibitors to treat endogenous depression. This treatment requires the administration of great doses during several months because, after prolonged use, these drugs trigger inhibition of the LC-NA system. Patients feel worse for weeks and months. Of course, at the end, NA uptake inhibitors produce an exhaustion of CNS-NA activity. It is like trying to reach heaven by passing through hell, or like Columbus seeking the Orient by sailing west. The increase of NA activity triggered by these drugs during the first weeks and months worsens the poor patients who become prey to seriously undesirable side effects. Inhibitors of NA uptake should be administered to dysthymic depressed and uncoping stressed patients and not to endogenous depressed subjects. For this reason, differential diagnosis must be made before starting neuropharmacological therapy.

Dysthymic Depression

In 1982 we published a research paper in the *Journal of Affective Disorders* showing that depressed patients can be differentiated into two types on the basis of their distal colon motility (low intestinal tone and high intestinal tone – IT). These two types of patients showed clinical differences when tested with the Hamilton Depression Rate Scale (HDRS). In 1983, we demonstrated that the low IT depressed patients were highly improved by clorimipramine (CMI = an inhibitor of serotonin uptake) whereas the high IT depressed patients were significantly improved by imipramine (but not by CMI). Imipramine is a NA uptake inhibitor, preferentially.

In 1985, we published two more research papers *(Neuroendocrinology)* demonstrating that low IT depressed patients were shown to have significantly higher NA plas-

Fig. 4.1. Major (endogenous) depression. LC = Locus coeruleus; DR = dorsal raphe; MR = median raphe; RM = raphe magnus; RO = raphe obscurus; RP = raphe pallidus; mcn = mesocortical nucleus; PVN = paraventricular nucleus; AH = anterior hypothalamus; PH = posterior hypothalamus; VMN = ventromedial nucleus; PRF = pontoreticular formation; PPN = pedunculopontine nucleus; CRF = corticotrophin-releasing factor; AP = area postrema; Na = noradrenaline; Ad = adrenaline; ACh = acetylcholine; 5HT = serotonin. → Excitation; –< inhibition. Concentric circles, bright and faded colors indicate neuronal activity. Dashed lines indicate reduced output.

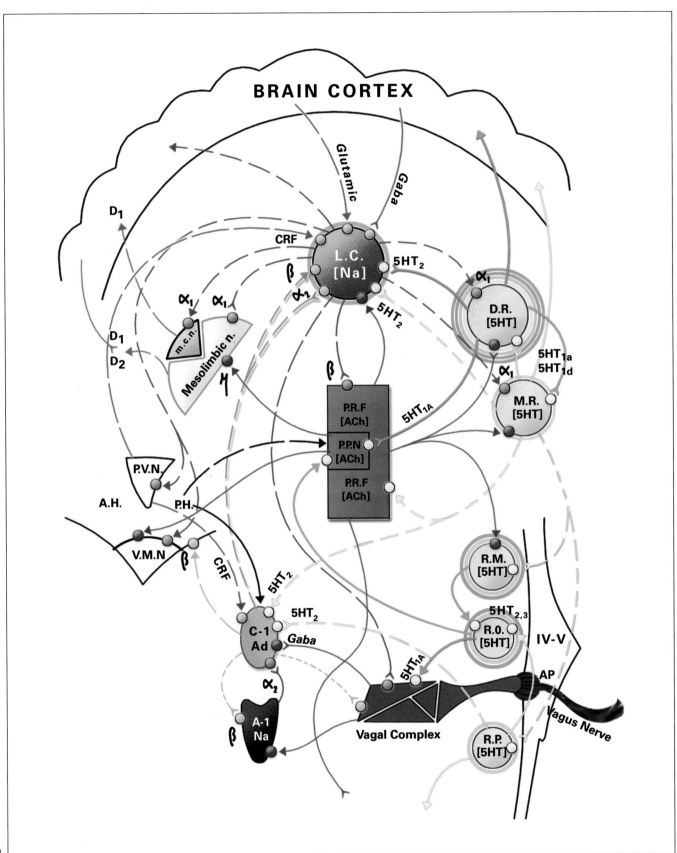

ma levels than high IT depressed patients. The two groups also showed significant differences according to their responses to clonidine (blood pressure, GH + CRT + prolactin secretion). Finally, in 1995 we published other two papers *(Biological Psychiatry)* demonstrating that the two reported types of depressed patients fit well with the diagnoses of endogenous (major), and dysthymic depressed patients.

The neurochemical, neurophysiological and neuropharmacological profile of dysthymic depressed patients will be defined and depicted in this chapter.

The dysthymic depression diagram is characterized by smaller than normal blue disk (NA system) plus a big DR-serotonergic system (yellow disk). The weak NA activity is responsible for low mesocortical DA activity (lilac), whereas excessive DR-5HT activity bridles mesolimbic DA activity (fig. 4.2).

The C1-Ad medullary nuclei (green) are depicted with low activity. These patients show poor adrenomedullary responsiveness to all kinds of stressors (orthostasis, exercise, glucose, buspirone). Two factors converge in this phenomenon: (1) the LC-NA → CRF → C1-Ad cascade is diminished, and (2) the disinhibited vagal complex (from LC-NA axons) exerts bridling effects on C1-Ad nuclei.

This parasympathetic (vagal) hyperactivity is responsible for the high platelet serotonin (p5HT) levels registered in these patients. In turn, the raised tryptophan plasma levels are consistent with high DR-5HT activity.

Fig. 4.2. Dysthymic depression. LC = Locus coeruleus; DR = dorsal raphe; MR = median raphe; RM = raphe magnus; RO = raphe obscurus; RP = raphe pallidus; mcn = mesocortical nucleus; PVN = paraventricular nucleus; AH = anterior hypothalamus; PH = posterior hypothalamus; VMN = ventromedial nucleus; PRF = pontoreticular formation; PPN = pedunculopontine nucleus; CRF = corticotrophin-releasing factor; AP = area postrema; Na = noradrenaline; Ad = adrenaline; ACh = acetylcholine; 5HT = serotonin. → Excitation; —< inhibition. Concentric circles, bright and faded colors indicate neuronal activity. Dashed lines indicate reduced output.

Chapter 5

....

Stress versus Depression

Abstract

Exhaustive evidence is cited showing that uncontrollable (uncoping) stress provoked in experimental mammals leads to depletion of central noradrenergic activity + adrenomedullary-cortical gland hyperactivity. These physiological disorders cause the typical neuroendocrine peripheral profile: (a) raised catecholamines (CA) in plasma [NA + Ad + DA]; (b) reduced NA/Ad ratio in plasma, and (c) raised plasma cortisol.

Exhaustive evidence is quoted which indicates that severely ill humans show peripheral neuroendocrine profile similar to that found in mammals submitted to uncontrollable stress situation. Further, the NA/Ad ratio does not increase but decreases during orthostasis and exercise stress challenges, as well as oral glucose stress (tolerance) test.

Exhaustive evidence is quoted which indicates that endogenous depressed subjects show a neuroendocrine profile opposite to that observed in stressed mammals and severely ill humans. This profile consists of central NA (neural sympathetic) hyperactivity + adrenomedullary glands hyporesponsivity. These disorders are reflected in a 3- to 10-fold increase of the NA/Ad ratio in plasma.

Exhaustive evidence is also cited showing that dysthymic depressed patients show low plasma catecholamines + low NA/Ad plasma ratio (<2) during supine-resting which becomes normal at orthostasis and exercise periods.

It is quoted evidence showing that whereas platelet serotonin is increased in dysthymics, the same is reduced in endogenously depressed subjects.

Further evidence shows that free serotonin in plasma is greatly raised in uncoping stressed mammals and in severely ill humans. The same parameter is normal or slightly increased in dysthymic and endogenous depressed humans. These findings are consistent with the increased platelet aggregability observed in uncontrollable stressed mammals and in severely ill, but not depressed patients.

Evidence also reveals that whereas parasympathetic activity is absent in uncontrollable stressed mammals and severely ill humans, the same is increased in both types of depressed humans.

According to the above, the authors postulate the existence of three distinct central plus peripheral neuroendocrine profiles describing endogenous depression, dysthymic depression, and maladaptation to stress syndrome. These different profiles should lead researchers to attempt different therapeutical approaches. In view of the fact that the authors found much clinical overlap among the three syndromes (endogenous depression, dysthymic depression and severely ill patients), they believe that a differential diagnosis should be based on neurochemical, neuroendocrine, physiologic, metabolic and neuropharmacological grounds.

The experimentally induced uncontrollable stress ('behavioral despair') syndrome in mammals is shown to be invalid as a model for human depressive syndrome.

Introduction

Great overlap and consequent confusion exists between the diagnosis of stress and that of depressive syndrome in humans. This has arisen from the mistaken belief that the inescapable (uncontrolled) stress syndrome, as experimentally induced in mammals, represents an adequate equivalent model for human depression. Further, the fact that both inescapable stress in animals and the human depressive syndrome are improved by so-called antidepressant drugs contributes to accentuate such confusion. Finally, the empirical finding that stressors can precipitate clinical features which resemble symptoms observed in depressed humans, reinforces the error [Aprison and Hingtgen, 1981; Aprison et al., 1982; Hellhammer 1983; Nagayama et al., 1981; Maier 1984; Porsolt et al., 1978; Weiss et al., 1981; Zimmerman et al., 1985].

Mounting evidence demonstrates that the neurochemical, neuroendocrine and physiologic disorders underlying inescapable stress in mammals and depression in humans are wholly different. Hence, the clinical signs shared by both syndromes (immobility, unresponsiveness to stimuli, etc.) are too weak to support the hypothesis that the two conditions are equivalent. Conversely, many findings support the hypothesis that opposite mechanisms underlie the two syndromes. Additionally, it should be remembered that there are not one but several clinical depressive syndromes that lay claim to the label of depression. For instance, endogenous depression is totally different to dysthymic depression. Hence, which of the depressive syndromes purportedly corresponds to the inescapable stress model experimentally induced in mammals: endogenous, dysthymic, or some other? [Anisman and Zacharko, 1982; Davies et al., 1981; Rubin et al., 1979; Schatzberg 1978; Schildkraut et al., 1977; Targum 1984; Von Zerssen et al., 1984].

Neurochemical Evidence

Depletion of central NA stores occurs in mammals submitted to inescapable stress situation [Misman et al., 1979; Fuxe et al., 1983; Glavin 1985; lrwin et al., 1986; Kobayashi et al., 1975]. This central NA depletion is responsible for the upregulation of α_2-receptors registered at the hypothalamic level in experimental animals [Eden et al., 1979; Eriksson et al., 1982; McWilliam and Meldrum, 1983; Siever and Uhde, 1984]. In addition, although both catecholamines NA and Ad rise in plasma during stress situation, the NA/Ad ratio is significantly lower than normal [Breier et al., 1987; Burchfield, 1979; De Boer et al., 1990; Sachser, 1987; Vesifeld et al., 1976]. This fact is consistent with adrenomedullary overactivity and reveals dissociation between peripheral (adrenal) and central (neural) sympathetic activities (table 5.1) [Anisman 1978; Anisman and Sklar, 1979; Anisman et al., 1980; Benarroch et al., 1983; Caramona and Soares Da Silva, 1985; Glavin, 1985; Kvetnansky et al., 1979; Sourkes, 1985]. Conversely, higher than normal NA plasma levels are observed in endogenous depressed subjects, thus their NA/Ad ratio is greatly raised [Azorin et al., 1988; Berger et al., 1982; Lake et al., 1982; Lechin F et al., 1988c, 1995b, 1993, 1991; Roy et al., 1985; Wyatt et al., 1971]. Taking into account that circulating NA reflects central noradrenergic activity mainly, this finding opposes the central NA depletion registered in stressed mammals [Lake et al., 1976; Ziegler et al., 1977].

Neuropharmacological Evidence

A blunted GH + CRT + NA + DBP (diastolic blood pressure) responses to clonidine are observed in endogenous depressed patients (fig. 5.1). This unresponsiveness to clonidine is interpreted as a downregulation of α_2-receptors at the hypothalamic level and is compatible with the raised central and plasmatic NA level (increased central NA activity) registered in these patients (fig. 5.2) [Charney et al., 1982; Checkley et al., 1981; Lechin F et

Table 5.1. Plasma NA, Ad, TRP, f5HT, CRT, and NA/Ad ratio in 55 major depressed patients, 41 dysthymic depressed patients, and their age- and sex-paired normal controls

	Major depression (MD)	Dysthymic depression (DD)	Controls (C)
NA, pg/ml	$523.0 \pm 52^{a,b}$	76.0 ± 21^{c}	273.0 ± 23
Ad, pg/ml	25.0 ± 07	29.0 ± 09	34.0 ± 08
NA/Ad	$12.0 \pm 03^{a,b}$	2.1 ± 02^{c}	5.1 ± 02
TRP, ng/ml	$3,583 \pm 54^{a,b}$	$12,528 \pm 25^{c}$	$8,085.0 \pm 36$
f5HT, ng/ml	$2.6 \pm 01^{a,b}$	7.5 ± 7.5^{c}	1.2 ± 04
CRT, µg/ml	$15.0 \pm 02^{a,b}$	9.0 ± 02	8.0 ± 02

Values are expressed as mean ± SEM. [a] MD vs. DD; [b] MD vs. C; [c] DD vs. C; $p < 0.001$ in all cases. Most decimals were omitted [Lechin F et al., Arch Ven Farm Terap 1988c;7(suppl 1):abstr 7].

al., 1985b, c; Matussek et al., 1980; Siever et al., 1982]. Conversely, hyperresponsiveness of GH to clonidine and upregulation of α_2-hypothalamic receptors are found in inescapable stressed mammals, which show central NA depletion [Blackard and Heidingsfelder, 1968; Day and Willoughby, 1980; Eden et al., 1979; Eriksson et al., 1982; Lechin F et al., 1987b; McWilliam and Meldrum, 1983; Siever and Uhde, 1984].

All 'antidepressant' drugs are able to revert the inescapable stress syndrome in experimental mammals [Anisman and Zacharko, 1982; Aprison and Hingtgen, 1981; Aprison et al., 1982; Davies et al., 1981; Hellhammer 1983; Leonard and Kafoe, 1976; Lucki and Frazer, 1985; Maier, 1984; Nagayama et al., 1981; Porsolt et al., 1978; Rodriguez-Echandia et al., 1987; Rubin et al., 1979; Schatzberg, 1978; Schildkraut et al., 1977; Sherman and Petty, 1980; Targum 1984; von Zerssen et al., 1984; Weiss et al., 1981; Zimmerman et al., 1985]. However, therapeutical improvement triggered in depressed patients by all these drugs is not the rule. On the contrary, failures are more frequent than successes [Carroll 1982; Kraemer and McKinney, 1979; Lechin F et al., 1983b; Morris and Beck, 1974; Przegalinski et al., 1981; Schatzberg, 1978].

The so-called 'antidepressant' drugs include a great diversity of neuropharmacological agents which act through different mechanisms. Some potentiate central NA activity [Huang, 1979; Roffman et al., 1977; Sulser and Mobley, 1981], others increase central 5HT [Ogren et al., 1982, 1979] and/or DA activity, while still others hamper 5HT neurotransmission [Clements-Jewery, 1978; Liang-Fu, 1979]. Most of these drugs trigger more than

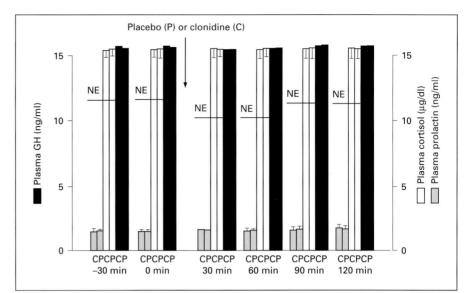

Fig. 5.1. Effects of i.m. clonidine (2.5 µg/kg) and placebo on plasmatic levels of GH, cortisol and prolactin in 26 high distal colon tone depressed patients. The drugs did not modify any mean ± SEM hormonal value at any time [Lechin et al., Neuroendocrinology 1985b;41:156–162].

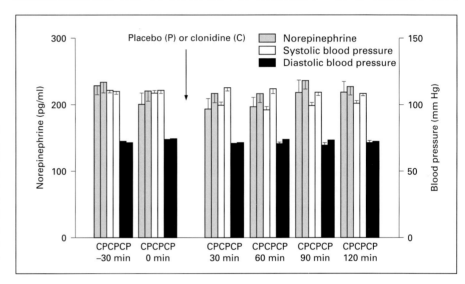

Fig. 5.2. Effects of i.m. clonidine (2.5 µg/kg) and placebo on norepinephrine plasma level, systolic and diastolic blood pressure in 26 high distal colon tone depressed patients. Systolic blood pressure was significantly reduced at 30, 60, 90 and 120 min. Neither diastolic blood pressure nor norepinephrine plasma levels were reduced at any period. Each bar represents mean ± SEM [Lechin et al., Neuroendocrinology 1985b;41:156–162].

one neuropharmacological mechanism and act upon more than one neurotransmitter system. For instance, desipramine and protryptiline are NA uptake inhibitors [Nielsen and Braestrup, 1977; Nybaeck et al., 1975]; amytryptiline, clorimipramine, imipramine and doxepin are NA + 5HT uptake inhibitors [Bower, 1972; Fuxe et al., 1977; Maj, 1978; Scuvee-Moreau and Dresse, 1979; Vetulani et al., 1984]; fluoxetine, sertraline and paroxetine act like 5HT uptake inhibitors [Benfield et al., 1986]; mianserin is an α2- + 5HT2-receptor blocking agent provoking NA + 5HT release from terminals [Klimek and Mogilnicka, 1978; Leonard and Kafoe, 1976; Przegalinski et al., 1981; Sugrue 1980]; tianeptine enhances the uptake of 5HT by terminals and reduces synaptic availability of this

neurotransmitter and in addition suppresses the stress-induced release of NA [Delbende et al., 1991]. Amineptine inhibits the uptake of DA [Sherman and Petty, 1980]. All these drugs are able to revert the uncontrollable stress syndrome induced by stressors in experimental mammals, but their antidepressant success in humans is variable, poor or nil [Fuxe et al., 1981, 1982; Kraemer and McKinney, 1979; Nagayama et al., 1981; Raiteri et al., 1976; Rosembaum et al., 1980; Wolfe et al., 1978].

We can observe that most of the 'antidepressants' potentiate one, two or more monoaminergic systems. This phenomenon fits well with the fact that all (NA, DA, and 5HT) neurotransmitters are exhausted during inescapable stress [Anisman, 1978; Anisman et al., 1981; Cabib et al.,

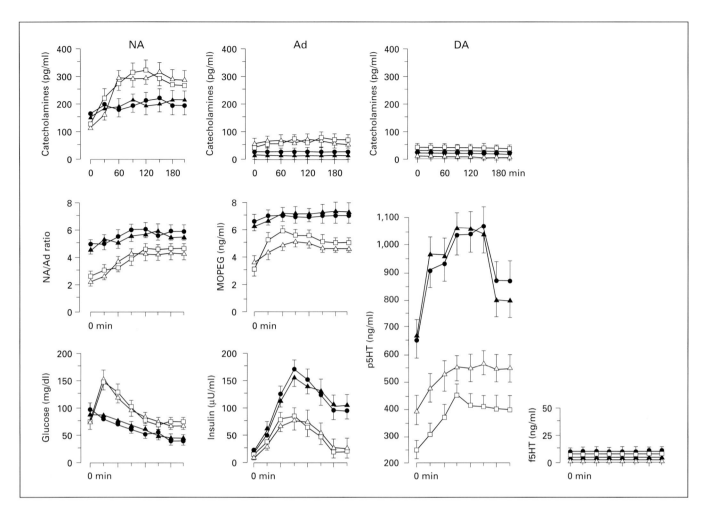

Fig. 5.3. Postprandial symptomatic hypoglycemic (depressed) patients. Three consecutive oral glucose tolerance tests (OGTT) were performed in each of the 12 patients and their age-sex paired controls (□); the first (▲) before placebo, the second (●) before doxepin therapy, and the third (△) after doxepin therapy. Large increases in NA, NA/Ad ratio, MOPEG and p5HT were observed. No glucose rise was registered during OGTT; on the contrary, a progressive reduction in plasma glucose was observed, which paralleled plasma insulin rise.

Reductions in heart rate, systolic + diastolic blood pressure (not presented data) as well as nonadrenergic symptoms were registered throughout OGTT. These symptoms disappeared quickly after i.m. injection of 10 mg of propantheline (a parasympathetic ganglionic blocking agent). Values are mean ± SEM. Neither DA nor plasma f5HT varied throughout OGTT [Lechin et al., Clin Sci 1991;80: 373–384].

1988; Dunn, 1988a; Fuxe et al., 1983; Glavin, 1985; Herman et al., 1982; Imperato et al., 1989; Kobayashi et al., 1975; Kvetnansky et al., 1976; Petty and Sherman, 1983; Roth et al., 1982; Tanaka et al., 1989; Thierry et al., 1976; Tissari et al., 1979]. On the other hand, antidepressants most often found to be useful are 5HT-potentiating drugs [Aberg-Wistedt et al., 1982; Baldessarini, 1984; Civeira et al., 1990; DeMontigny and Blier, 1984; Fuxe et al., 1982; Geerts et al., 1994; Guelfi et al., 1992; Koyama and Meltzer 1986; LaPierre, 1994; Paykel, 1990; Quitkin et al., 1991; Rimon et al., 1993]. Taking into account that

circulating serotonin and tryptophan levels are decreased in endogenous depressed patients, who at the same time show central NA overactivity, the therapeutic improvement induced by these drugs is compatible with their ability to reduce central NA activity through the strengthening of its antagonic 5HT system [Banki et al., 1991; Baraban and Aghajanian, 1980; Gibbons and Davis, 1986; Heninger et al., 1984; Kahn et al., 1990; Lechin F et al., 1979a, 1989a; Meltzer and Lowy, 1987; Murphy et al., 1978; Pujol et al., 1978].

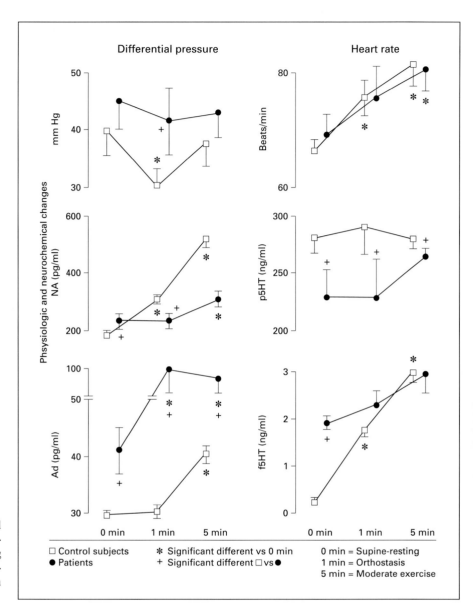

Fig. 5.4. Physiological and neurochemical changes induced by orthostasis and moderate exercise in 35 severely ill (uncoping stress) patients and their age-sex paired controls [Lechin et al., Psychother Psychosom 1996b;65:129–136].

Physiological and Metabolic Evidence

Inescapable stress, experimentally induced, is characterized by adrenomedullary plus cortical gland hyperactivity [Anisman, 1978; Anisman et al., 1979; Breier et al., 1987; Burchfield, 1979; De Boer et al., 1990; Dimsdale and Moss, 1980; Fuxe et al., 1983; Glavin, 1985; Hendley et al., 1988; Segal, 1979; Sourkes, 1985; Vesifeld et al., 1976]. Conversely, endogenous depressed subjects show adrenomedullary hypoactivity [Lechin F et al., 1988c, 1991, 1995b]. Such patients do not show the Ad peak during postprandial hypoglycemia or during orthostasis or

moderate exercise. This adrenal sympathetic hypoactivity is consistent with the high parasympathetic tone found in depressed patients. In effect, throughout the oral glucose tolerance test (OGTT), they show progressive blood pressure reduction paralleled by plasma glucose decrease (fig. 5.3). The parasympathetic nature of these phenomena is supported by the fact that atropine prevents both blood pressure and glucose decreases [Lechin F et al., 1991]. Atropine, injected before orthostasis and exercise challenges in these patients, also prevents the pulse pressure (systolic less diastolic) fall normally registered during orthostasis [Lechin F et al., 1996a]. This pulse pressure

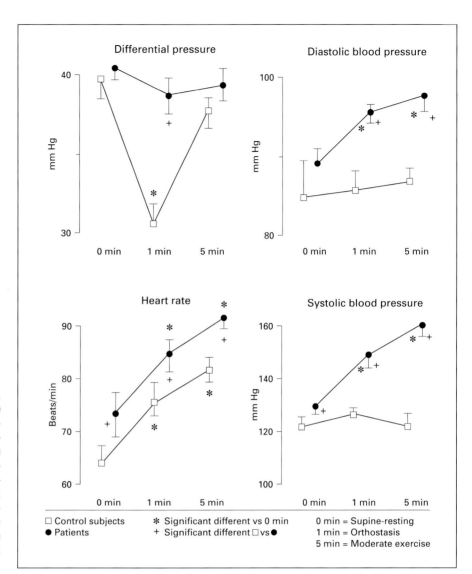

Fig. 5.5. Mean ± SEM values for heart rate, systolic, diastolic and differential (pulse) pressure measured in 36 healthy humans before (□ = control) and after atropine administration (● = atropine). The two tests were performed at 2-week intervals. The anticholinergic drugs suppressed the normal differential (pulse) pressure fall at orthostasis. In addition, atropine provoked abnormal increases of heart rate, systolic and diastolic blood pressure at orthostasis and exercise periods [Lechin et al., Res Commun Biol Psychiatry 1994a;21:55–72].

fall is more accentuated in depressed than normal subjects (fig. 5.4, 5.5) and is compatible with the higher than normal parasympathetic tone they present. This hyperparasympathetic activity that endogenous depressed patients show is consistent with their poor adrenal sympathetic responsiveness [Dilsaver and Coffman, 1989; Lechin F et al., 1989a, 1995b; Siever et al., 1981]. Similar hyperparasympathetic plus poor adrenomedullary activity was observed in dysthymic depressed patients who differ from endogenous depressed subjects because they show neither the greater than normal neural sympathetic activity nor the higher than normal platelet serotonin levels registered in the latter group. On the contrary, dysthymics show increased tryptophan plasma levels and de-

creased platelet serotonin levels when compared with normals.

Summarizing, whereas stressed animals present central NA depletion + adrenal gland sympathetic hyperresponsiveness, endogenous depressed patients show increased neural (central) NA activity plus adrenal sympathetic hypoactivity [Lechin F et al., 1995b; Natelson et al., 1987; Stoddard et al., 1986; Swenson and Vogel, 1983; Yoshimatsu et al., 1985; Young et al., 1984]. On the other hand, dysthymics show poor adrenomedullary activity plus high tryptophan plasma levels plus increased platelet serotonin level. Other physiologic disorders presented by stressed mammals are absent in depressed subjects, for example increased platelet aggregability [Ardlie et al.,

1984; Haft and Arkel, 1976; Hsu et al., 1979; Larson et al., 1989; Lechin F et al., 1990a, 1994b; Levine et al., 1985]. This platelet disorder is consistent with the raised f5HT in the plasma observed in stressed mammals but not in depressed subjects [Dunn, 1988b; Lechin AE et al., 1994a, b; Lechin F et al., , 1988c, d, 1989c, 1990a, 1992b, 1993, 1994a, b].

Clinical Evidence

A great many papers have been devoted to the relationship of somatic diseases, stress and depression. Basing their approach on clinical grounds, most of these papers fail, in our opinion, to differentiate depression from stress. All psychometric scales addressed to measuring stress quantify the magnitude of the stressors and/or their acute effects on the subjects. However, these clinical approaches do not take into account individual response to the challenge of chronic stress. It is known that the application of acute stressors to mammals provokes short-lived and reversible changes in them. Further, prolongation of acute stress and/or repetition of stressor application provokes either adaptation (coping) or maladaptation (uncoping) phenomena. Adapted mammals are able to accept stressors with minimal or nonsignificant neurochemical, physiologic or behavioral changes. Such adapted mammals are characterized by greater than normal central NA stores. Their adrenal glands respond poorly to the acute presentation of stressors, thus they do not show plasma Ad increase during stressful situation. Conversely, maladapted mammals are characterized by the depletion of central NA stores and hyperresponsiveness of adrenal glands to acute stress challenge [Anisman et al., 1980; Cabib et al., 1988; Breier et al., 1987; Gamallo et al., 1986; Heinsbroeck et al., 1991; lrwin et al., 1986; Kobayashi et al., 1975; Konarska et al., 1989; Natelson et al., 1988; Ottenweller et al., 1989; Roth et al., 1982; Swenson and Vogel, 1983; Tanaka et al., 1989]. In both coping and uncoping mammals there is a dissociation of the two branches of the sympathetic system: central (neurosympathetic) and peripheral (adrenal-sympathetic). In one type of dissociation, NA > Ad and in the other NA < Ad [Anisman, 1978; Anisman and Sklar, 1979; Anisman et al., 1980; Benarroch et al., 1983; Caramona and Soares Da Silva, 1985; Ellsworth et al., 1982; Glavin, 1985; Kvetnansky et al., 1979; Sourkes, 1985; Yoshimatsu et al., 1985].

Behavioral responses to stressor presentation in coping and uncoping mammals are easily observed under ex-

perimental conditions. However, behavioral responses (symptoms) in humans are frequently obscured by complex psychological mechanisms (repression, denial, neurotic exaggeration, etc.), thus the clinical diagnosis of maladaptation to stress in humans is not easy to assess. To the best of our knowledge, there exists no validated psychometric tool addressed to evaluate stress adaptation in human subjects. The use of the magnitude of anxiety and/or stressors as a measure of maladaptation to stress in subjects has neither adequate scientific support nor convincing clinical validity.

According to the above, the assessment of uncontrollable stress situation in humans should be made on neurochemical, hormonal, pharmacological, physiological but not clinical grounds.

Human Model of Maladapted to Stress Situation

Experimental animal procedures cannot be employed to provoke uncontrollable stress situation in humans. We cannot apply stressors to humans and then obtain brain slides to investigate neurochemical changes. However, we can measure many neurochemical, physiological, metabolic, and hormonal disorders that are well known to be invariably observed in experimental mammals during inescapable-induced stress situation. Following this procedure, the authors either find the typical peripheral uncontrollable stress profile, or fail to find it. In the first case, they are obliged to consider maladaptation to stress as a possible diagnosis. Furthermore, if an accurate psychiatric investigation is able to discard endogenous depression and dysthymic depression, we would have additional support favoring a diagnosis of maladaptation to stress syndrome. This syndrome is based on the following findings: (1) increased catecholamines (CA) plasma levels; (2) reduced NA/Ad ratio in plasma; (3) increased cortisol (CRT) in plasma; (4) increased platelet aggregability, and (5) increased f5HT in plasma. These findings should arise during supine resting conditions and/or after challenge to stressors.

Although some of these findings are observed in other syndromes, only maladaptation to stress syndrome includes all. For instance, while high CRT plasma levels are found in endogenous depressed and uncoping stressed patients [Davies et al., 1981; Lechin F et al., 1983a, 1985b; Rubin et al., 1979]; only endogenous depressed subjects present a great increase in NA/Ad plasma ratio [Lechin F et al., 1988c, 1991, 1995b]. Similarly, although dysthymics show low resting NA/Ad plasma ratio like

Table 5.2. Plasma neurotransmitters and cortisol in chronic illness and normal controls

	Ast (n = 12)	CB (n = 6)	UC (n = 10)	CD (n = 12)	CAH (n = 6)	CRP (n = 6)	MS (n = 11)	TN (n = 13)	SLE (n = 6)	RA (n = 6)	GM (n = 88)	Nm (n = 88)
Exacerbation												
NA, pg/ml	411±25*,+	389±21*,+	415±24*,+	417±26*,+	413±19*,+	398±15*,+	393±19*,+	391±22*,+	397±25*,+	427±26*,+	405±23*,+	279±14
Ad, pg/ml	323±22*,+	312±17*,+	327±21*,+	326±25*,+	328±22*,+	301±14*,+	298±13*,+	296±20*,+	303±24*,+	300±29*,+	316±21*,+	38±13
p5HT, ng/ml	35±14*,+	38±13*,+	41±12*,+	43±11*,+	33±10*,+	34±12*,+	40±15*,+	39±13*,+	41±12*,+	34±13*,+	37±15*,+	227±24
f5HT, ng/ml	9.6±1*,+	5.4±0.9*,+	10±2*,+	11±2*,+	9.9±2*,+	7.6±0.9*,+	6.4±0.9*,+	13±2*,+	14±3*,+	11±1*,+	12±2*,+	0.9±0.8
NA/Ad ratio	1.1±0.9*,+	2.0±1*,+	0.92±0.9*,+	0.65±0.9*,+	0.55±0.8*,+	0.98±1*,+	2.0±1*,+	1.4±1*,+	1.5±2*,+	0.7±0.6*,+	0.8±0.8*,+	5.7±1
CRT, µg/dl	34.4±4*,+	29.6±3*,+	41.6±5*,+	40.3±6*,+	42.7±6*,+	38.3±5*,+	29.1±4*,+	29.7±3*,+	39.3±4*,+	37.7±4*,+	37.6±4+	9.9±1
Improvement												
NA, pg/ml	299±6+	301±7+	312±16+	316±14+	343±14+	340±10+	308±5+	342±13+	357±17+	354±19+	332±19+	279±14
Ad, pg/ml	116±17+	98±8+	124±23+	127±13+	125±16+	117±13+	97±6+	95±17+	98±15+	102±21+	109±25+	38±13
p5HT, ng/ml	106±12+	115±9+	76±9+	74±8+	81±9+	109±10+	111±13+	100±5+	67±17+	72±11+	89±13+	227±24
f5HT, ng/ml	3.6±2+	3.1±1+	5.5±2+	5.7±4+	5.3±2+	5.2±02+	3.0±0.8+	3.2±0.8+	4.3±1+	4.2±1+	4.2±1.9+	0.9±0.8
NA/Ad ratio	2.2±1+	2.3±1+	1.7±1+	1.1±0.9+	1.7±1+	1.4±1+	2.7±0.8+	2.6±0.8+	1.8±0.9+	1.7±0.9+	2.1±1.1+	5.7±1
CRT, µg/dl	19±2+	16±1+	27±3+	28±2+	27±3+	25±2+	18±2+	18±1+	22±3+	23±3+	23.6±2.1+	9.9±1

General mean ± SE. Nm = Normal controls. * Exacerbation vs. improvement, $p < 0.001$; + exacerbation or improvement vs. Nm, $p < 0.001$. Nonsignificant differences were found between patients groups. Ast = Asthmatics; CB = chronic bronchitis; UC = ulcerative colitis; CD = Crohn's disease; CAH = chronic active hepatitis; CRP = chronic relapsing pancreatitis; MS = multiple sclerosis; TN = trigeminal neuralgia; SLE = systemic lupus erythematosus; RA = rheumatoid arthritis. Several decimals were omitted or approximated.

stressed subjects, the dysthymic group show increased tryptophan plasma levels, normal free serotonin levels, normal platelet aggregability, adrenomedullary hypoactivity, etc., all of which differentiate this dysthymic profile from the other two groups. Psychiatric investigation will provide, respectively, negative or positive additional information to support maladaptation to stress or depression syndromes.

Over the past 25 years the authors have investigated this matter in thousands of patients (psychiatric, psychosomatic and somatic), reporting the results in many published papers. Our findings may be summarized as follows:

(1) All severely diseased patients presented uncoping stress profile (table 5.2), accentuated during relapse and attenuated during remission (fig. 5.6–5.11).

(2) While an uncoping stress profile was observed in subjects other than severely diseased (fig. 5.12; table 5.2), these severely diseased patients never lacked the uncoping stress profile.

(3) All acutely diseased subjects presented the uncoping stress profile, which totally disappeared after healing. However, only attenuation (but not total disappearance) of the uncoping stress profile was observed during remission of chronic severe diseased subjects (table 5.2).

(4) Psychosomatic patients (headache, nervous diarrhea, some bradyarrhythmias and tachyarrhythmias, labile hypertension, adult respiratory distress syndrome,

etc.) as well as some psychiatric (nondepressed) subjects (anxiety, insomnia disorders, etc.) usually present the uncoping stress profile.

(5) Some psychosomatic (spastic colon syndrome, headache, reflux esophagitis, somatoform disorders, etc.) and some psychiatric patients did not show the uncoping stress profile during the supine resting condition but presented it throughout the orthostasis-moderate exercise challenge.

(6) All patients presenting the uncoping stress profile also showed: (a) adrenal gland hyperresponsiveness to oral glucose load; (b) growth hormone hyperresponsiveness to intramuscular clonidine injection; (c) great diastolic blood pressure fall after clonidine; (d) deep sleep after clonidine; (e) absence of distal colon tone plus distal colon motility suppressed by clonidine; (f) increased platelet aggregability, and (g) high f5HT in plasma.

Psychiatric investigation ruled out endogenous and dysthymic depression in all subjects showing the maladptation to stress profile. Conversely, depressed patients presented the neurochemical, hormonal, physiologic, metabolic and clonidine test profile typical of depression.

Up to the present, the authors have investigated a great many severe chronic diseases: cancer [Lechin F et al., 1987a, 1988b, 1989d, 1990b; Lechin S et al., 1988; van der Dijs et al., 1988b, c; Vitelli et al., 1988], ulcerative colitis [Lechin F et al., 1982d, 1985a], Crohn's disease [Lechin F et al., 1989d, 1994b], duodenal ulcer (fig. 5.6–

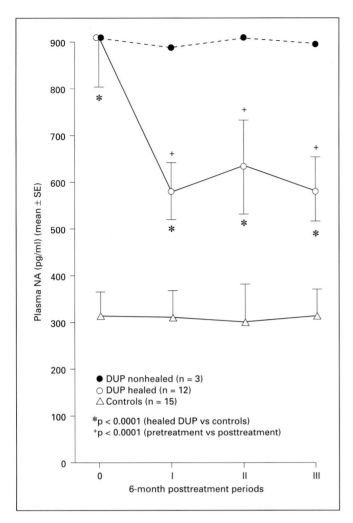

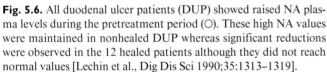

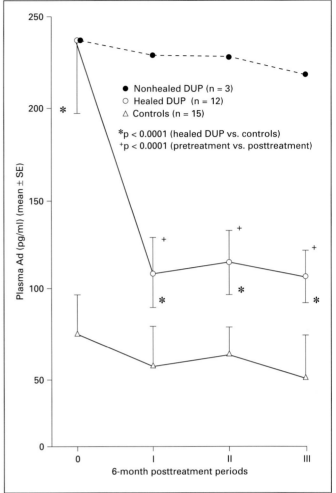

Fig. 5.6. All duodenal ulcer patients (DUP) showed raised NA plasma levels during the pretreatment period (O). These high NA values were maintained in nonhealed DUP whereas significant reductions were observed in the 12 healed patients although they did not reach normal values [Lechin et al., Dig Dis Sci 1990;35:1313–1319].

Fig. 5.7. All duodenal ulcer patients (DUP) showed raised adrenaline plasma levels during the pretreatment period (O). These elevated values were maintained in nonhealed DUP whereas significant reductions were observed in the 12 healed DUP, although they did not reach normal values [Lechin et al., Dig Dis Sci 1990a;35:1313–1319].

5.11) [Jara et al., 1988; Lechin F et al., 1990a], bronchial asthma [Lechin AE et al., 1988c, 1994a, b; Lechin F, 2000; Lechin and van der Dijs, 2001; Lechin F et al., 1998a, b, 1996c], systemic lupus erythematous [Lechin F et al., 1994b], rheumatoid arthritis [Lechin F et al., 1994b], trigeminal neuralgia [Lechin F et al., 1988a, 1989c], postprandial hypoglycemia [Lechin F et al., 1991], hypertensive syndrome [Lechin F et al., 1993], multiple sclerosis [Lechin F et al., 1994b], relapsing pancreatitis [Lechin F et al., 1992b], chronic bronchitis [Lechin F et al., 1994b], chronic active hepatitis [Lechin F et al., 1994b]. These patients were investigated during exac-

erbation as well as remission periods (table 5.2). We also have investigated many acutely diseased patients who were controlled after healing (acute pancreatitis, acute appendicitis, acute hepatitis, pneumonia, acute cholecystitis, acute viral infection, acute myocardial infarction, etc.). In addition, psychosomatic patients (irritable bowel syndrome, headache, reflux esophagitis, somatoform disorders, and others) [Lechin AE et al., 1988b; Lechin F et al., 1977a, b, 1978, 1994a, c; Lechin and van der Dijs, 1977, 1980; Lechin ME et al., 1988a–d; van der Dijs et al., 1988a] and psychiatric patients [Gomez et al., 1988; Lechin and van der Dijs, 1981a–d, 1982; Lechin F et al.,

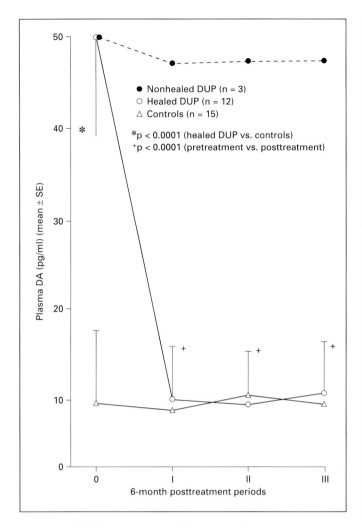

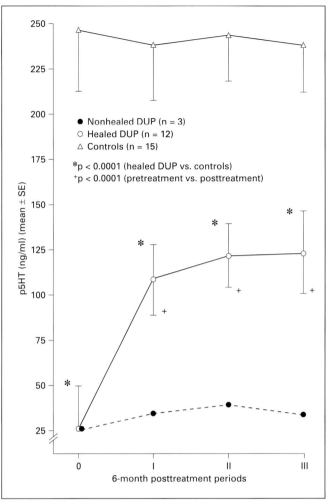

Fig. 5.8. All DUP showed raised DA plasma levels during the pretreatment period (○). These high DA values remained unchanged in non-healed DUP whereas they became totally normal in the 12 healed patients [Lechin et al, Dig Dis Sci 1990a;35:1313–1319].

Fig. 5.9. All DUP showed decreased platelet serotonin values during the pretreatment period. These values remained low in nonhealed patients while they rose significantly throughout the 3 posttreatment periods (I, II, III) in healed DUP when compared with pretreatment values (○), although remaining significantly lower than controls [Lechin et al., Dig Dis Sci 1990a;35:1313–1319].

1980a, b, 1982a–c, 1983a–c, 1995a, b] were also investigated according to the same protocol.

Questions arise as to the cause-effect sequence between diseases and the maladaptation to stress profile. Obviously, exacerbation of all diseases should provoke neurochemical, hormonal, metabolic and physiological disorders compatible with uncoping stress. In most cases, the uncoping stress profile does not disappear totally during chronic disease remission periods. Interestingly, in some cases we detected the uncoping stress profile before the appearance of exacerbation periods. Hence, the authors believe both statements to be true: (1) uncoping stress

favors the appearance of disease, and (2) exacerbations aggravate the uncoping stress profile (table 5.2, 5.3).

The authors also found that some chronic diseases are associated with the endogenous depression profile (autoimmune diseases, malignant hypertension, some types of headache, and some types of postprandial hypoglycemia, spastic colon syndrome, etc.) (fig. 5.3, 5.13). However, some of these diseases may present a stress profile during severe exacerbations.

The authors also routinely investigated the peripheral immunological profile of all patients. We found that immunological disorders paralleled neurochemical, hor-

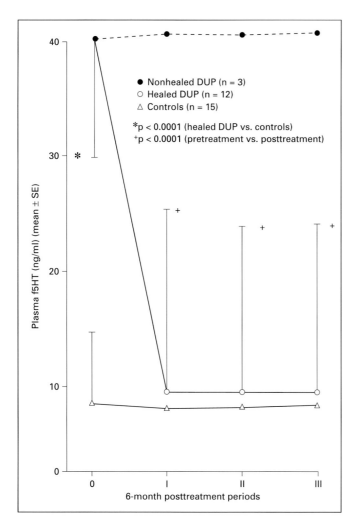

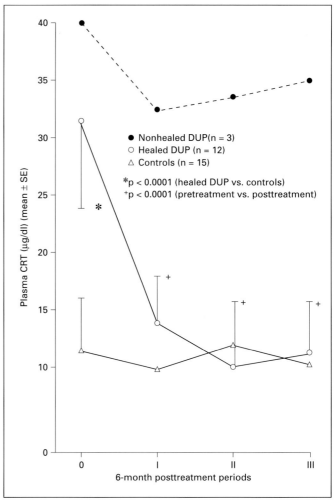

Fig. 5.10. All DUP showed high p5HT values during the pretreatment period (○). These values remained unaltered in nonhealed patients, whereas they became completely normal after the first 6-week posttreatment period (I) in the 12 healed patients [Lechin et al., Dig Dis Sci 1990a;35:1313–1319].

Fig. 5.11. All DUP showed raised cortisol plasma values during the pretreatment period (○). These values remained high in nonhealed patients, whereas they became totally normal in the 12 healed patients after the first 6-week post-treatment period (I) [Lechin et al., Dig Dis Sci 1990a;35:1313–1319].

monal and metabolic disorders. While uncoping stress profile was found to be associated with immunosuppression, endogenous depression profile was associated with normal immunity or hyperimmunity. We believe that the conflicting reports dealing with this matter may be attributed to a lack of accurate differential diagnosis distinguishing the two types of patients (uncoping stressed or endogenous depressed) [Andreoli et al., 1992; Cabrera et al., 1988; Croiset et al., 1987; Cross and Roszman, 1988; Dantzer and Kelley, 1989; Darko et al., 1988; Khansari et al., 1990; Lechin F et al., 1985b, 1987b, 1989b, 1990b, 1994b, 1995a, b; Maes et al., 1993, 1994; Mormede et al.,

1988; Pavlidis and Chirigos, 1980; Steplewski et al., 1985; Tecoma and Huey, 1985; Tonnesen et al., 1984; Weisse et al., 1990; Weizman et al., 1994].

The authors are aware that the stress profile they have demonstrated in humans is a peripheral profile which cannot be linked with certainty to the central neurochemical disorder occurring during uncontrollable stress in mammals. However, we believe that the peripheral approach to this issue is strongly supported by ample scientific evidence, permitting it to meet clinical and therapeutic requirements.

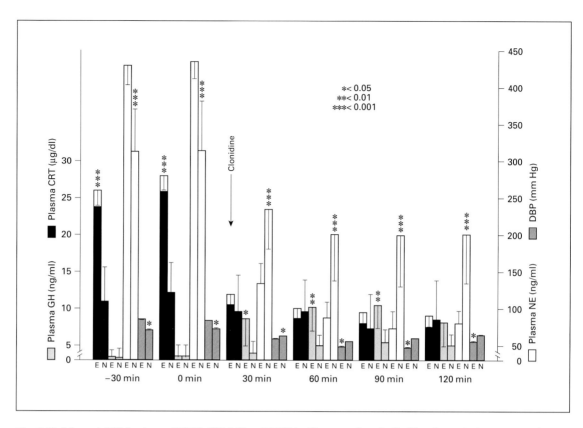

Fig. 5.12. Mean ± SEM values of CRT, GH, NE and DBP in 92 severe chronically ill patients during exacerbation (E) and nonexacerbation (N) periods, before and after the administration of clonidine (2 µg/kg, i.m.). p Values are shown for comparison of E with N mean values at each time (paired t test for preclonidine and ANOVA for postclonidine times). Clonidine provoked significantly greater reduction of NE, DBP, and CRT during E than N periods. In addition, the drug induced significantly greater increase of GH during E than N periods [Lechin et al., Psychoneuroendocrinology 1987b;12:117–129].

Table 5.3. Plasma NA, Ad, f5HT, p5HT, platelet aggregability (pAgg), CRT, peripheral blood lymphocytes (lymphocytes %), natural killer cell activity (NK), and CD4/CD8 lymphocytes subset ratio in 23 long-term (≥ 4 years) symptomless cancer patients, 56 exacerbated cancer patients, and their age- and sex-paired normal controls

	Symptomless patients	Control subjects	Exacerbated patients	Control subjects
NA, pg/ml	427.0 ± 15.0[a]	253.0 ± 9.0	97.0 ± 18.0[b]	267.0 ± 8.0
Ad, pg/ml	86.0 ± 8.0[a]	52.0 ± 6.0	134.0 ± 15.0[b]	49.0 ± 5.0
NA/Ad	4.5 ± 0.4	5.1 ± 0.6	1.4 ± 0.8[b]	5.2 ± 0.7
p5HT, ng/ml	253.0 ± 29.0	248.0 ± 25.0	107.0 ± 31.0[b]	225.0 ± 22.0
f5HT, ng/ml	1.1 ± 0.4	1.2 ± 0.3	7.4 ± 2.0[b]	1.2 ± 0.5
CRT, µg/ml	9.7 ± 2.0	9.5 ± 2.0	19.0 ± 3.0[b]	9.4 ± 2.0
Lymphocytes, %	42.0 ± 1.0[a]	31.0 ± 2.0	17.0 ± 4.0[b]	33.0 ± 3.0
NK cells, %	44.0 ± 3.0[a]	35.0 ± 2.0	22.0 ± 3.0[b]	34.0 ± 2.0
CD4/CD8	2.4 ± 0.1[a]	2.0 ± 0.1	1.2 ± 0.1[b]	2.0 ± 0.1
pAgg, %	17.0 ± 2.0	19.0 ± 2.0	43.0 ± 5.0[b]	18.0 ± 2.0

Values are expressed as mean ± SEM. [a] Symptomless vs. control; $p < 0.001$; [b] exacerbated vs. control; $p < 0.001$. Only exacerbated patients showed hyperresponsiveness to i.m. clonidine injection. No depression was registered in patients and controls. Many decimals were omitted [Lechin F et al., Psychoneuroendocrinology 1987b;12:117–129]

Human Model of Maladapted to Stress
Situation

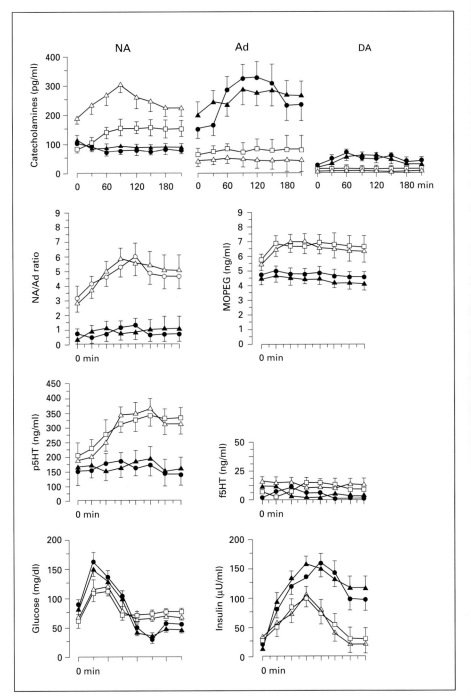

Fig. 5.13. Three consecutive oral glucose tolerance tests were performed in 11 postprandial symptomatic hypoglycemic (nondepressed) patients and their age-sex paired healthy controls (□). The first (▲) before placebo; second (●) before doxepin therapy, and third (△) after 3-week doxepin therapy. Large increases in Ad (coincident with adrenergic symptoms = tachycardia, anxiety, etc.), as well as elevation of DA values were registered during tests in untreated patients. On the contrary, no changes in NA/Ad ratio, MOPEG, p5HT or f5HT were observed after doxepin therapy. The nadir in glucose occurred at 150 min. All disordered variables were normalized and all symptoms disappeared after doxepin therapy. Values are mean ± SEM [Lechin et al., Clin Sci 1991;80:373–384].

Dysthymic Depression and Endogenous Depression

The changes of systolic, diastolic and differential (pulse) pressure (SBP, DBP and PP) as well as heart rate (HR) and plasma neurotransmitters provoked by ortho-stasis and moderate exercise in 17 dysthymic depressed patients and their age-sex paired controls were investigated (fig. 5.14, 5.15). Also, the plasma CRT and platelet aggregability values were reported. No significant differences between the two groups were observed in resting (0-min) values of BP, HR, Ad, DA, CRT, and platelet

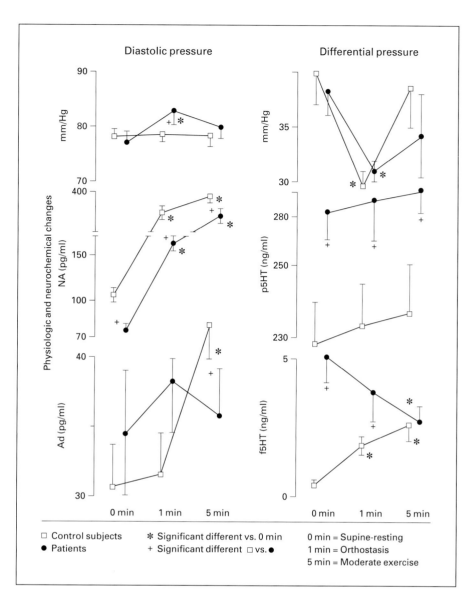

Fig. 5.14. Physiologic and neurochemical changes provoked by orthostasis and moderate exercise in 17 dysthymic depressed patients and their age-sex paired controls [Lechin et al., Biol Psychiatry 1995a;37: 884–891].

□ Control subjects   ＊ Significant different vs. 0 min   0 min = Supine-resting
● Patients   ＋ Significant different □ vs. ●   1 min = Orthostasis
                                                            5 min = Moderate exercise

aggregability. On the other hand, dysthymic subjects showed significantly greater TRP and f5HT plasma levels and significantly lower NA and NA/Ad ratios than normals. Although dysthymic patients showed the normal differential PP reduction at orthostasis (1 min), this was not prevented by atropine as in the case of controls (fig. 5.16). This PP fall is due to the fact that patients but not normals showed significant rises of DBP throughout the test which paralleled and were positively correlated with NA and NA/Ad rises. Furthermore, elevated resting (0 min) f5HT values registered in patients (suppressible by atropine) showed progressive and significant reductions throughout the test, and were negatively correlated

with DBP, NA, and NA/Ad values. Ad did not show the normal exercise (5-min) peak. The above findings strongly suggest that dysthymic patients show inhibition of adrenal gland sympathetic activity. Conversely, evidence of hyperparasympathetic activity in dysthymic subjects was obtained [Lechin F et al., 1988c, 1995a].

The inhibition of adrenal glands + weakness of neural sympathetic activity + high parasympathetic activity (raised TRP + f5HT plasma levels) suppressible by atropine, registered in dysthymics contrast with the high neural (NA) sympathetic + low TRP profile registered in major (endogenous) depression patients. In turn, both groups differ from uncoping stressed subjects who show

---

Dysthymic Depression and Endogenous
Depression

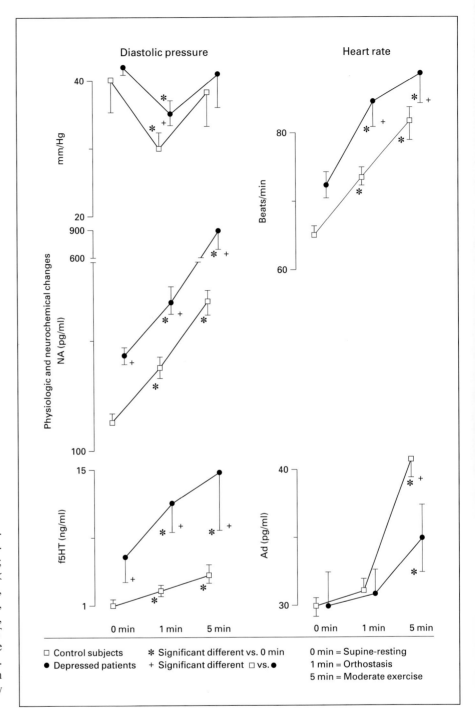

Fig. 5.15. Supine-resting depressed vs. control values (mean ± SE): differential pressure = 43.3 ± 2.1 vs. 40.4 ± 4.0, p = NS; heart rate = 73.1 ± 2.6 vs. 65.2 ± 2.2, p < 0.02; NA = 362.4 ± 33.3 vs. 112.4 ± 28.2, p < 0.001; Ad = 29.4 ± 2.0 vs. 29.3 ± 1.9, p = NS; f5HT = 5.9 ± 1.0 vs. 0.9 ± 0.2, p < 0.001. The heart rate, NA, and f5HT rises at orthostasis and exercise periods were greater in depressed than in normal subjects. The 5′-Ad rise was smaller in patients than in normals [Lechin et al., Biol Psychiatry 1995;38:166–173].

high adrenal gland sympathetic activity + hypoactivity of the parasympathetic system + total exhaustion of neural (NA) sympathetic system. These three different profiles registered in dysthymic depression, endogenous depression and uncoping stress favor the understanding of their underlying pathophysiologic mechanisms and, consequently, their diagnostic and therapeutical approach. Furthermore, the weak central (NA) system registered in dysthymics during supine resting periods suggests that these patients are more easily thrown into uncoping stress situations than normals or, of course, than endogenous depressed subjects.

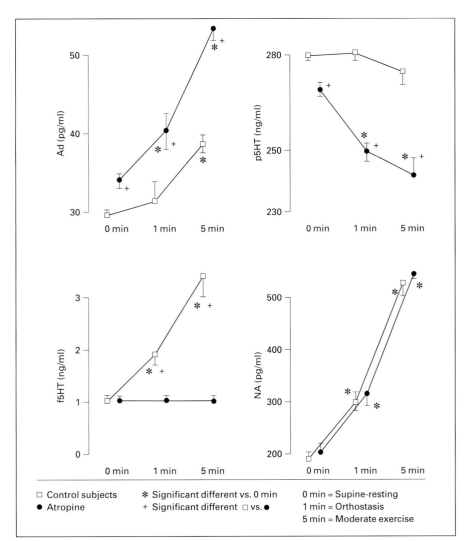

Fig. 5.16. Plasma NA, Ad, f5HT, heart rate, and differential (pulse) pressure during supine-resting, orthostasis and moderate exercise in 35 endogenous depressed patients and their age-sex paired controls. Whereas NA rose at the 1-min and 5-min periods, Ad showed a slight 5-min peak only. f5HT was higher than normal at the 0-min period and experienced greater than normal rises at the 1-min and 5-min periods. Differential pressure reduction at 1 min was registered in both groups. The same was prevented by atropine in both groups (not presented data). The 1-min and 5-min heart rate peaks were greater in depressed patients than in normals [Lechin et al., Biol Psychiatry 1995b;38: 166–173].

□ Control subjects   * Significant different vs. 0 min   0 min = Supine-resting
● Atropine   + Significant different □ vs. ●   1 min = Orthostasis
                                                         5 min = Moderate exercise

Biological Markers Differentiating Endogenous and Dysthymic Depressed Patients from Maladapted to Stress Patients

Up to the present, our research group has developed the following biological markers which have proved to behave differently in endogenous and dysthymic depressed and supposedly stressed patients:

(1) Plasma dosification of neurotransmitters (NA, Ad, DA, p5HT, f5HT, TRP), CRT, and platelet aggregability during the supine-resting-fasting condition [Cabrera et al., 1988; Gomez et al., 1988; Jara et al., 1988; Lechin AE et al., 1988b, c, 1994a; Lechin F et al., 1988a–d, 1989d, 1990a, b, 1992b, 1994b; Lechin ME et al., 1988a–d; van der Dijs et al., 1988a–c; Vitelli et al., 1988].

(2) Plasma neurotransmitters, DBP (fig. 5.2), CRT, GH (fig. 5.1, 5.2, 5.12) and distal colon motility (fig. 5.17) before and after intramuscular clonidine injection [Lechin F et al., 1985b, c, 1987b, 1989a].

(3) Plasma neurotransmitters, plasma glucose, plasma insulin, blood pressure (BP) and heart rate (HR) throughout an oral glucose tolerance test (OGTT) (fig. 5.3, 5.13) [Lechin AE et al., 1988a; Lechin F et al., 1991, 1992a, 1993].

(4) Plasma neurotransmitters, BP, and HR during supine-resting-fasting, orthostasis and moderate exercise conditions (fig. 5.4, 5.5, 5.14–5.16) [Lechin AE et al., 1994b; Lechin F et al., 1995a, b, 1996a, b].

Endogenous depressed (fig. 5.18), maladapted to stress (fig. 5.19), and dysthymic depressed patients (fig. 5.20) showed three distinct profiles (fig. 5.21).

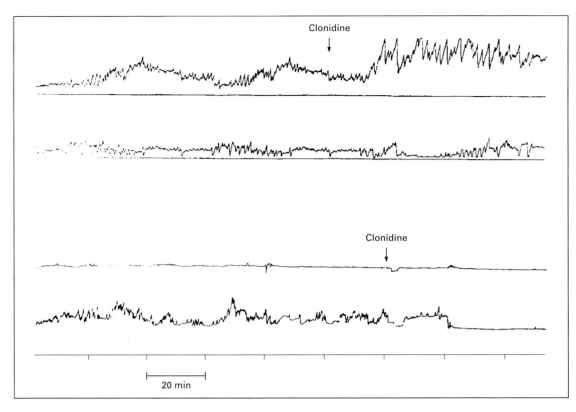

Fig. 5.17. Clonidine (2 µg/kg, i.m.) increased sigmoidal tone and phasic activity (waves) in the upper case (depressed subjects). On the contrary, the drug reduced rectal colon motility in the lower case (severely ill stressed patient) and provoked deep sleep, but not in the former subject. In addition, DBP showed great reduction in the stressed but not in the depressed patient [Lechin et al., The Autonomic Nervous System: Physiological Basis of Psychosomatic Therapy. Barcelona, Editorial Científico-Médica, 1979b].

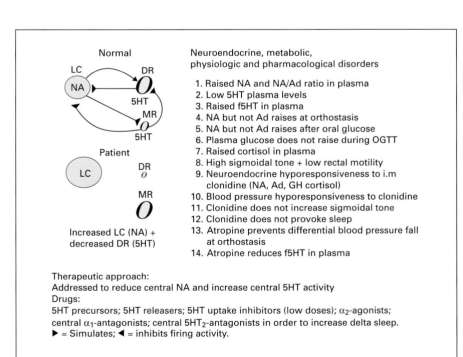

Normal

Neuroendocrine, metabolic, physiologic and pharmacological disorders

1. Raised NA and NA/Ad ratio in plasma
2. Low 5HT plasma levels
3. Raised f5HT in plasma
4. NA but not Ad raises at orthostasis
5. NA but not Ad raises after oral glucose
6. Plasma glucose does not raise during OGTT
7. Raised cortisol in plasma
8. High sigmoidal tone + low rectal motility
9. Neuroendocrine hyporesponsiveness to i.m clonidine (NA, Ad, GH cortisol)
10. Blood pressure hyporesponsiveness to clonidine
11. Clonidine does not increase sigmoidal tone
12. Clonidine does not provoke sleep
13. Atropine prevents differential blood pressure fall at orthostasis
14. Atropine reduces f5HT in plasma

Patient

Increased LC (NA) + decreased DR (5HT)

Therapeutic approach:
Addressed to reduce central NA and increase central 5HT activity
Drugs:
5HT precursors; 5HT releasers; 5HT uptake inhibitors (low doses); α_2-agonists; central α_1-antagonists; central $5HT_2$-antagonists in order to increase delta sleep.
▶ = Simulates; ◀ = inhibits firing activity.

Fig. 5.18. Endogenous depression. Hyperactivity of central NA system plus exhaustion of 5HT activity [Lechin et al., Prog Neuro-Psychopharmacol Biol Psychiatry 1998;20: 899–950].

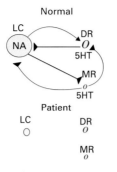

Normal

LC   DR
(NA)   O
           5HT
             MR
              o
             5HT

Patient
LC   DR
O   O

             MR
              o

LC (NA), DR (5HT) and
MR (5HT)
activities are exhausted

Neuroendocrine, metabolic,
physiologic and pharmacological disorders

1. Raised Ad in plasma
2. Low NA/Ad plasma ratio
3. Low p5HT levels
4. Raised f5HT plasma levels
5. Raised cortisol plasma levels
6. The normal NA peak at orthostasis is absent
7. An abnormal Ad peak at orthostasis is present
8. The raised supine-resting f5HT does not
   show the normal orthostasis + exercise increase
9. Ad + DA but NA rise after oral glucose
10. Low sigmoidal tone + rectal hypermotility
11. Neuroendocrine hyperresponsiveness to i.m
    clonidine (NA, Ad, GH, CRT)
12. Blood pressure hyperresponsiveness to clonidine
13. Clonidine suppresses rectal hypermotility
14. The normal differential blood pressure reduction
    during orthostasis is not observed
15. Clonidine provokes deep sleep
16. Atropine does not provoke f5HT reduction
17. Increased platelet aggregability

Therapeutic approach:
Addressed to reduce adrenal glands hyperactivity
+ increase central NA + 5HT activity and parasympathetic activity.
Enhancement of SWS
Drugs:
5HT, NA, DA uptake inhibitors; 5HT precursors; α_2-agonists; central α_1-antagonists;
central $5HT_2$ antagonists; GH stimulating drugs

Fig. 5.19. Maladaptation to stress. Exhaustion of both central NA and 5HT activity [Lechin et al., Prog Neuro-Psychopharmacol Biol Psychiatry 1998;20:899–950].

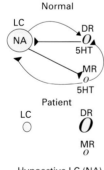

Normal

LC   DR
(NA)   O
           5HT
             MR
              o
             5HT

Patient
LC   DR
O   O

             MR
              o

Hypoactive LC (NA) +
hyperactive DR (5HT)

Neuroendocrine, metabolic,
physiologic and pharmacological disorders

1. Low NA and NA/Ad ratio in plasma
2. Raised p5HT plasma levels
3. Raised f5HT in plasma
4. Plasma Ad does not show the normal rise
   during moderate exercise (adrenals hyporesponsiveness)
5. NA show the normal orthostasis + exercise peaks
6. f5HT does not show the normal orthostasis
   + exercise peaks. Instead, it shows reductions
7. DBP peaks at orthostasis + exercise. The peaks are
   positively correlated with NA peaks. And both DBP-Na
   are negatively correlated with f5HT reductions
8. Atropine reduces the resting raised f5HT
9. Atropine does not prevent the differential blood
   pressure orthostasis fall, as occurs in normal
   and major depressed subjects

Therapeutic approach:
Addressed to increased central NA activity and to reduce central 5HT activity.
Drugs:
Catecholamine precursors and releasers; cathecholamine uptake
inhibitors (low doses); 5HT uptake enhancers; 5HT depleting agents;
5HT1a agonists parasympathetic ganglionic-blocking drugs

Fig. 5.20. Dysthymic depression. Central 5HT hyperactivitiy plus NA hypoactivity [Lechin et al., Prog Neuro-Psychopharmacol Biol Psychiatry 1998;20:899–950].

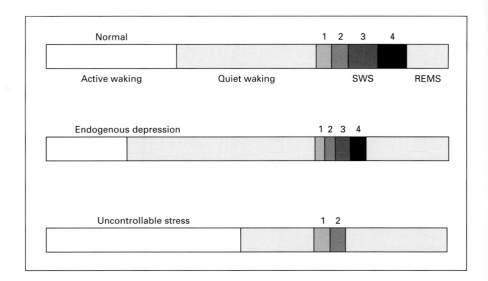

Fig. 5.21. SWS = Stages 1, 2, 3, and 4.

Hypothesis

According to the experimental findings presented above, the authors propose three different models of central neurochemical disorders as seen in the syndromes of endogenous depression (fig. 5.18), maladaptation to stress (fig. 5.19) and dysthymic depression (fig. 5.20). These models are based on neuroanatomical, neurophysiological, neurochemical and neuropharmacological findings and have been amply demonstrated in experimental mammal studies as enumerated here.

The NA neurons of the locus coeruleus (LC = A6 nucleus) rule central sympathetic activity. Stimulation of this nucleus provokes a release of NA from central noradrenergic terminals as well as peripheral sympathetic nerves, thus increasing the levels of circulating NA. The locus coeruleus neurons send excitatory axons to serotonergic nuclei of DR = (B7) and MR = (B8). In turn, both DR and MR neurons send inhibitory axons to NA neurons in the locus coeruleus. DR and MR neurons are more active during waking periods. However, all three types of neurons are silent during REM sleep. Furthermore, DR and MR neurons interchange inhibitory axons. [Lechin F et al., 1979b, 1989a; Lechin and van der Dijs, 1984].

Although exhaustion of NA (A6) + 5HT (B7-B8) nuclei has been shown in experimentally stressed mammals,

exact information as to the physiological activity of these nuclei has not been ascertained for endogenous and dysthymic depressed humans. However, indirect evidence supports the inference that whereas NA (A6) overactivity + 5HT (B7-B8) inhibition underlie endogenous depression, the opposite profile of NA (A6) hypoactivity + 5HT (B7-B8) hyperactivity would exist in dysthymic depression.

Our hypothesis receives additional support from the finding that whereas sleep deprivation induces maladaptation to stress syndrome, the same procedure is able to improve depression [Vogel, 1975].

Conclusions

Evidence is presented showing the existence of three distinct syndromes in humans: (1) endogenous depression; (2) dysthymic depression, and (3) maladaptation to stress. Although these syndromes may present clinical overlap, they can be differentiated throughout their neuroendocrine, neurochemical, physiologic, metabolic and neuropharmacological profiles. These findings should lead to trials of more specific therapeutical approaches. Theoretical pathophysiological models are postulated for the three syndromes.

Chapter 6

....

Bipolar Syndrome

We will attempt to delineate the two phases of this syndrome: manic and depressive.

Manic Stage

The very low levels of TRP in the plasma registered in manic patients are indicative of their poor midbrain serotonergic activity. This neurochemical deficiency is consistent with an unbalanced neurocircuitry showing predominance of both the DA + the NA systems. Although the plasma NA levels registered in these patients are not as high as those found in endogenous depressed patients these NA values show significant rise during orthostasis, moderate exercise, oral glucose and buspirone stress challenges.

Although it is not possible to correlate mesocortical-mesolimbic DA activity with a plasma neurotransmitter profile, both clinical and experimental data strongly suggest that such activity is highly increased during manic stage syndrome. Intellectual, emotional, affective, reward, sexual and motor hyperactivities are always present in manic patients. In addition, the overt predominance of DA over the serotonergic system is consistent with the insomnia registered in these patients.

The absence of anxiety observed in manic patients is compatible with the poor adrenomedullary responsiveness registered in them. In effect, plasma Ad did not rise during the different stress tests we used routinely. For this reason, we have depicted a normal (size and color) C1-Ad medullary nuclei (fig. 6.1). We hypothesize that these patients present an unbalanced excitatory (glutamic acid) plus a low inhibitory (GABA) profile. Both the VTA-DA and the LC-NA nuclei receive excitatory glutamic inputs. On the contrary, the DR-5HT nucleus receives only gabaergic input, which arises from the habenula nucleus.

For this reason, manic patients did not respond to gabamimetic drugs (benzodiazepines) over long-term periods.

Neuropharmacologic manipulations usually administered to manic patients seek to increase serotonin release at both cortical and subcortical areas. Lithium salts, carbamazepine and other serotonin-releasing agents are administered in progressively higher doses. However, these treatments tend to lose effectiveness due to two causes: exhaustion of serotonin stores and downregulation of postsynaptic 5HT receptors. Dopaminergic antagonists are also used for treating manic syndrome. In our experience, sulpiride is the most useful DA antagonist to treat these patients. This DA_2 + DA_3 antagonist is, in addition, a moderate 5HT releaser and does not provoke extrapyramidal side effects.

Fig. 6.1. Bipolar – manic stage. LC = Locus coeruleus; DR = dorsal raphe; MR = median raphe; RM = raphe magnus; RO = raphe obscurus; RP = raphe pallidus; mcn = mesocortical nucleus; PVN = paraventricular nucleus; AH = anterior hypothalamus; PH = posterior hypothalamus; VMN = ventromedial nucleus; PRF = pontoreticular formation; PPN = pedunculopontine nucleus; CRF = corticotrophin-releasing factor; AP = area postrema; Na = noradrenaline; Ad = adrenaline; ACh = acetylcholine; 5HT = serotonin. → Excitation; −< inhibition. Concentric circles, bright and faded colors indicate neuronal activity. Dashed lines indicate reduced output.

Fig. 6.2. Bipolar – depressive stage. LC = Locus coeruleus; DR = dorsal raphe; MR = median raphe; RM = raphe magnus; RO = raphe obscurus; RP = raphe pallidus; mcn = mesocortical nucleus; PVN = paraventricular nucleus; AH = anterior hypothalamus; PH = posterior hypothalamus; VMN = ventromedial nucleus; PRF = pontoreticular formation; PPN = pedunculopontine nucleus; CRF = corticotrophin-releasing factor; AP = area postrema; Na = noradrenaline; Ad = adrenaline; ACh = acetylcholine; 5HT = serotonin. → Excitation; −< inhibition. Concentric circles, bright and faded colors indicate neuronal activity. Dashed lines indicate reduced output.

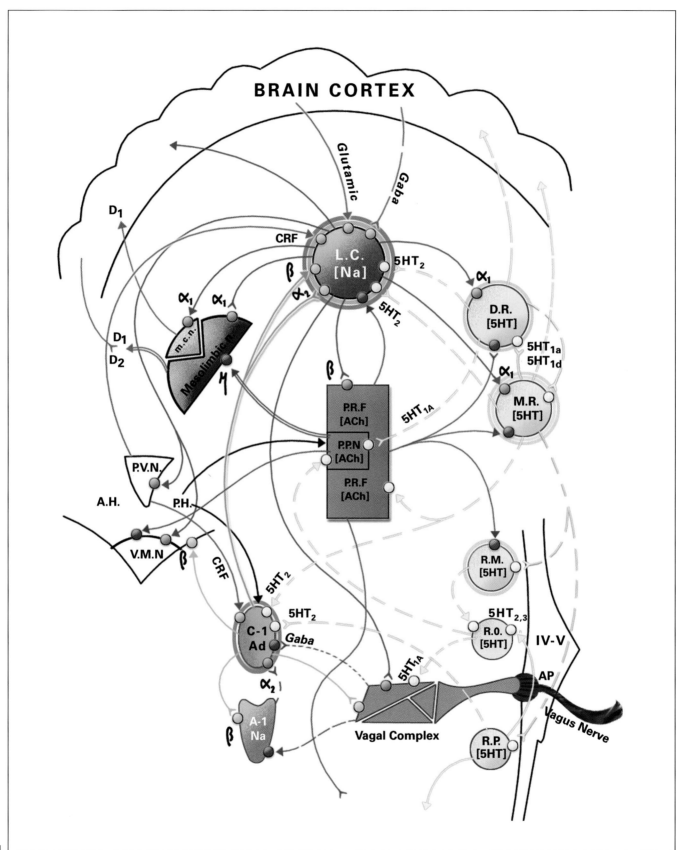

Bipolar Syndrome

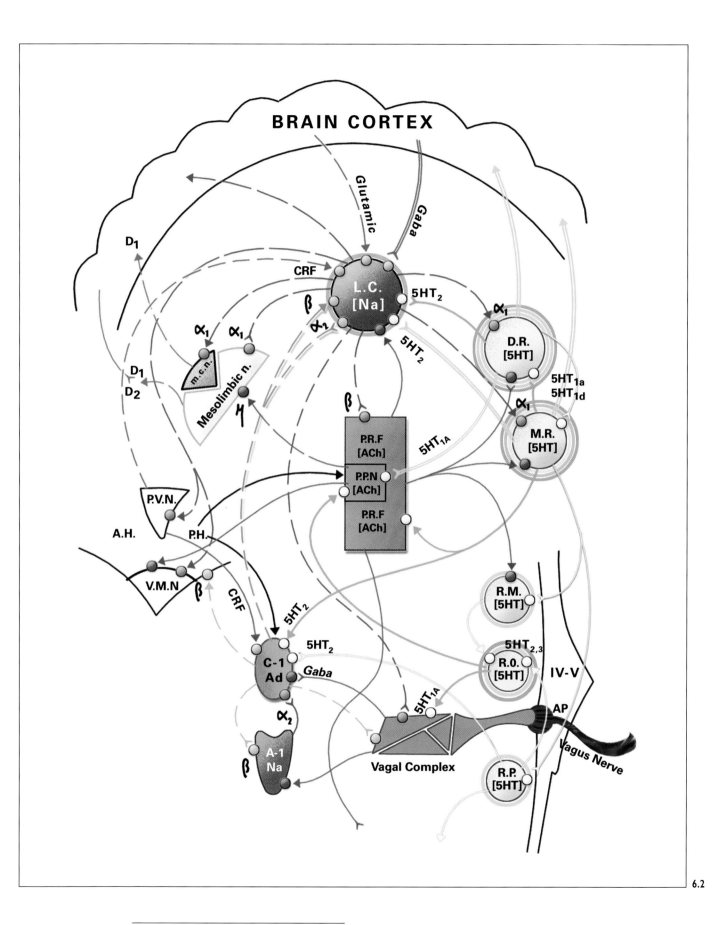

In our experience, the 5HT precursor 5-OH-TRP is the most useful drug for treating manic patients. We have treated hundreds of these patients with this drug without observing any undesirable side effects. Neither were relapses observed in patients receiving this treatment. Progressive reduction of the drug is usually employed, until reaching its total and/or maximal suppression. Progressive reduction of lithium doses should be made in patients receiving this treatment.

Depressive Stage

Absence of mesolimbic dopaminergic activity + restoration of serotonergic activity are the main neurochemical changes postulated in the brain neurochemical circuitry of these patients, once they change from manic to depressive stage (fig. 6.2). We depict an MR-5HT predominance over the DR-5HT, because the firing activity of DR neurons depend on excitatory NA-α_1 input arising from the LC-NA axons. However, this excitatory input depends on the GABA interposed neuron, presynaptically located at the DR-5HT neuron. If we accept that manic patients have a deficit of the GABA system, the DR-5HT system would always be deficient. In addition, the MR-5HT nucleus would be disinhibited from the DR-5HT inhibitory axons. Other data may be observed in the diagram.

In our long experience of treating these patients, best results were obtained with administration of low doses of an NA-uptake inhibitor (desipramine, maprotyline, doxepin, etc.), no more than 25 mg before breakfast, along with an NA precursor (*L*-phenylalanine or *L*-tyrosine 50 mg) + an NA-releasing agent such as yohimbine (2.5–5 mg). This therapy should be balanced once the patient overcomes depression, when 5-OH-TRP should be added at night (25–50 mg) before bed. Further, most of our patients are maintained with very low doses of clomipramine (25 mg) before bed. This drug is a 5HT uptake inhibitor (75%) and its metabolite (desmethylimipramine) is an inhibitor of NA uptake. In addition, there are several experimental and clinical researchers who have demonstrated that clomipramine triggers neuroautonomic balance while also displaying DA antagonistic activity.

According to our wide experience, we cannot support the simplistic therapeutic approaches based on high doses of lithium during manic stages and 'antidepressants' during depressive stages. Physicians treating these patients should be supplied with appropriate neurochemical + neuropharmacological information.

Chapter 7

....

Psychotic Syndrome

The so-called dopaminergic hypothesis of schizophrenia was based on two statements: (1) All or most antipsychotic drugs were DA-blocking agents (DA antagonists). (2) Brain DA receptors were found to be increased in postmortem studies of schizophrenia.

Objections to this simplistic hypothesis arose from well-known neurophysiological and pharmacological findings showing that upregulation and not downregulation of DA receptors is secondary to a deficiency but not an excess of dopamine in the brain. Further, prolonged administration of DA-blocking agents triggers upregulation instead of downregulation of DA brain receptors. We discussed this issue in several published papers [J Clin Pharmacol 1980a, 1980b; Am J Psychiatry 1981; Br J Psychiatry 1981; Res Comm Psychol Psychiat Behav 1983]. In these papers and in our book [Neurochemistry and Clinical Disorders: Circuitry of Some Psychiatric and Psychosomatic Syndromes, Boca Raton, CRC Press, 1989], we postulate that noradrenergic plus serotonergic disorders should be included along with the DA mesolimbic overactivity + DA mesocortical deficit as pathophysiologic factors in psychotic patients. In effect, some recent hypotheses involve the 5HT brain system in causes of schizophrenia. Many experimental findings support this hypothesis. For instance, increased utilization of dopamine in the nucleus accumbens but not in the cerebral cortex was registered after lesions to the DR-5HT axons. This would explain the reduced cortical + increased mesolimbic DA activity postulated as the main neurochemical disorder in psychotic syndromes. In effect, experimental mammals whose mesocortical DA axons have been previously destroyed present a psychotic profile. With respect to this, it has been demonstrated that mesocortical DA activity displays a modulatory control over subcortical (mesolimbic) DA activity. In addition, experimental rats submitted to this type of lesion are being used as a reliable model of hyperkinetic (hyperactive) behavior.

The MR serotonergic nucleus has also been associated with the psychotic profile. Electrolytic lesions of the MR-5HT nucleus are responsible for opposite changes in dopamine utilization (increased) in the mesolimbic accumbens nucleus and decreased in the frontal cortex. In other words, the MR-5HT nucleus is positively associated with mesolimbic DA activity and negatively associated with mesocortical DA activity. This MR-5HT-DA interaction is antagonistic to that demonstrated by DR-5HT-DA interaction. Summarizing, MR-5HT would be positively associated with a psychotic profile whereas the DR-5HT nucleus would display an antagonism to the former. These findings are consistent with the demonstration that MR-5HT activity is associated with 'killing' (aggressive) behavior.

Nonmedicated schizophrenic patients show greater than normal p5HT values. This parameter would be associated with excessive activity of the adrenergic system plus hypoparasympathetic activity (low levels of cicuulating ACh). It is known that ACh interferes with platelet uptake which favors the increase of p5HT.

The demonstration by us in 1980 concerning the beneficial effects displayed by clonidine (α_2-antagonist drug) on suppression of acute psychotic episodes gave rise to the adrenergic hypothesis of schizophrenia. Similar effects were observed by others with the administration of β-adrenergic blocking agents; however, these drugs were unable to maintain their therapeutic effects during nonacute psychotic stages.

Further, it was demonstrated that psychotic patients show increases of basal and stimulated adrenergic activity. In effect, they show a dissociation of peripheral sympathetic activity: increased Ad + decreased NA plasma lev-

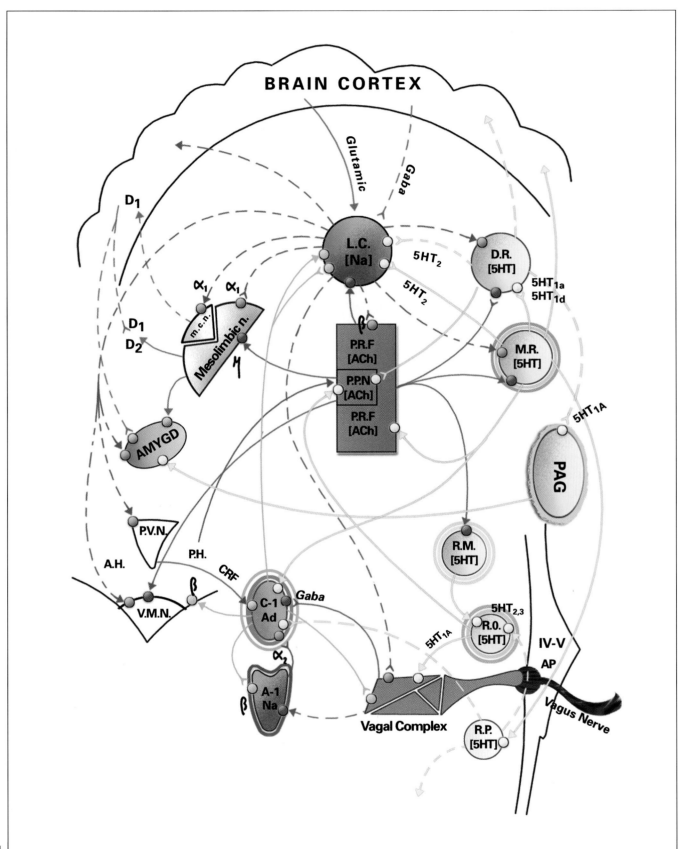

BRAIN CORTEX

els. The NA/Ad ratio falls to less than 2 during supine-resting condition. This NA/Ad ratio shows further reductions throughout all types of stress tests (orthostasis, moderate exercise, oral glucose, and buspirone). These findings are consistent with the ability of clonidine to suppress acute psychotic attacks. Overactivity of adrenal glands fits well with evidence showing that psychotic patients usually present an immunological profile of the Th2 type. The Th2 immunological profile is registered when humoral but not tissue immunity predominates. This Th2 > Th1 profile is registered during uncoping stress situation and is associated with excessive adrenergic (adrenomedullary) activity. A bulk of evidence ratifying the above continues to grow. The well-known fact that the C1-Ad medullary nucleus and not the LC-NA nucleus, is the main target of clonidine is consistent with all the above.

Recent findings, revealing that the quantity of LC-NA (locus coeruleus) neurons is diminished in the postmortem brain of untreated schizophrenic patients, supports the hypothesis that a deficiency of cortical NA activity is present in the psychotic syndrome.

Summarizing, accumulated evidence converges for the postulation that the neurocircuitry of the psychotic brain will include the following: (a) deficiency of LC-NA, DR-5HT + deficiency of DA mesocortical activities; (b) predominance of DA-mesolimbic, MR-5HT and C1-Ad functioning; (c) increased activity of the medullary serotonergic nuclei (fig. 7.1).

In addition to all the above, reduction of both DR-5HT and LC-NA activity favors the disinhibition of the serotonergic periaqueductal gray nucleus. Hyperactivity of the PAG-amygdala system has been found responsible for panic attacks, frequently observed in psychotic patients.

The above postulated disordered circuitry receives strong support from neuropharmacological findings demonstrating that all new antipsychotic drugs share the following properties: they enhance DA mesocortical activity + enhance NA mesocortical activity + antagonize DA mesolimbic receptors, and, finally, they display $5HT_2$ receptor antagonism at the level of the mesolimbic structures.

Fig. 7.1. Psychotic syndrome. LC = Locus coeruleus; DR = dorsal raphe; MR = median raphe; RM = raphe magnus; RO = raphe obscurus; RP = raphe pallidus; mcn = mesocortical nucleus; PVN = paraventricular nucleus; AH = anterior hypothalamus; PH = posterior hypothalamus; VMN = ventromedial nucleus; PRF = pontoreticular formation; PPN = pedunculopontine nucleus; CRF = corticotrophin-releasing factor; AP = area postrema; Na = noradrenaline; Ad = adrenaline; ACh = acetylcholine; 5HT = serotonin. → Excitation; —< inhibition. Concentric circles, bright and faded colors indicate neuronal activity. Dashed lines indicate reduced output.

Chapter 8

Panic Attacks

We have carried out the only scientific research dealing with this syndrome in which all plasma neurotransmitters were assessed during both resting and stimulated conditions. We also tested the effects of buspirone, a drug which is able to trigger the increase of both central NA activity + central DA activity. The LC noradrenergic neurons and the ventral tegmental (VTA) or A10 DA neurons are both excited by buspirone. In addition, this drug depresses central 5HT activity. In effect, buspirone is a $5HT_{1A}$ agonistic drug that inhibits the firing activity of those serotonergic neurons endowed with $5HT_{1A}$ inhibitory somatodendritic autoreceptors. $5HT_2$ inhibitory autoreceptors which are located at 5HT-terminal axons also exist.

Considering that $5HT_{1A}$ autoreceptors are located mainly at the DR 5HT nucleus, these serotonergic neurons are the main target of the low doses of buspirone we used in our research. In effect, MR 5HT neurons are not crowded with $5HT_{1A}$ receptors. Finally, caudal serotonergic nuclei (raphe magnus, raphe obscurus and raphe pallidus) are inhibited by buspirone only when great doses of this drug are microinjected directly onto these nuclei. In light of all the above, the oral dose of buspirone (10–20 mg) we administered to panic patients would act mainly at the DR-5HT nucleus. These buspirone doses were able to trigger panic attacks in all our patients. It is a very well-stated fact that panic attacks are associated with disinhibition of the periaqueductal gray (PAG-5HT)-amygdala pathway. Furthermore, this pathway is bridled by 5HT axons arising from DR-5HT neurons, thus, panic attacks have been associated with the failure of the DR-PAG inhibitory pathway. Our finding that TRP plasma levels are very low in panic patients is consistent with the above. The low TRP plasma levels were registered both during the attack and during the nonattack periods.

Many authors have reported that NA and/or Ad are raised in panic patients, thereby originating great confu-sion among readers. These plasma catecholamines have been investigated during both panic and nonpanic periods. However, we have shown, throughout the last 20 years, that only systematic assessment of all plasma neurotransmitters during both resting and stressed situations (orthostasis, exercise, glucose, buspirone, etc.) can reveal the particular participation of both central (neural) and peripheral (adrenal) sympathetic activity. We and many other researchers have exhaustively demonstrated that these two branches of the sympathetic system can act independently or in associated or dissociated ways. It is a great mistake to continue dwelling on 'sympathetic' activity as if it were self-contained. For a start, central sympathetic activity depends on firing by the LC A6 group of NA neurons, whereas peripheral (adrenomedullary) sympathetic activity is dependent on C1 Ad neurons located at the rostral ventral lateral area of the medulla. Further, it has been shown that ACh preganglionic axons innervating the adrenal medulla, located at the thoracic segments of the intermediolateral spinal column, receive modulatory axons arising from the C1-Ad neurons. In effect, stimulation of C1-Ad neurons triggers adrenaline release from

Fig. 8.1. Panic attacks. LC = Locus coeruleus; DR = dorsal raphe; MR = median raphe; RM = raphe magnus; RO = raphe obscurus; RP = raphe pallidus; mcn = mesocortical nucleus; PVN = paraventricular nucleus; AH = anterior hypothalamus; PH = posterior hypothalamus; VMN = ventromedial nucleus; PRF = pontoreticular formation; PPN = pedunculopontine nucleus; CRF = corticotrophin-releasing factor; AP = area postrema; Na = noradrenaline; Ad = adrenaline; ACh = acetylcholine; 5HT = serotonin. → Excitation; —< inhibition. Concentric circles, bright and faded colors indicate neuronal activity. Dashed lines indicate reduced output.

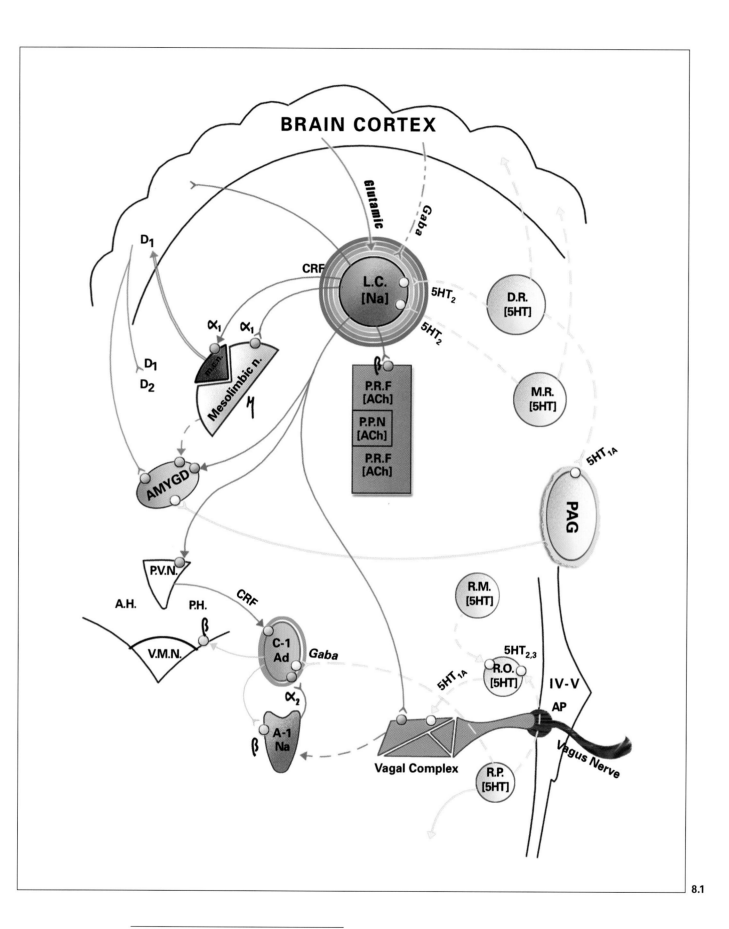

8.1

the adrenomedullary glands. Conversely, stimulation of the A6-NA (LC) neurons can stimulate and/or inhibit adrenaline secretion. There are several polysynaptic pathways that explain the association or dissociation of these two sympathetic activities. For instance, one pathway is the LC-PVN hypothalamic-C1; another pathway links the LC-posterior hypothalamus-C1; another is the LC-medullary vagal motor nuclei-C1; yet other pathways, more complex, include connections through DR and MR 5HT nuclei. Conversely, although there is no direct LC-C1 connection, there is a direct C1-LC pathway. These adrenergic axons reaching the LC-NA neurons are able to excite them through β-adrenergic receptors located at the LC-NA neurons, and also to inhibit the latter by releasing adrenaline at the α_2-receptors located at NA neurons. According to all the above, we consider it anti-scientific to continue referring to 'sympathetic activity' in a simplistic fashion. It is imperative to determine which of the three possibilities are active at any circumstance.

We found that panic attack patients present normal NA and normal NA/Ad ratio plasma values during nonattack periods. However, they show very high NA and NA/Ad values during attack periods. These findings are consistent with the interpretation that LC-NA is highly excited at these periods. Although the Ad plasma values also rise during panic attacks, the NA/Ad ratio increase indicates that neural sympathetic activity predominates over the adrenomedullary activity. This central over peripheral sympathetic predominance is opposed to that registered in anxiety patients and in uncoping stressed subjects, in whom central NA activity is exhausted. Considering that LC-NA neurons excite and inhibit the mesocortical and mesolimbic dopaminergic systems, respectively, we infer that NA and DA are increased at the cortical levels. Conversely, serotonin disappears from the cortical levels because pontine serotonergic nuclei are exhausted. The disinhibited PAG-5HT nucleus is depicted as increased. The C1-Ad medullary nucleus is activated during panic attacks, whereas the parasympathetic activity is totally absent because of the strong added NA plus Ad bridle.

Some research papers have associated panic attacks with epilepsy. Indeed, our findings are in agreement with such studies showing that LC-NA activation plays a predominant role among physiologic disorders underlying convulsive syndromes. The above pathophysiologic mechanisms underlying both panic and epileptic attacks are consistent with our findings showing that anti-epileptic drugs are very useful for treating panic attacks: for instance, lamotrigine (25 mg), serotonin-releasing agents such as carbamazepine, and serotonin precursors such as 5-OH-TRP (25–50 mg). Lamotrigine inhibits the release of glutamic acid. This excitatory amino acid exerts strong activity on LC-NA neurons. This effect is opposite to that exerted by GABA axons. GABA axons exert inhibitory influence on LC-NA, DR-5HT, VTA-DA and C1-Ad neurons and, in addition, GABA-mimetic drugs including benzodiazepines are commonly employed in the treatment of both epileptic and panic syndromes. However, we have learned that although all GABA-mimetic drugs are useful under acute circumstance, they are very dangerous when consumed over prolonged periods. In our experience, some 70% of patients consulting our institute consume benzodiazepines; we find that BDZ addiction is one of the most severe and hard to cure disorders at the present time.

Summarizing, the model of panic syndrome we postulate is based on an unbalanced glutamic vs. GABA functioning. This would favor epileptic discharges of the LC-NA neurons, which are not mitigated by exhausted DR-5HT neurons. PAG-5HT neurons, disinhibited from the DR-5HT axons, trigger activation of the PAG-amygdala pathway (fig. 8.1). Our model of panic attack fits well with the successful therapies based on administration of any drug able to inhibit the uptake of 5HT. However, these 5HT-potentiating drugs take too long to produce beneficial effects. This is probably due to the fact that all enhancers of 5HT uptake act first upon those 5HT systems that are most active; in this case, they would act first at the PAG-5HT system. For this reason, panic patients may be worsened during the first 2–3 weeks of taking these drugs.

....

Chapter 9

Neuroautonomic, Neuroendocrine and Neuroimmune Interactions

The central nervous system (CNS) circuitry, the peripheral autonomic nervous system (ANS), the endocrine system, and the immune system maintain permanent crosstalk, in such a way that every physiologic or pathophysiologic change affecting one of them triggers signals perceived by the others. True advances in biomedicine will occur when scientific and clinical researchers as well as practitioners become aware of the fact that there are no diseases which affect only a single organ or isolated system. For instance, cardiologists should know that atherosclerosis, myocarditis, arteritis, Raynaud and Takayashu diseases are included among autoimmune disorders. Pulmonary hypertension, thrombophlebitis and arterial thrombosis occur because aggregated platelets are disrupted and stores of 5HT are released into the plasma (f5HT). f5HT triggers vasospasms and favors thrombosis. Moreover, platelets aggregate because excessive Ad is released from adrenomedullary glands, specifically during acute stress and chronic (noncompensated or uncoping) stress situations. Gastroenterological, endocrinological, neurological, dermatological and other diseases also show neuroimmunological disorders. In light of the above, it becomes urgent that physicians can and do obtain basic immunological, neurochemical, and physiological information. Moreover, the practice of scientific neuropharmacological therapy requires that doctors know the appropriate CNS drugs that are able to prevent, restore and/or control physiological disorders.

Neuroautonomic Interactions

Both monoaminergic (NA, Ad, DA and 5HT) and ACh circuitries maintain close two-way communications (fig. 9.1).

NA System: Pontine (LC-A6, A7, A5) NA nuclei and medullary (A1 and A2) NA nuclei send and receive monosynaptic as well as polysynaptic connections with the peripheral sympathetic and parasympathetic systems through the ventromedial and posterior hypothalamic areas, as well as through pre-sympathetic and pre-parasympathetic (medullary and spinal) neurons.

Pontine, midbrain and medullary 5HT neurons display autonomic influences through hypothalamic, medullary and spinal pre-sympathetic and pre-parasympathetic nuclei. Both NA and 5HT systems exert a close modulatory influence on the vagal complex as well as on nuclei with controlling roles in deglutory, respiratory, and cardiovascular functioning, etc.

The mesolimbic, mesocortical, incertohypothalamic, tuberoinfundibular and medullary-spinal DA systems also exert important modulatory influences (direct and indirectly) on the autonomic nervous system.

The hystaminergic system, also extensively distributed in the CNS, modulates NA, 5HT and DA systems.

This complex central monoaminergic circuitry receives information not only from peripheral, visceral changes, but also from external stimuli and conscious plus unconscious events, through deep and extensive brain cortex connections. For instance, DR-5HT neurons display firing activity while the test animal is moving but stop firing when it stops walking. Conversely, MR-5HT neurons show increased activity at these moments. Both DR and MR serotonergic nuclei innervate different nonoverlapping brain areas. Some cortical brain areas would be free of 5HT in those circumstances when the animal is alert; on the other hand, 5HT released into other nuclei facilitates some specific functions (defense or attack).

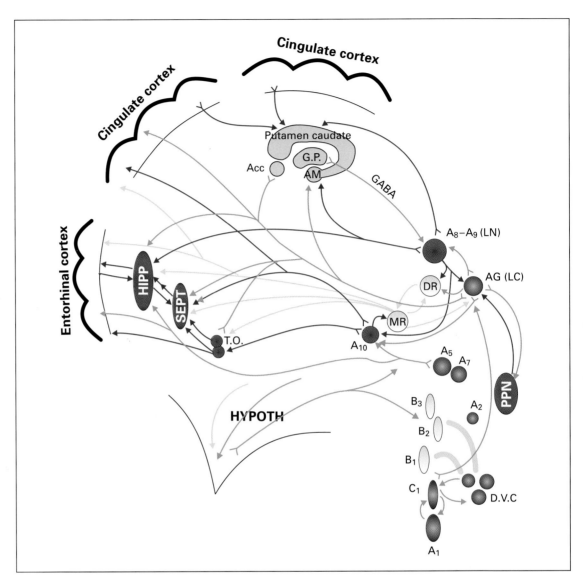

Fig. 9.1. Anatomical integration model of the central autonomic nervous system. Putamen caudate and amygdala integrate the mesostriatic system (MS); these structures receive NE, DA and 5HT innervation from LC, LN and DR nuclei, respectively. OT and septi nuclei belong to the mesolimbic system (ML); this system receives NE, DA and 5HT innervation from A5–A7, A10 and MR neuronal nuclei, respectively. Structures innervated by mixed (MS + ML) monoaminergic neuronal groups belong to the mixed system (M), hippocampus and accumbens nucleus. Dorsal vagal complex (DVC) antagonizes the C1 nucleus. B1, B2 and B3 5HT nuclei excite DVC parasympathetic neurons whereas they bridle C1 Ad neurons. C1 axons inhibit LC-NA neurons. A5, A7 = Noradrenergic neurons; GP = globus pallidus; Hypoth = hypothalamus; A10 = dopamine neurons; B1, B2, B3 = medullary serotonergic neurons; AM = amygdala; DR = dorsal raphe (5HT neurons); AC = accumbens nucleus; DVC = dorsal vagal complex; ACh = acetylcholine; PPN = pedunculopontine nucleus (ACh); HIPP = hippocampus; LC = locus coeruleus (NA neurons); LN = locus niger (DA neurons); MR = medium raphe (5HT neurons); OT = olfactory tubercle.

Neuroimmune Interactions

Complex and intense crosstalk is maintained between the CNS and the immune system. All significant CNS changes reverberate on the immune system and, conversely, all immunological events are noticed by the CNS. This two-way communication is accentuated during pathophysiological situations. For instance, anxiety, aggression, depression, rewarding activity and stressful situations (uncoping and coping) show correlated immuno-

Neuroautonomic, Neuroendocrine and
Neuroimmune Interactions

logical changes. In turn, the CNS receives information about immunological changes occurring during all types of sepsis, tissue damage, metabolic disorder, anoxia, and other pathologic states. Cytokines, substances secreted from lymphocytes, become messengers which cross the BBB and act at specific receptors located at different CNS areas.

Peripheral and central catecholamine systems are involved in neural-immune interactions. Regions in which lymphocytes (mainly T cells) reside, and through which they recirculate, receive direct sympathetic neural input. The immune system can, therefore, be considered 'hard-wired' to the brain. These lymphocytes possess receptors for catecholamines (NA and DA). A wide range of research shows that the CNS can influence the immune system. In addition to NA, Ad secreted by adrenal medulla and serotonin derived from platelets can be taken up into sympathetic nerve terminals and released as classical neurotransmitters following appropriate neural stimulation. Such findings point to a role for the adrenal medulla and sympathetic nerves in regulating events in the dissemination of cells and products of an immune response, as the potential mechanisms by which stress can influence the immune system.

Catecholamines, when increased in the blood during stressful situations, trigger platelet aggregation and secondary release of 5HT stored in them. This immunosuppressive amine is taken up by macrophages which then lose their immunological competence. In effect, it has been shown that pharmacological enhancement of 5HT metabolism suppresses the immune response in vivo. This immunosuppressive influence occurs peripherally, not centrally. Macrophages inhibit microbial infections by producing the indoleamine 2,3-dioxygenase (IDO), which catabolizes TRP, the precursor of 5HT. According to this, it has been proposed that IDO-producing cells represent an ancient mechanism adapted to suppressing T-cell responses in vivo.

Not only 5HT but also Ad inhibits macrophage activity through β_1- and β_2-adrenergic receptors but not through α-receptors. These findings are consistent with the anti-Th1 (anti-inflammatory) activity registered in experimental and clinical conditions during stress situations, when both Ad and f5HT are raised in the plasma.

NA is accepted as an immunoenhancing neurotransmitter. Animals primarily immunized with SRBC, 48 h after administration of 6-hydroxy-dopamine (6-OHDA = a drug which interferes with noradrenergic synthesis), have a markedly impaired primary antibody response whose effects persist for at least 1 month. These animals showed almost total disappearance of NA in both the brain stem and hypothalamus. Conversely, the administration of 5-OH-TRP, which increases brain 5HT stores, results in significant suppression of the primary antibody response, whereas diminished serotonin levels induced by PCPA (p-chlorophenylalanine) administration augment the response.

Other research has demonstrated that sympathetic nervous system (SNS) denervation enhances the synthesis and production of peripheral IL-1 and IL-6 cytokines, showing that SNS exerts a tonic inhibitory control over these inflammatory cytokines. Other studies examining the effect of chemical NA denervation on the immune system have shown that SNS inhibits a number of immune functions including cell proliferation in lymph nodes, spleen and bone marrow; it also reduces lymphocyte migration into lymph nodes, B-cell proliferation and differentiation, interleukin-2 (IL-2) and IL-4 production by splenocytes and macrophage function.

Other studies have demonstrated that increased activity of the LC-NA occurs during peak immune response.

Th1/Th2 Paradigm

On the basis of this paradigm most autoimmune diseases have been differentiated. Although much overlap exists, this model is useful for understanding pathological findings and some physiological mechanisms underlying autoimmune diseases. In table 13.9 we present several diseases around which some consensus exists as to their grouping into Th1 or Th2 disorders. For example, Th1 disorders present predominance of hyperactivity of immunity at tissue level, whereas Th2 presents humoral immune hyperactivity, mainly. However, there are many diseases which present both types of autoimmune activity. As a further complication, Th1/Th2 alternation is often observed.

Helper lymphocytes (Th) included among type 1 are characterized by producing the following cytokines: interferon-γ, TNFβ and IL-2 , mainly. On the other hand, Th2 lymphocytes secrete IL-4, IL-5, IL-6, and IL-10 cytokines.

Neurochemical research carried out in our laboratory on several thousand autoimmune diseased patients showed us that patients labeled as Th1 type present raised NA/Ad ratio plus low TRP levels. Conversely, type Th2 autoimmune diseased patients showed decreased NA/Ad ratio + raised f5HT + increased platelet aggregability. In other words, Th1 autoimmune patients showed a major depression neurochemical profile, while type 2 presented an uncoping stress neurochemical profile. These findings have received support from many research papers.

Chapter 10

Neuroendocrine-Immune Interactions

All neurochemical, neuroautonomic and immunological changes are paralleled by physiological or pathophysiological endocrine changes. Together these systems make up the neuroautonomic-endocrine-immunology network.

Cells that synthesize CRH or CRF are located at the PVN of the hypothalamus. They receive excitatory drives from LC-NA and DR-5HT + MR-5HT axons. In turn, CRH neuroendocrine cells send excitatory axons to the LC and excitatory-inhibitory axons to serotonergic nuclei. CRH-paraventricular cells interchange axons with the medullary C1-Ad nuclei. CRH released into portal circulation excites vasopressinergic cells at the posterior hypophysial lobe, which release vasopressin and oxytocin. Both hormones display an important immunoactivating role. Vasopressin is also released when excited by Ad axons arriving from the C1-Ad medullary group.

CRH initiates the ACTH → cortisol cascade, which results in an increase of cortisol circulating levels. Cortisol displays an important immunomodulatory role that results in enhancement of humoral and reduction of tissue immunity activity. The rises of both adrenaline and cortisol registered during acute and chronic (uncontrollable/ uncoping) stress situation cooperate to the same end: activation of humoral (Th2) host immunity.

GH is one of the most powerful immune-stimulating agents. Activation of the CRH → ACTH → cortisol cascade is accompanied by suppression of the GHRH → GH cascade and of gonadotropin secretion. The latter will explain why infertility in women is frequently observed during uncoping stress situations. Conversely, somatostatin secretion is increased during acute and chronic (uncoping) stress situations. Prolactin is another hormone released from the hypophysis during acute and chronic (uncoping) stress. Serotonin released from DR- + MR-5HT, and DA released from DA axons, exert excitatory and inhibitory influences on prolactin secretion, respectively. DA axons arise from the incertohypothalamic and tubero-infundibular DA neurons located at this level. Prolactin, contrary to cortisol, is an important Th1-stimulating factor.

Thyrotropin-stimulating hormone (TSH) is a neuroendocrine hormone also released during acute stress situations. This hormone fills an important function as an endogenous regulator within the immune system.

Activation of the CRH cascade registered during acute and chronic uncontrollable (uncoping) stress situations is paralleled by adrenomedullary and glucagon secretions. On the other hand, insulin secretion is inhibited during these periods. Insulin secretion increases during parasympathetic activation. Moreover, insulin crosses the BBB and stimulates central NA and 5HT activities. Insulin also triggers further parasympathetic activation by exciting the RO-5HT-vagal complex circuit.

The endocrine system is modulated by CNS circuitry. In turn, hormones provoke different changes in the immune system depending of this system's release of distinct types of cytokines. Cytokines are polypeptide regulators which in addition can cross the BBB; they can alter neurotransmission both at presynaptic and postsynaptic levels. They interfere in the regulation of the hypothalamic pituitary adrenal axis.

Glucocorticoid suppression by means of adrenalectomy results in an increase of plasma concentrations of noradrenaline released from the sympathetic nerves. On the other hand, glucocorticoid administration to normal humans provokes the opposite effect, decreasing NA release from the sympathetic nerves. Glucocorticoids regulate molecular mechanisms involved in Th1/Th2 pathways by regulating inflammatory cytokines, absent during the Th2 response.

Cortisol interferes with delayed-type hypersensitivity (Th1 activity). This phenomenon occurs during acute and chronic-uncoping stress situations when cortisol is raised in the plasma, as well as adrenaline and f5HT. All these factors are associated with predominance of the Th2 immunological profile. This profile favors anti-inflammatory activity and decreased surveillance of tumor-producing agents. These cortisol effects on the immune system are mediated by the thymus, mainly. Conversely, during chronic-coping stress situation, cortisol and adrenaline levels are reduced, whereas plasma NA levels are raised. An enhancement of Th1 immune activity is registered during these circumstances.

Glucocorticoids have been shown to shift the balance of macrophage progenitors to granulocyte progenitors. In addition, cortisol interferes with the differentiation of the monocyte cell line to macrophage cell line. Cortisol induces apoptosis of the immune cells (immature T lymphocytes) but not of immature B cells, this phenomenon occurring in the thymus, mainly. For this reason, the thymus is very sensitive to adrenal glucocorticoids. This explains why glucocorticoids favor humoral (Th2) immunity, and interfere with Th1 (cell-mediated) immunity, and display anti-inflammatory (tumoral favoring) activity. For these reasons, glucocorticoids administration to humans provokes T-cell depletion. This is the same profile registered during acute and chronic (uncoping) stress situations. It is amply accepted that neurohormonal disorders (cortisol, adrenaline, free serotonin, etc.) registered during uncontrollable (uncoping) stress are important factors which favor tumor progression and metastasis. Conversely, these factors favor the reduction and amelioration of the inflammatory process affecting Th1 autoimmune diseases.

Growth hormone is not secreted during acute stress and chronic (uncontrollable or uncoping) stress situations. Progressive reduction of GH secretion by the hypophysis is observed with aging. Exhaustion of NA neurons of the LC occurs during uncontrollable stress when neural sympathetic activity is diminished or absent. The quantity of LC-NA neurons shows progressive reduction throughout aging. This phenomenon is responsible for the very low NA/Ad ratio registered in the plasma of elder people. In effect, although older subjects usually show greater than normal plasma catecholamine levels, their NA/Ad ratio is low (less than 2), a fact indicating that plasma catecholamines arise from the adrenal medulla, mainly. GH is a thymopoietic factor. Both the thymus and GH fade progressively with aging, resulting in fewer naive T cells (memory T cells remain normal). Now, it has been demonstrated that GH is able to trigger thymopoiesis in adults and elder people. This favors reappearance of naive T cells. In our institute, we have successfully used GHRH and GH in the treatment of many stress-associated (Th2) diseases. We have also demonstrated that neuropharmacological manipulations addressed to enhancing central NA activity are able to increase GH responses to GHRH, arginine, clonidine and pyridostigmine stimuli.

Lymphocytes have receptors for GH. Administration of GH augments antibody synthesis, increases IL-2 synthesis, stimulates proliferation of human lymphoblastoid cells, and increases activity of cytotoxic T lymphocytes and NK cells.

Not only GH but also prolactin are able to increase the secretion of thymulin, a thymic hormone. In vitro studies have shown that prolactin antisera blocked a number of immune reactions. This led to the discovery that cells involved in immunity appear capable of producing prolactin and GH, although the physiological significance of these observations has not been explored. The immune-augmenting role displayed by prolactin has been studied showing that this hormone also displays pro-inflammatory properties. With respect to this, the circadian worsening of rheumatic arthritis disease has been positively correlated with normal prolactin peaks occurring at 2:00–3:00 a.m. Finally, there is recent evidence showing that prolactin could be a marker of rejection in heart transplant recipients.

Ovarian hormones, both estradiol and progesterone, are associated with Th2 immunity. They are responsible for the well-known Th2 profile registered during pregnancy. This effect is not only mediated peripherally but also centrally. In effect, it has been shown that estrogens cross the BBB and antagonize DA receptors. Estrogens act in a similar way to the DA-blocking agents employed in the treatment of schizophrenia. Thus, they are able to counteract the recognized immunoenhancing effects of central DA systems. This issue should be thoroughly investigated now that an increase in the incidence of mammary and ovarian cancer has been registered in women taking estrogens to improve menopause symptoms.

Chapter 11

Stress, Depression and Immunity

It is worth repeating that the word 'stress' has been oversimplified and manipulated in public usage. Moreover, psychiatrists and psychologists are responsible for a great overlap and consequent confusion between the definition and diagnosis of stress and that of depression in humans. This arises from the mistaken belief that the inescapable (uncontrollable) stress syndrome, as experimentally induced in mammals, can be taken as an appropriate model for human depression. Compounding this error are empirical observations that stressors can precipitate clinical features resembling symptoms seen in depressed humans. Adding to the confusion, both inescapable stress in animals and the human depressive syndrome are improved by so-called 'antidepressant' drugs. Accumulated evidence demonstrates conclusively that the neurochemical, neuroendocrine and physiologic disorders underlying inescapable stress are wholly different to those marking depression (see chapter 5). Clinical signs shared by both syndromes (immobility, unresponsiveness to stimuli, etc.) are too weak to support the hypothesis that the two conditions are equivalent. In fact, many findings give evidence of opposite mechanisms underlying the two syndromes. Additionally, it should be remembered that there are not one but several clinical syndromes that lay claim to the label of depression. Hence, which of the depressive syndromes purportedly correspond to the inescapable stress model experimentally induced in mammals: endogenous, dysthymic, or some other?

Neurochemical Evidence

Depletion of central NA stores occurs in mammals submitted to inescapable stress situation. This central NA depletion is responsible for the upregulation of α_2-receptors registered at the hypothalamic level in experimental animals. In addition, although the catecholamines NA and Ad rise in plasma during stress situation, the NA/Ad ratio is significantly lower than during resting state. This fact is consistent with adrenomedullary glands overactivity and reveals dissociation between peripheral (adrenal) and central (neural) sympathetic activities. Conversely, higher than normal NA plasma levels are observed in endogenous (major) depression, thus their NA/Ad ratio is greatly raised. Taking into account that circulating NA reflects central noradrenergic activity mainly, this finding opposes the central NA depletion registered in stressed mammals.

Neuropharmacological Evidence

A blunted GH + CRT + NA + DBP response to clonidine is observed in endogenous depressed patients. This unresponsiveness to clonidine is interpreted as downregulation of α_2-receptors at the hypothalamic level and is compatible with the raised central and plasmatic NA levels registered in these patients (increased central NA activity). Conversely, hyperresponsiveness of GH to clonidine and upregulation of α_2-hypothalamic receptors are found in inescapably stressed mammals which show central NA depletion.

All 'antidepressant' drugs are able to revert the inescapable stress syndrome in experimental mammals. However, therapeutic improvement triggered in depressed patients by such drugs is not the rule. On the contrary, failures are more frequent than successes.

The so-called 'antidepressant' drugs include a great diversity of neuropharmacological agents which act through different mechanisms. Some potentiate central

NA activity, others increase central 5HT and/or DA activity, while still others hamper 5HT neurotransmission. Most of these drugs trigger more than one neuropharmacological mechanism and act upon more than one neurotransmitter system. For instance, desipramine, protryptiline, clorimipramine, imipramine and doxepin are NA + 5HT uptake inhibitors. Fluoxetine, sertraline, and paroxetine act like 5HT uptake inhibitors; mianserin is an α_2- + $5HT_2$-receptor blocking agent provoking NA + 5HT release from terminals; tianeptine enhances the uptake of 5HT by terminals and reduces synaptic availability of this neurotransmitter and in addition, suppresses the stress-induced release of NA. Amineptine inhibits DA uptake. All these drugs are able to revert the uncontrollable stress syndrome in experimental mammals, but their antidepressant success in humans is variable, poor or nil.

We can observe that most of such 'antidepressants' potentiate one, two or more monoaminergic systems. This phenomenon fits well with the fact that all (NA, DA and 5HT) neurotransmitters are exhausted during inescapable stress. Indeed, the drugs most often found to be useful in cases of depression are 5HT-potentiating drugs. Taking into account that circulating TRP levels are decreased in endogenous depressed patients, who at the same time show central NA overactivity, the therapeutic improvement induced by these drugs is compatible with their ability to reduce central NA activity through the strengthening of its antagonic 5HT system.

Physiological and Metabolic Evidence

Inescapable stress, experimentally induced, is characterized by adrenomedullary + cortical gland hyperactivity. Conversely, endogenous depressed subjects show adrenomedullary gland hypoactivity. Such patients do not show an Ad normal peak during postprandial hypoglycemia or during orthostasis, moderate exercise, oral buspirone, etc. This adrenal sympathetic hypoactivity is consistent with the high parasympathetic tone found in depressive patients. In effect, throughout the oral glucose test (OGTT), they show progressive blood pressure reduction paralleled by plasma glucose decrease. The parasympathetic nature of these phenomena is supported by the fact that atropine prevents both blood pressure and glucose decreases. Atropine, injected before orthostasis and exercise challenges in these patients, also prevents the differential pulse pressure (differential = systolic less diastolic) fall normally registered during orthostasis. This pulse pressure fall is more accentuated in depressed than nor-

mal subjects and is compatible with the higher than normal parasympathetic tone they present. This hyperparasympathetic activity shown by endogenous depressed patients is consistent with their poor adrenomedullary activity. A similar hyperparasympathetic plus poor adrenomedullary responsiveness was observed in dysthymic depressed patients who differ from endogenous depressed subjects because they show neither greater than normal neural sympathetic activity nor the lower than normal TRP plasma levels registered in the latter group. On the contrary, dysthymics show increased TRP plasma levels when compared with normals. TRP plasma levels are parameters positively correlated with 5HT and parasympathetic activities. Finally, dysthymic depressed patients showed lowered central NA and peripheral Ad activities.

Clinical Evidence

A great many papers have been devoted to the relationship of somatic diseases, stress and depression. Basing their approach on clinical grounds, most of these papers fail, in our opinion, to differentiate depression from stress. All psychosomatic scales addressed to measuring stress quantify the magnitude of the stressors and/or their acute effects on the subjects. However, these clinical approaches do not take into account individual response to the challenge of chronic stress. It is known that the application of acute stressors to mammals provokes short-lived and reversible changes in them. Further, prolongation of acute stress and/or repetition of stressor application provokes either adaptation (coping) or maladaptation (uncoping) phenomena. Adapted mammals are able to accept stressors with minimal or non-significant neurochemical, physiological and behavioral changes. Such adapted mammals are characterized by greater than normal central NA stores. Their adrenal glands respond poorly to the acute presentation of stressors, thus they do not show plasma Ad increase during stressful situations. Conversely, maladapted mammals are characterized by the depletion of central NA stores and hyperresponsiveness of adrenal glands to acute stress challenge. In both coping and uncoping mammals there is dissociation of the two branches of the sympathetic system: central (neurosympathetic) and peripheral (adrenal-sympathetic). In one type of dissociation (coping) NA > Ad, and in the other (uncoping) Ad > NA.

Behavioral responses to stressor presentation in coping and uncoping mammals are readily observed under experimental conditions. However, behavioral responses (symptoms) in humans are frequently obscured by complex psychological mechanisms (repression, denial, neurotic exaggeration, etc.), thus the clinical diagnosis of maladaptation to stress in humans is not easy to assess. To the best of our knowledge, there exists no validated psychometric tool addressed to evaluating stress adaptation in human subjects. The use of the magnitude of anxiety and/or stressors as a measure of maladaptation to stress in subjects has neither adequate scientific support nor convincing clinical validity. Conversely, careful investigation carried out in our institute showed that psychological tests were not able to differentiate patients presenting the neurochemical profile of endogenous depression (raised NA + low TRP plasma levels) from patients having a profile of maladapted (uncoping) stress (low NA + high Ad + normal TRP + raised f5HT + increased platelet aggregability). In our opinion, the dogma identifying human depression with the 'behavioral despair' or 'inescapable' stress syndrome observed in experimental rats has been promoted by researchers of the pharmaceutical industry for commercial motives. Human beings are not rats. Rats are not affected by depression. Assessment of inescapable, uncontrollable stress situation vs. depression in humans should be made on neurochemical, hormonal, pharmacological and physiological, but not clinical, grounds.

Acute Stress and Immunity

Acute stress is marked by increased catecholamines (adrenaline = Ad, noradrenaline = NA, and dopamine = DA) plasma levels. During this situation, both neural sympathetic activity (90% of NA + 10% of DA) and adrenomedullary activity (80% of Ad + 10% of NA + 10% of DA) are increased. p5HT is reduced whereas f5HT is increased because of adrenaline-induced platelet aggregation.

The immune profile during acute stress includes: (a) raised humoral immunity (Th2); (b) increased B-lymphocytes and natural killer (NK) cells; (c) decreased NK cytotoxicity against target cells (K-562), and (d) increased plasma Th2 cytokines such as IL-4, IL-5, IL-6 and IL-10.

All these inflammatory cytokines are raised in the plasma during this period. Obviously, this situation is much more complex than stated above, but these are the minimal immune changes found. Short-lived acute stress allows mammals to restore normality. Restoration is paralleled by reduction of central NA, DA, 5HT and Ad activities. The firing activity of monoaminergic circuitry returns to normal. The exacerbated CRH-ACTH-cortisol

and somatostatin secretions show fading. On the other hand, disappearance of the GHRH-GH bridling is registered. Antistress mechanisms predominate during resting, postprandial and sleep periods. Maximal parasympathetic + GH secretion is registered during the deepest stages (3 and 4) of slow wave sleep.

The above-mentioned neurochemical + neuroautonomic + neuroedocrine reversions are responsible for total recovery from stress situation. It follows that normalization of the sleep pattern is the most important antistress mechanism. For this reason benzodiazepines (BDZ) should be avoided. These drugs interfere with normalization of sleep; they suppress SWS (3 and 4) and REM sleep periods. In our long experience investigating this matter, we registered systematically that BDZ consumers always show raised adrenaline and cortisol plasma levels. In addition, these patients invariably present a stress profile of immunity (Th2 type).

Chronic Uncoping Stress and Immunity

Prolonged or repeated application of stressors to mammals interferes with recovery from stress situation. Accentuation of ensuing changes (neuroendocrine, neuroautonomic and neuroimmune) is observed. At the CNS level, all monoaminergic circuits become exhausted. Central NA stores are depleted and C1-Ad medullary nuclei are freed from the LC-NA bridle. All or almost all evidences of peripheral sympathetic activity are registered. Adrenal glands secrete maximal doses of adrenaline. Sympathetic nerves do not release NA or it is reduced to a minimum. The NA/Ad plasma ratio is dramatically low. Platelet aggregability is increased and reaches maximal level. f5HT in the plasma is permanently raised. Immunological changes show maximal reduction of Th1 immunity. This immunological profile favors the appearance of Th2 hetero and/or autoimmune diseases.

Chronic Coping Stress and Immunity

Chronic and dosified presentation of stressors (experimental and clinical) to mammals and humans may lead to stress adaptation. When this happens, central (neural sympathetic) activity predominates over peripheral (adrenomedullary) sympathetic activity. Plasma NA levels remain elevated. The NA/Ad ratio is high (more than 5). The subject responds with NA to stressor application, showing further NA/Ad increases during these periods.

Plasma cortisol levels are normal. The GHRH $\rightarrow$ GH cascade predominates over CRH $\rightarrow$ ACTH $\rightarrow$ cortisol cascade. p5HT and f5HT levels are normal. At the CNS level, high NA stores are registered. LC-NA activity is high whereas C1-Ad activity is almost silent. LC-NA and vagal complex activity bridle C1-Ad activity. The high LC-NA activity plus the parasympathetic preponderance are responsible for enhancement of GH release. All these neurochemical, neuroautonomic and neuroendocrine profiles favor the predominance of Th1 over Th2 immune activity.

Endogenous (Major) Depression and Immunity

We have investigated some 400 endogenous depressed patients. They routinely show greater than normal NA/Ad ratio + low TRP plasma levels. From the autonomic nervous system standpoint, they also showed increased parasympathetic activity plus poor adrenomedullary responsiveness when they were tested with stressors.

Although plasma GH basal levels are normal or elevated, these patients also showed a poor response to stimuli such as clonidine, arginine, and pyridostigmine, due to down-regulation of α_2-hypothalamic receptors. Immunological profiles are consistent with a Th1 profile, showing raised CD4/CD8 ratio, increased CD45 RO (memory) lymphocytes, increased CD8 (cytotoxic) lymphocytes, etc. A significant percentage of these patients show positive antinuclear antibodies in the absence of any autoimmune disease. These patients do not show the normal increases of IL-6 when submitted to acute stress. Both clinical and neurochemical profiles of endogenous depression are frequently observed in patients affected by Th1 autoimmune disease. Furthermore, neuropharmacological treatment addressed to improving endogenous depressed patients provokes significant improvement of autoimmune diseases (Crohn's enteritis, Sjögren's disease, rheumatoid arthritis, psoriasis, Raynaud's disease, scleroderma, etc.).

Although Th1 autoimmune diseases can only suggest a Th1 immune profile, one thing is definitely clear: all well-established Th1 autoimmune diseases present the neurochemical profile of major depression, specifically raised NA/Ad ratio plus low TRP levels.

Through our long experience in dosifying plasma neurotransmitters and investigating immunological parameters, it has been clearly established that 'uncoping stress' and 'major depression' present two opposite neurochemical and immunological profiles. These findings allow us to outline successful neuropharmacological treatments for both types of diseases.

Schizophrenia and Immunity

We have clearly stated that these patients show neurochemical and immunological profiles similar to those found in 'uncoping stress' subjects: low NA/Ad plasma ratio plus Th2 immune profile. In addition, platelet 5HT is found to be higher than normal.

Chapter 12

Bronchial Asthma

The treatment of bronchial asthma with tianeptine, a drug which enhances the uptake of 5HT from plasma to platelets has been tested in more than 16,000 patients: 3.125 mg (1/4 tablet) to 12.5 mg (one tablet). We used this treatment in patients aged from 6 months to 58 years, 2 or 3 times daily during days or weeks. The dose of tianeptine can be adjusted according to age and severity of symptoms. Usually, we administered tianeptine every day during 6–10 days. Further, the drug is taken when necessary. The administration of tianeptine at the beginning of attacks cut them suddenly. Furthermore, the administration of tianeptine during attacks provokes suppression 45–60 min after drug ingestion. We have never registered undesirable side effects. Progressive disappearance of asthma attacks are observed in all cases.

In 1996, Lechin and coworkers published a paper in *Annals of Allergy, Asthma and Immunology,* reporting findings showing that symptomatic asthma patients have increased levels of NA, Ad, DA, f5HT and CRT. They also demonstrated, that f5HT plasma levels but not the other parameters correlated significantly with clinical severity and, in addition, both f5HT and clinical rating correlated negatively with all parameters of pulmonary functioning (FEV_1, FVC, etc.). The plasma neurotransmitter profile registered during symptomatic asthma periods as well as the increased platelet aggregability they found in these patients during these periods, are consistent with the association of asthma attacks with uncoping stress

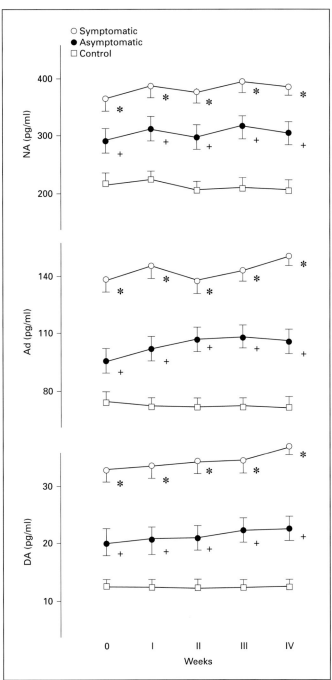

Fig. 12.1. Graphs show levels of NA, Ad, and DA in symptomatic asthmatic patients, and control patients at the start of study (week 0) and at 4-weekly intervals. Mean ± SEM. * Symptomatic vs. asymptomatic; +asymptomatic vs. control: p < 0.005 in all cases [Lechin et al., Ann Allergy Asthma Immunol 1996;77:245–253].

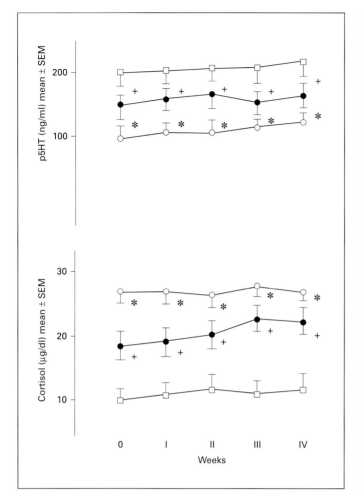

Fig. 12.2. Graphs show levels of p5HT and CRT in symptomatic asthmatic patients, asymptomatic asthmatic patients, and control patients at the start of the study (week 0) and at 4-weekly intervals. * Symptomatic vs. asymptomatic; + asymptomatic vs. control: p < 0.005 in all cases. Nonsignificant differences among weeks [Lechin et al., Ann Allergy Asthma Immunol 1996;77:245–253].

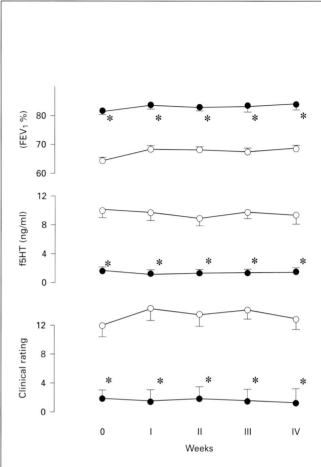

Fig. 12.3. Graphs show FEV_1, plasma f5HT, and clinical rating in symptomatic asthmatic patients, asymptomatic asthmatic patients, and control patients at the start of study (week 0) and at 4-weekly intervals. Mean values ± SEM. * Symptomatic vs. symptomless: p < 0.0001. Nonsignificant differences were registered among weeks [Lechin et al., Ann Allergy Asthma Immunol 1996;77:245–253].

situation. Finally, the association of asthma with uncoping stress situation is consistent with the inclusion of this disease among the Th-2 autoimmune diseases. Although the published paper [Lechin et al., 1996] appeared in September 1996, Lechin's group had previously published one abstract in *Am J Respir Crit Care Med* [Lechin AE et al., 1994].

In 1998, Lechin's group published two research papers showing that tianeptine provoked a dramatic and sudden decrease of both clinical rating and f5HT plasma levels and an increase in pulmonary functioning [Lechin et al., 1998a, b]. In addition, there are two other related articles

dealing with this issue by Cazzola and Matera [2000] and Lechin F [2000], both published in *Trends in Pharmacological Sciences*.

Finally, Dupont et al. [1999] demonstrated that 5HT facilitates cholinergic contraction in human airways in vitro through stimulation of both prejunctional 5-HT₃ and 5-HT₄ receptors. These findings ratified the etiopathogenic role of plasma 5HT in bronchial asthma and, in addition, strongly suggest that not only 5HT uptake enhancers but also 5HT₃ and 5HT₄ antagonists should be considered as powerful tools in the treatment of this disease.

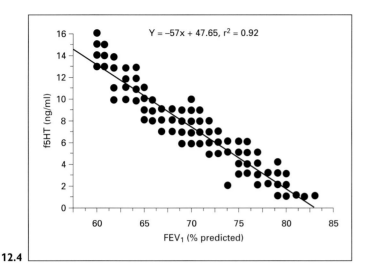

12.4

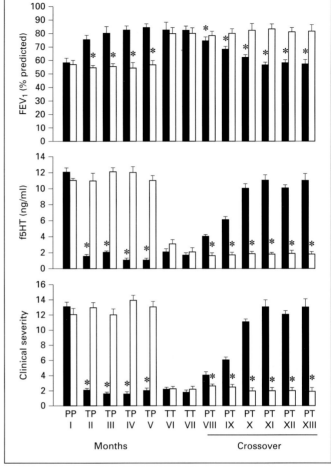

12.5

Fig. 12.4. Regression analysis showing a negative correlation between FEV_1 and f5HT levels in 57 symptomatic patients with asthma [Lechin et al., Ann Allergy Asthma Immunol 1996;77:245–253].

Fig. 12.5. Effects of tianeptine in 69 symptomatic patients with asthma, measured in three different parameters: FEV_1, clinical severity, and plasma f5HT. Solid bars = group that received placebo (P) for 4 weeks, tianeptine (T) for 24 weeks, and placebo again for 24 weeks. White bars = group received placebo for 20 weeks and tianeptine for 32 weeks. During the last 2 months the patients represented by the white bars did not take oral prednisone. * p < 0.005 [Lechin et al., Clin Pharmacol Ther 1998;64:223–232].

Pulmonary Hypertension

Plasma serotonin (f5HT) has found to be raised in primary pulmonary hypertension [Hervé et al., 1995]. Other findings demonstrated that fenfluramine, a 5HT-releasing agent, is responsible for pulmonary vasoconstriction. In addition to the above, Lechin's group found that several types of pulmonary hypertension patients – vasculitis (1 case), primary pulmonary hypertension (1 case), chronic bronchitis (3 cases), chronic asthma (7 cases), and obesity (1 case) – showing greatly raised f5HT plasma levels were much improved by tianeptine administration and that clinical improvement paralleled a normalization of plasma levels [Lechin, 2001; Lechin and van der Dijs, 2002; Lechin et al., 2002]. All the above support the etiopathogenic role played by f5HT.

Chapter 13

··

Concluding Remarks

The data and points of view presented in this book arise from the routine neurochemical and immunological investigation of more than 25,000 normal and diseased subjects. We understand that we have the only laboratory of plasma neurotransmitters in which all are routinely assessed both in basal and stimulated conditions. From their results we design specific neuropharmacological treatments. It is our earnest hope that other research groups will test this procedure. We are sure that they will be gratified by therapeutic results. In addition, patients will also be thankful, and indeed grateful, as attested by thousands of successfully treated cases of cancer and autoimmune diseases including multiple sclerosis, myositis, Sjögren disease, and myasthenia gravis, as well as our No. 1 MG case, Dr. Fuad Lechin (table 13.1–13.3). We also want to make available such effective, low-cost treatments as tianeptine for bronchial asthma, and clonidine for acute pancreatitis. We never found failures with these treatments. We hope that after Dr. Fuad Lechin dies mankind will benefit from this knowledge as he was never able to disseminate it widely enough.

We are successfully treating Takayashu disease, pulmonary hypertension and cerebrovascular accidents with ketanserine plus tianeptine. The former is a drug that blocks endovascular receptors ($5HT_2$- and α_1-receptors), while tianeptine is a drug that enhances serotonin uptake by platelets and reduces levels of f5HT in the plasma. Tianeptine has also proved to be the most powerful anti-asthmatic drug, reverting bronchospasms triggered by the plasma f5HT rises that follow increased platelet aggregation, prior to the onset of asthma attacks. Further, excessive plasma f5HT triggers a shift of immune activity to Th2 predominance. For this reason, bronchial asthma has been included among the Th2 autoimmune diseases. These findings teach us that pharmacological knowledge provides the only approach to scientific therapy. Yet tianeptine is still labeled as an antidepressant drug!

The previous examples illustrate the postulation of Claude Bernard that the three milestones of medical sciences are: (1) physiology (normal functioning); (2) pathophysiology (disordered functioning), and (3) pharmacology (knowledge of the drugs able to revert physiological disorders).

Gastric, small intestinal, colonic, hepatic and pancreatic diseases have proven to be underlain by severe neurochemical, neuroautonomic, neuroendocrine and immunological disorders. Some of the latter are included among the Th2 type (gastroduodenal ulcer, gastric cancer, maltoma, hepatitis C), whereas others are considered to be Th1 autoimmune disorders (Crohn's enteritis, pancreatitis, cholangiohepatitis, celiac sprue). Finally, yet others such as ulcerative colitis belong to a type of autoimmune disorder presenting alternating Th1 and Th2 periods. Such findings explain why severe rheumatological, dermatological, and hematological disorders may accompany the mentioned gastroenterological diseases.

Sjögren disease consists of inflammation and later atrophy of the lachrymal glands. It is a Th1 autoimmune disease that frequently presents damages at many levels or tissues (arthritis, neuritis, skin disorders, etc.). Our research group found successful neuropharmacological treatment which reverted the Th1 dominance (neuroimmune profile) to a Th1 ↔ Th2 balance. Because they lacked knowledge of neurochemistry, neuroimmunology

Table 13.1. Clinical characteristics and therapeutic responses to neuropharmacologically induced NA stimulation in 52 myasthenia gravis patients (cases 1–17)

Patient No.	sex	age	Since month/year	Osserman classification	Crisis before	Crisis after	Thymectomy date	Mestinon, mg/day before	Mestinon, mg/day after	Plasmapheresis before	Plasmapheresis after	Improvement, % acute	Improvement, % late
1	M	71	11/96	II-a	0	0	no	0	0	0	0	100	100
2	F	58	07/90	II-b	3	0	no	360	0	3	0	100	80
3	F	65	08/91	II-b	4	0	no	420	0	6	0	80	90
4	F	36	09/93	II-a	0	0	1995	180	0	0	0	100	100
5	F	66	06/97	II-a	0	0	no	180	0	0	0	100	100
6	M	63	08/89	II-a	0	0	no	240	0	0	0	100	100
7	M	61	05/97	II-b	1	0	no	240	0	1	0	100	100
8	M	70	01/95	II-a	0	0	no	180	0	0	0	100	100
9	F	50	05/91	II-a	0	0	1992	180	60	0	0	80	80
10	F	35	05/93	II-b	1	0	1995	180	0	4	0	100	100
11	F	41	02/94	I	0	0	no	60	0	0	0	100	100
12	M	31	07/87	IV	13	0	1989	240	60	15	0	70	50
13	M	13	04/96	II-a	0	0	no	0	0	0	0	80	80
14	F	53	06/92	II-b	3	0	1994	360	60	6	0	60	60
15	F	50	10/93	III	0	0	1994	180	0	2	0	100	80
16	F	32	07/69	III	2	0	1992	240	0	0	0	100	70
17	F	31	01/84	II-b	3	0	1984	600	0	7	0	100	80

Mestinon doses: Before = at the first visit; after = after late improvement. Improvement: acute = at the second visit (15 days); late = ≥ 3 months. No relapse was observed in any case [Lechin et al., J Med 2000;31:1–30].

Table 13.2. Clinical characteristics and therapeutic responses to neuropharmacologically induced NA stimulation in 52 myasthenia gravis patients (cases 18–34)

Patient No.	sex	age	Since month/year	Osserman classification	Crisis before	Crisis after	Thymectomy date	Mestinon, mg/day before	Mestinon, mg/day after	Plasmapheresis before	Plasmapheresis after	Improvement, % acute	Improvement, % late
18	F	20	03/79	IV	24	0	1980	300	0	22	0	90	90
19	M	27	05/98	II-a	0	0	no	210	0	0	0	100	100
20	F	18	11/96	I	0	0	no	0	0	0	0	100	100
21	M	38	03/95	II-a	0	0	1993	180	0	0	0	100	70
22	F	39	02/86	I	0	0	no	240	0	0	0	100	100
23	F	18	03/99	II-b	0	0	no	180	0	0	0	100	100
24	F	27	10/94	IV	14	0	1996	360	120	5	0	70	70
25	F	56	09/99	II-b	2	0	1990	240	0	4	0	100	80
26	F	62	07/81	II-b	1	0	no	480	0	0	0	80	100
27	F	44	10/85	II-b	0	0	no	1,020	240	0	0	50	90
28	F	32	02/92	II-a	0	0	no	180	60	0	0	70	70
29	F	64	08/75	II-a	0	0	1976	0	0	0	0	80	80
30	F	40	07/83	II-b	1	0	no	240	120	2	0	60	60
31	F	32	09/94	III	12	0	1995	360	180	12	0	80	80
32	F	16	06/97	II-b	0	0	no	360	0	0	0	100	100
33	F	36	06/79	III	15	0	1979	300	0	18	0	70	50
34	M	21	04/94	III	6	1	1995	360	120	3	0	40	80

Mestinon doses: Before = at the first visit; after = after late improvement. Improvement: acute = at the second visit (15 days); late = ≥ 3 months. No relapse was observed in any case [Lechin et al., J Med 2000;31:1–30].

Table 13.3. Clinical characteristics and therapeutic responses to neuropharmacologically induced NA stimulation in 52 myasthenia gravis patients (cases 35–52)

Patient			Since month/year	Osserman classification	Crisis		Thymectomy date	Mestinon mg/day		Plasmapheresis		Improvement, %	
No.	sex	age			before	after		before	after	before	after	acute	late
35	F	24	03/96	II-a	1	0	1997	480	0	2	0	100	80
36	F	50	04/71	III	12	0	1993	1,260	630	19	0	50	50
37	M	36	04/98	IV	4	0	no	600	300	4	0	70	50
38	F	46	03/93	II-a	1	0	1999	360	120	0	0	80	80
39	F	15	03/94	II-b	0	0	1994	0	0	0	0	100	90
40	F	51	07/74	II-a	8	0	1995	720	120	0	0	80	70
41	F	41	04/83	II-a	1	0	no	240	60	0	0	80	80
42	F	35	06/86	II-b	0	0	1988	480	120	0	0	90	70
43	F	36	09/98	III	1	0	1999	360	0	1	0	100	80
44	M	47	07/97	II-a	2	0	no	120	0	10	0	70	80
45	F	44	02/92	II-b	0	0	1992	360	90	3	0	80	90
46	F	36	03/98	II-a	1	0	no	480	90	1	0	70	80
47	F	76	10/91	II-b	2	0	no	240	0	1	0	80	100
48	F	59	04/96	II-b	0	0	no	360	120	0	0	80	80
49	M	62	06/89	II-b	0	0	1993	240	0	0	0	70	70
50	M	64	11/97	II-a	1	0	no	240	0	1	0	90	100
51	M	65	04/95	II-a	0	0	no	240	120	0	0	90	90
52	M	48	08/97	II-a	3	0	1998	300	60	2	0	80	70

Mestinon doses: Before = at the first visit; after = after late improvement. Improvement: acute = at the second visit (15 days); late = ≥ 3 months. No relapse was observed in any case [Lechin et al., J Med 2000;31:1–30].

and neuropharmacology, ophthalmologists had previously prescribed artificial tears and ultimately eye extirpation for one Sjögren patient who fortunately turned them down. This treatment protocol was employed in this study which constituted the post-doctoral dissertation by Dr. Siony Piedra, presented at the Ophthalmology Department of the Faculty of Medicine, Universidad Central de Venezuela, 2000). Two other Sjögren-afflicted patients could no longer walk (they used wheel chairs) because of severe arthritis. They recovered from this disability at the same time that their ophthalmic disease was cured. The treatment employed to cure these patients included: small doses of an inhibitor of 5HT uptake (paroxetine) + very small doses of trifluoperazine (a DA$_2$ blocking agent) + small doses of 5-OH-TRP (a serotonin precursor). Our 7 patients were cured after 2–3 months of therapy. All had been previously treated unsuccessfully with corticosteroids (at the Rheumatological Department of the Central University Hospital, Caracas). Neither ophthalmologists nor rheumatologists possessed the neurochemical, neuroimmunological and neuropharmacological knowledge to understand and adequately treat the poly-physiological disorders underlying Sjögren disease.

Sjögren disease, Crohn's enteritis, rheumatoid arthritis, multiple sclerosis, psoriasis, etc. are all Th1 autoimmune diseases presenting a similar neurochemical disorder: raised NA/Ad ratio + low plasma TRP and low Ad levels. This is the neurochemical profile we found in major (endogenous) depression. The fact that both Th1 autoimmune diseases and endogenous depressed patients are improved by the same neuropharmacological therapy, addressed to decreasing central NA activity and increasing central 5HT activity, gives strong support to the postulation that these diseases share common CNS, ANS and immune system disorders.

Conversely, Th2 autoimmune diseases present a neurochemical disorder characterized by low NA/Ad ratio + increased f5HT plasma levels. This is the same profile we routinely register in chronic, maladapted (uncoping) stress situation. Both the excessive Ad secretion from adrenomedullary glands as well as the increased f5HT plasma levels trigger inhibition of Th1 immunity (tissue level) and predominance of humoral immunity (Th2).

GHRH, GH, prolactin and androgens have proven to favor Th1 immunity whereas somatostatin, CRH, ACTH, cortisol and estrogens favor Th2 immunity. Thus, specialists including gastroenterologists, cardiolo-

Concluding Remarks 71

Table 13.4. Immunological parameters (mean ± SEM) in 57 normal humans, BDZ users and 15 days after BDZ withdrawal (pBDZ)

	N	BDZ	p-BDZ	p values		
				N vs. BDZ	N vs. pBDZ	BDZ vs. BDZ
PBL	38.0±1.3	36.8±1.6	42.7±1.9	NS	NS	<0.05
CD3	67.1±2.3	62.9±1.7	68.3±4.5	<0.05	NS	<0.05
CD4	48.3±1.7	39.1±1.5	46.7±2.7	<0.02	NS	<0.02
CD8	23.9±0.9	23.4±1.0	20.2±3.4	NS	NS	NS
CD4/CD8	1.91±0.1	1.31±0.1	2.71±0.5	<0.05	<0.02	<0.001
CD20	13.1±3.2	12.7±0.9	9.91±1.4	NS	<0.05	<0.05
CD57	8.61±0.6	14.4±0.7	5.62±0.5	<0.001	<0.05	<0.05
CD11b	17.9±5.2	25.1±1.4	18.7±4.6	<0.05	NS	<0.05
CD16	7.39±2.0	3.78±0.6	3.92±0.8	<0.02	<0.02	NS
G-D	7.12±1.3	4.55±0.3	9.72±4.9	<0.02	NS	<0.01
NK %	40.3±2.0	48.2±2.8	40.2±4.3	<0.02	NS	<0.02

PBL = Peripheral blood lymphocytes; CD3 (anti-leu4) = T cells; CD4 (anti-leu3a) = T-helper/inducer cells; CD8 (anti-leu2a) = T-cytotoxic/suppressor cells; CD20 (anti-leu16) = B cells; CD57 (anti-leu7) = T-cell subset + NK-cell subset; CD11b (anti-leu15) = T-cell subset + NK cells + monocytes; CD16 (anti-leu11) = NK cells; G-D = γ-δ-cells; NK % = cytotoxicity against target cells; NS = nonsignificant [Lechin F et al., Clin Neuropharmacol 1994;17:63–72].

Table 13.5. Plasma neuroendocrine parameters (mean ± SE) in 43 normal younger (<45 years) BDZ consumers (BDZY), 39 normal elderly (>65 years) BDZ consumers (BDZE) and their age- and sex-matched non-BDZ-consuming controls (NY and NE, respectively)

	NY	NE	BDZY	BDZE
NA, pg/ml	233±15	292±18	129±13	89±17
Ad, pg/ml	29±3	67±5	41±10	89±7
NA/Ad	6.2±0.9	3.7±0.8	2.9±0.9	0.9±1.2
DA, pg/ml	17.1±1.2	14.9±1.6	15.2±0.9	13.8±2.6
p5HT, ng/ml	196±9	141±6	152±7	101±13
f5HT, ng/ml	0.9±0.2	3.4±1.1	4.6±0.9	9.4±1.7
TRP, ng/ml	14,060±21	9,634±17	10,403±23	6,771±34
CRT, µg/ml	8.9±1.3	18.6±2.2	19.4±2.1	29.5±3.3

Many values were rounded off [Lechin et al., Psychother Psychosom 1996;65:171–182].

gists, rheumatologists, dermatologists, neurologists, hematologists, ophthalmologists, etc. should be aware of and informed about pertinent interdisciplinary knowledge in order to prescribe appropriate treatments and avoid iatrogenia.

The scientific findings above are backed by successful therapeutic results obtained by our research group in numerous diseases. Many of these results have been published (pancreatitis, Crohn's enteritis, duodenal ulcer, irritable bowel syndrome, ulcerative colitis, biliary dysky-nesia, postprandial hypoglycemia, hypertension, trigeminal neuralgia, myasthenia gravis, non-Hodgkin lymphoma, malignant diseases, Gilles de la Tourette disorder, psychogenic infertility, bronchial asthma, Sjögren disease, headache syndromes, acute psychosis, manic syndrome, depressive disorders, anxiety, social phobia, panic attacks). Other results await publication (rheumatoid arthritis, granulomatous lung disease, psoriasis, penphigus, atopic dermatitis, Takayashu disease, cerebrovascular accidents, pulmonary hypertension, multiple sclerosis,

Table 13.6. p values between plasma neuroendocrine parameters in 43 normal younger (<45 years) BDZ consumers (BDZY), 39 normal elderly (>65 years) BDZ consumers (BDZE) and their age- and sex-matched non-BDZ consuming controls (NY and NE, respectively)

	NE[1]	BDZY[1]	BDZE[1]	BDZY[2]	BDZE[2]	BDZY vs. BDZE
NA	<0.05	<0.01	<0.001	<0.001	<0.001	<0.05
Ad	<0.001	<0.05	<0.001	<0.05	<0.01	<0.001
NA/Ad	<0.02	<0.01	<0.001	NS	<0.002	<0.02
DA	NS	NS	NS	NS	NS	NS
p5HT	<0.05	<0.05	<0.001	NS	<0.05	<0.02
f5HT	<0.01	<0.005	<0.001	NS	<0.01	<0.01
TRP	<0.001	<0.001	<0.001	NS	<0.01	<0.05
CRT	<0.005	<0.005	<0.001	NS	<0.01	<0.01

Multivariate analysis of variance, paired and unpaired t tests were employed for statistical analysis. Most values were rounded off. NS = Nonsignificant.

[1] Compared to NY.
[2] Compared to NE [Lechin et al., Psychother Psychosom 1996;65:171–182].

Guillain Barré disease, dermatomyositis, sleep disorders, carcinoid syndrome, uveitis and osteoporosis).

The sections of Neurochemistry, Neuroimmunology and Neuropharmacology at the Institute of Experimental Medicine (Faculty of Medicine, Universidad Central de Venezuela) are headed by Dr. Fuad Lechin (MD, PhD), emeritus professor of the Department of General Pathology and Pathophysiology. This Institute (IME) is provided with the only neurochemical laboratory existing in the world (at hospital level) in which all plasma neurotransmitters (NA, Ad, DA, p-5HT, f5HT and plasma TRP) are routinely assessed in all normal and diseased subjects as well as experimental mammals. Some 25,000 subjects have been investigated with this procedure both during supine-resting condition and after different types of stress challenges (orthostasis, moderate walking, oral glucose, buspirone administration, clonidine, tianeptine, amino acids, etc.). This type of laboratory, not available at any hospital in the world, exists only at high level neurochemistry research institutes because plasma neurotransmitter assays are a very expensive procedure requiring sophisticated technology. Equipment and supplies are also costly and demand constant maintenance, making these types of neurochemical assays unprofitable from a financial standpoint. Other financial obligations include the acquisition of drugs for treating patients. These drugs, often exorbitantly expensive, should be administered free of charge to patients enrolled in therapeutic trials.

A sleep laboratory was recently installed in our institute. This expensive lab was bought in the US through a long-term credit. All types of sleep disorders are being investigated in our sleep lab. In addition, neurochemical investigation is carried out parallel to electroencephalographic studies, so as to register the neurochemical variations occurring during the different phases of sleep.

Table 13.7. Peripheral immunological parameters (mean ± SE) in 43 normal younger (<45 years) BDZ consumer (BDZY), 39 normal elderly (>65 years) BDZ consumers (BDZE) and their age- and sex-matched non-BDZ consuming controls (NY and NE, respectively)

	NY	NE	BDZY	BDZE
PBL	37.6±1.2	32.2±1.1	31.4±1.0	24.2±1.3
CD3	68.1±2.4	59.1±1.9	60.4±1.8	51.4±2.1
CD4	28.5±1.7	24.6±1.6	24.2±1.2	21.9±0.9
CD4/CD8	2.1±0.1	1.7±0.1	1.7±0.2	1.3±0.1
CD20	13.9±3.1	12.8±2.9	12.8±0.9	12.6±1.4
CD57	8.7±0.7	13.6±0.8	14.3±1.1	17.3±1.0
CD11b	16.8±4.9	22.4±1.9	23.4±2.1	26.4±3.6
CD16	7.4±1.1	4.8±0.7	4.7±1.3	3.7±0.9
NK %	42.1±2.1	49.3±2.9	47.8±1.8	51.4±2.2

PBL = Peripheral blood lymphocytes; CD3 (anti-leu4) = T cells; CD4 (anti-leu3a) = T-helper/inducer cells; CD8 (anti-leu2a) = T-cytotoxic/suppressor cells; CD20 (anti-leu16) = B cells; CD57 (anti-leu7) = T-cell subset + NK-cell subset; CD11b (anti-leu15) = T-cell subset + NK cells + monocytes; CD16 (anti-leu11) = NK cells; NK % = cytotoxicity against K562 target cells [Lechin et al., Psychother Psychosom 1996;65:171–182].

Table 13.8. p values between peripheral immunological parameters in 43 normal younger (<45 years) BDZ consumers (BDZY), 39 normal elderly (>65 years) BDZ consumers (BDZE) and their age- and sex-matched non-BDZ consuming controls (NY and NE, respectively)

	NE[1]	BDZY[1]	BDZE[1]	BDZY[2]	BDZE[2]	BDZY vs. BDZE
PBL	<0.05	<0.05	<0.01	NS	<0.02	<0.02
CD3	<0.05	<0.05	<0.01	NS	<0.02	<0.02
CD4	<0.05	<0.05	<0.02	NS	NS	<0.05
CD4/CD8	<0.05	<0.05	<0.02	NS	<0.05	<0.05
CD20	NS	NS	NS	NS	NS	NS
CD57	<0.01	<0.01	<0.005	NS	<0.05	<0.05
CD11b	<0.05	<0.05	<0.01	NS	<0.05	<0.05
CD16	<0.05	<0.05	<0.05	NS	NS	NS
NK %	<0.05	<0.05	<0.02	NS	NS	NS

Multivariate analysis of variance, paired and unpaired t tests were employed for statistical analysis. Most values were rounded off. PBL = Peripheral blood lymphocytes; CD3 (anti-leu4) = T cells; CD4 (anti-leu3a) = T-helper/inducer cells; CD8 (anti-leu2a) =T-cytotoxic/suppressor cells: CD20 (anti-leu16) = B cells, CD57 (anti-leu7) = T-cell subset + NK-cell subset; CD11b (anti-leu15) = T-cell subset + NK cells + monocytes; CD16 (anti-leu11) = NK cells; NK % = cytotoxicity against K562 target cells. NS = Nonsignificant.
[1] Compared to NY.
[2] Compared to NE [Lechin et al., Psychother Psychosom 1996;65:171–182].

Sleep disorders should not be treated with BDZ. These dangerous drugs trigger exhaustion of the GABAergic system and, finally, lose effectivity and provoke addiction. They adversely affect memory, intellectual and sexual activities, and immunity (table 13.4–13.8), and favor the appearance of many mental and somatic diseases (Parkinson, Alzheimer, malignant tumors, etc.). For a start, they interfere with the normal sleep pattern. This is constituted by four SWS stages + REM sleep. Benzodiazepines are antiphysiologic and dangerous because they induce sleep lacks from stages 3 and 4 of SWS as well as REM sleep. Hence, they interfere with immunity because GH, which is responsible for recovery from stress situation and stimulates immunity, is secreted only during stages 3 and 4 of the slow wave sleep.

In the past our institute has received financial support from two private foundations, Funda-IME (Fundación para el Instituto de Medicina Experimental) and Funda-Neuroinmunologia. However, leading supporters of these foundations have died or are absent from Venezuela. At present, our research work is sustained by those patients who are able to pay (totally or partially) for the tests performed. Other patients are examined and treated free of charge. As we enter the new millennium, our research work is further limited because we are devoting large resources to a program for 'Bronchial asthma eradication'

Table 13.9. Pathophysiological conditions associated with prevalent Th1 and Th2 responses

Th1	Th2
Hashimoto thyroiditis	Transplantation tolerance
Grave's ophthalmopathy	Successful pregnancy
Sjögren syndrome	Reduced protection against
Type 1 diabetes mellitus	intracellular pathogens
Multiple sclerosis	Measles virus infection and
Crohn's disease	vaccination
Rheumatoid arthritis	SLE
HCV-induced chronic hepatitis	Myasthenia gravis
Primary sclerosis cholangitis	Some idiopathic eosinophilic
Acute allograft rejection	syndromes
Unexplained recurrent	Atopic dermatitis
abortions	Thrombocytopenic purpura
Aplastic anemia	Hemolytic anemia
	Progression to AIDS in HIV
	infection
	Bronchial asthma

which we have launched in the state of Aragua, Venezuela. Up to the present, we have successfully treated more than 10,000 asthmatic children living in the cities and small towns of this state.

Chapter 14

··

Illustrations of Some Therapeutic Results

According to our paradigm, all diseases showing a Th1 autoimmune profile (excessive cellular immune activity) present a neurochemical profile similar to endogenous depression: high NA + normal Ad = raised NA/Ad ratio values (greater than 5) + low TRP plasma levels. On the contrary, all diseases showing a Th2 autoimmune profile (excessive humoral immunity) present a neurochemical profile similar to that registered in chronic uncoping stress patients: low NA + high Ad + low NA/Ad ratio values (less than 2) + raised or normal TRP + raised f5HT plasma levels.

The Th1 (endogenous or major depression) profile would express the following CNS neurochemical profile: hyperactivity of the LC NA neuronal group + hypoactivity of the pontine serotonergic nuclei DR and MR + hypoactivity of the C1-adrenergic medullary nuclei.

The Th2 (chronic uncoping stress) profile would express the following CNS neurochemical profile: hypoactivity of the LC-NA + DR-5HT + MR-5HT nuclei + hyperactivity of the C1-Ad medullary nuclei. Both those 5HT nuclei send excitatory axons to the two vagal motor nuclei, nucleus tractus solitary and nucleus ambiguus. Vagal nerves are the excitatory drive responsible for the release of 5HT by enterochromaffin cells. Intestinal 5HT constitutes the only source of blood serotonin. Ninety percent of blood 5HT is stored in the platelets (p-5HT). For this reason, p-5HT shows significant rise during postprandial periods and during sleep, at which time hyperparasympathetic activity is registered. According to all the above, adrenomedullary-sympathetic and parasympathetic activities are liberalized from the pontine NA-5HT control and would display alternating predominances. Two factors cooperate to maintain the increased free serotonin (f-5HT) in the plasma of uncoping stressed mammals: (a) adrenaline-triggered platelet aggregation during hypersympathetic predominance, and (b) acetylcholine-induced inhibition of platelet uptake during parasympa-

thetic activation. The raised Ad + raised f-5HT converge to suppress Th1 immune activity and favor Th2 predominance.

Neuropharmacological therapy of Th2 immune disorders is the treatment we prescribe for all uncoping-stress associated diseases. Malignant diseases are included among this group. However, Hodgkin's lymphoma and pancreatic adenocarcinoma are not included in this group. Neuropharmacological manipulations are addressed to increasing central noradrenergic (neural sympathetic) activity. The following drugs are routinely administered:

(1) NA precursors (L-tyrosine, L-phenylalanine).

(2) NA-releasing agents (α_2-antagonists) such as yohimbine.

(3) Small doses of β-blocking agents (propranolol).

(4) NA uptake inhibitors (desipramine, maprotyline, doxepin, etc.).

(5) NA + dopamine enhancer drug (buspirone). These NA-potentiating drugs should be administered early in the morning.

(6) Small doses of 5HT precursor (5-OH-tryptophan = 25 mg) + a 5HT-releasing agent like trazodone 25–50 mg before bed.

(7) GH-releasing agents such as GH-RH hormone and arginine should also be administered before bed. GH is the most powerful Th-1-activating agent. However, GH itself should not be administered in cancer patients. This factor provokes macrophage accumulation around tumoral cells and granulomas are induced. These granulomas simulate tumor growth in which biopsies, however, detect nontumor cells. In some cases, tumoral cells are found in the deepest zones of such GH-induced granulomas.

(8) Dopaminergic agonists like amantidine in small doses (100 mg two times weekly). This drug should be used in good sleepers only.

(9) Levamisole (50 mg), twice weekly.

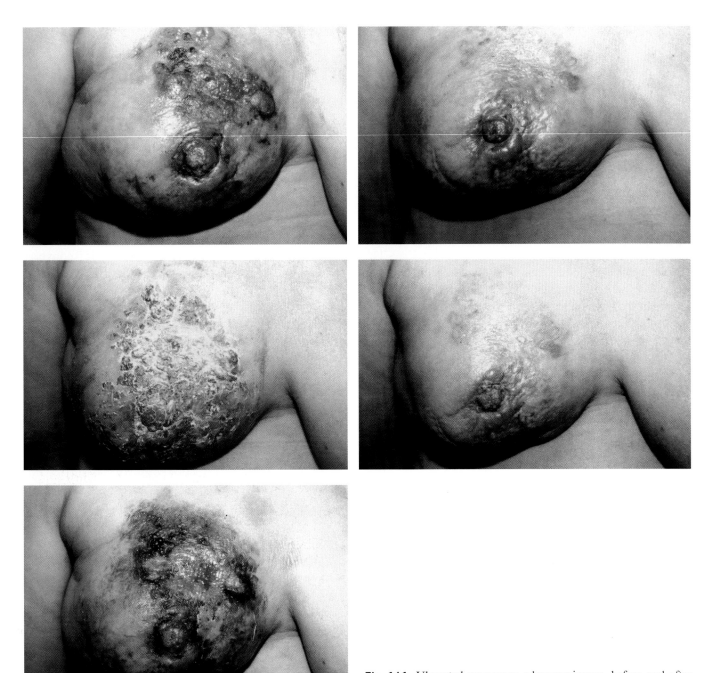

Fig. 14.1. Ulcerated mammary adenocarcinoma, before and after 4 months of neuropharmacological therapy. The great improvement registered in this patient permitted surgical resection (she died 7 years later).

Up to the present we have treated some 3,000 advanced cancer patients. Most came to our institute when all conventional therapies had failed. We have presented our results in the most important cancer hospitals of the US (see references).

We present here a small sample of various cured or greatly improved malignant tumors. It is not our intention to announce a cure for malignant diseases, but to demonstrate the close association existing between uncoping stress situation, Th-2 immune profile, and malignant dis-

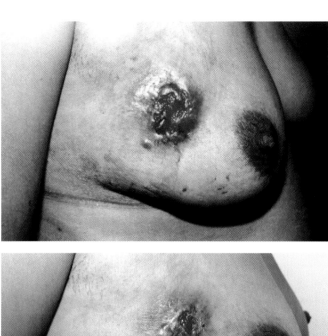

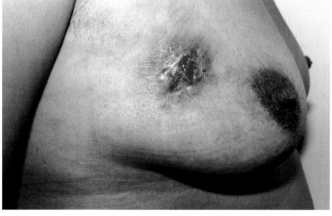

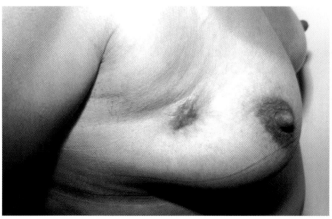

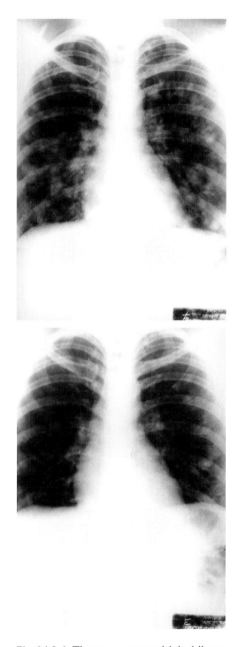

Fig. 14.2. b The same case: multiple, bilateral pulmonary metastasis almost disappeared also.

Fig. 14.2. a Ulcerated mammary adenocarcinoma, before and after 5 months of neuropharmacological therapy.

ease. When we lectured, by invitation at conferences in several US oncology hospitals and universities, oncologists were greatly impressed. However, they asked us for a package treatment like chemotherapy and radiotherapy. They could not accept treatments based on neuropharmacological, neuroendocrinological or neuroimmunological manipulations. Their hospitals are not provided with neurochemical laboratories. These specialists felt unable to design appropriate neuropharmacological therapy according to neurochemical + immunological findings. Unfortunately, this obstacle is still present. For our part, we continued applying our therapeutical approach on cancer

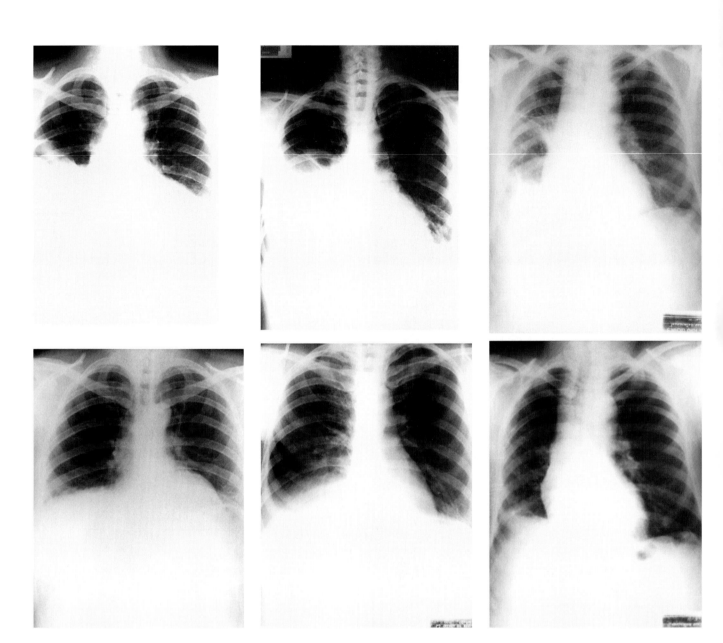

Fig. 14.3. Pulmonary metastasis in the right lung, secondary to previously resected mammary gland. Total disappearance was observed within 4 months of neuropharmacological therapy. No relapses occurred.

Fig. 14.4. Right pleuropulmonary metastasis, secondary to previously resected mammary gland. Total disappearance was observed after 3 months of neuropharmacological therapy.

Fig. 14.5. Breast metastasic lung cancer before and after 5 months of neuropharmacological therapy (mammary adenocarcinoma).

patients attending our institute and gave up reporting our experience to medical journals because they lacked adequate reviewers and asked for double-blind studies. Sadly, the great majority of our patients are short-term survivors of chemo- and radiotherapy who have been informed that their days are numbered. They visit our institute to alleviate pain and perhaps prolong their lifespan. After they leave the institute they are in God's hands. In our long experience, the low percentage of patients having previously received neither chemotherapy nor radiotherapy, show the best response to neuropharmacological treatment.

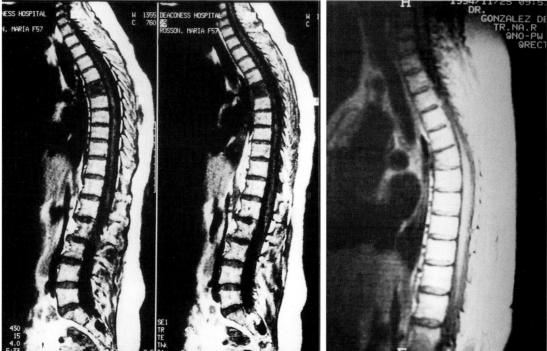

14.6 a

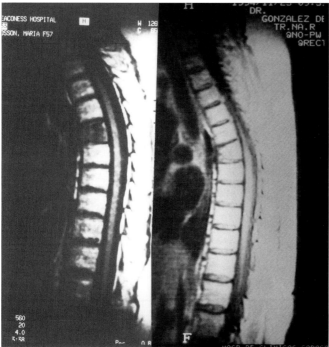

14.6 b

Fig. 14.6 a–c. Bone metastasis at the 6th thoracic vertebra. After 5 months of neuropharmacological therapy the bone was healed. The primary tumor, a pulmonary adenocarcinoma, was resected 1 month before at the Deaconess Hospital in Boston (USA), where post-surgical radiotherapy was suggested to alleviate pain. No radiotherapy was applied.

(Fig. 14.6 c, see next page.)

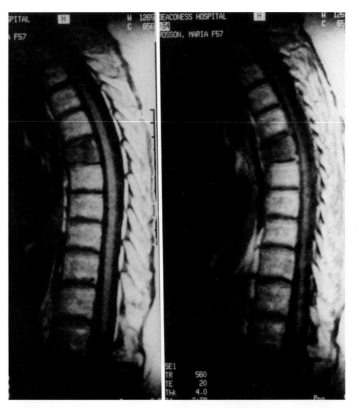
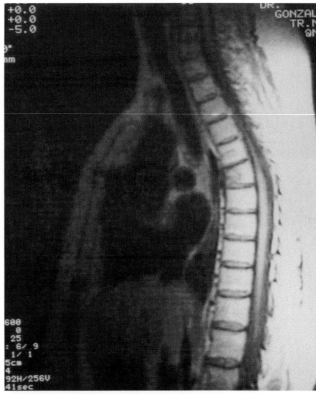
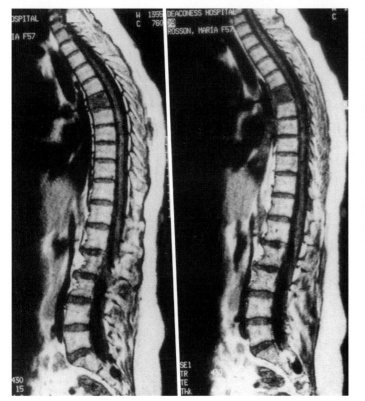
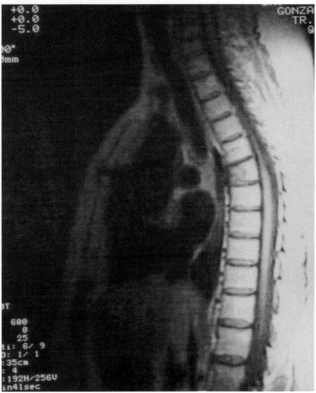

14.6 c

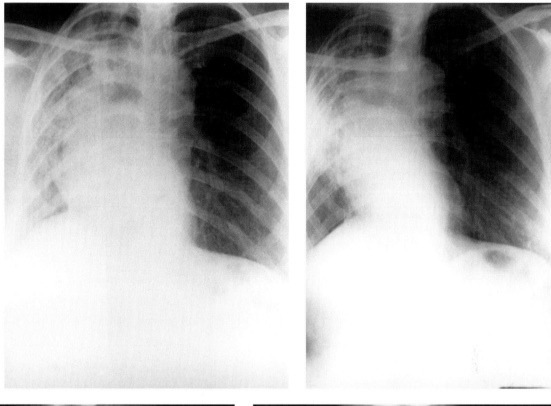

14.7

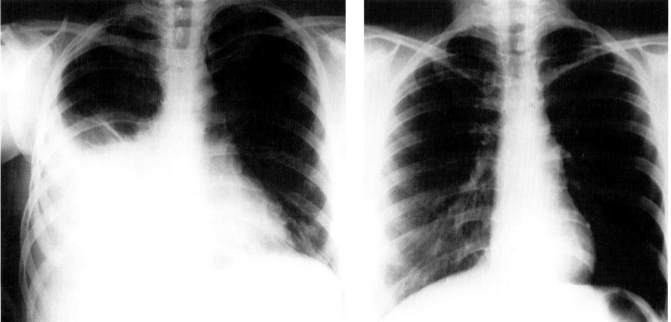

8

Fig. 14.7. Lung cancer (adenocarcinoma) + supraclavicular metastasis. Eight months after chemotherapy + radiotherapy courses, cancer symptoms reappeared and the patient entered neuropharmacological therapy. Within 2 years, significant reduction of tumoral images was obtained and the patient was discharged symptomless. She then traveled to San Francisco (USA) where she attended her severely diseased mother, night and day, for several months. She died 2 months after her mother's funeral.

Fig. 14.8. Right pleuropulmonary metastases from a previously resected mammary adenocarcinoma. Normalization was obtained after 4 months of neuropharmacological therapy.

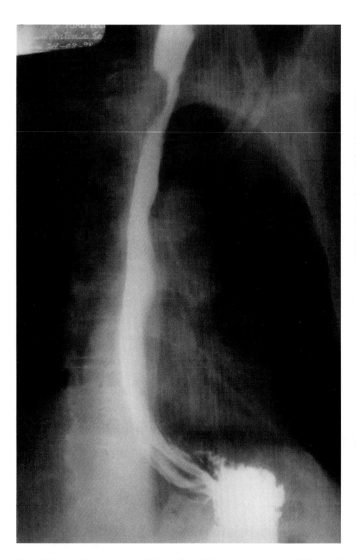

Fig. 14.9. a Carcinoma epidermoid of the esophagus (radiological plus endoscopic diagnosis).

Fig. 14.9. b Total disappearance (endoscopic + radiological) of the tumor was obtained within 7 months of neuropharmacological therapy. The patient was absent and without medication during 13 months. The tumor reappeared and he entered neuropharmacological therapy again in October 2000 continuing this up to the present.

Other Diseases Associated with Uncoping Stress Profile (Th2 Autoimmune Diseases)

We have treated many other patients showing a neurochemical profile of uncoping stress and a Th-2 immune profile. These patients received neuropharmacological therapy addressed to increasing central noradrenergic activity and to bridling peripheral adrenomedullary activity. To date we have successfully treated patients suffering from myasthenia gravis (over 800 cases), thrombocytopenic purpura, Guillain-Barré, atopic dermatitis, stress-associated female infertility, gastric malthoma, and non-Hodgkin lymphoma.

Neuropharmacological Therapy of Endogenous Depression Neurochemical Profile Diseases (Th1 Autoimmune Diseases)

These diseases frequently present a Th-1 immune profile. Rheumatoid arthritis, Sjögren disease, psoriasis, scleroderma, Raynaud disease, multiple sclerosis, Crohn's enteritis, dermatomyositis and pemphigus are included among the Th-1 profile diseases. In the following section,

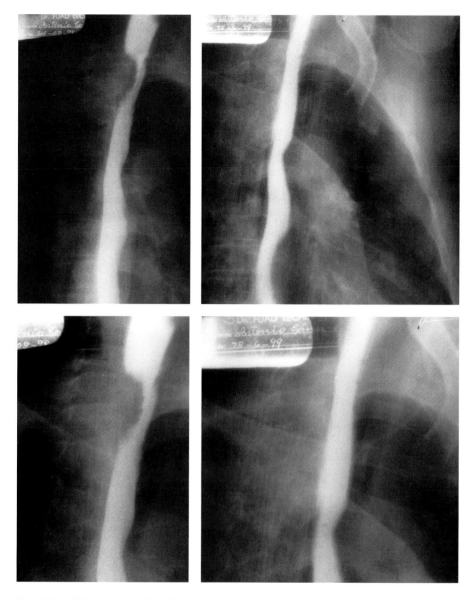

Fig. 14.9. c The same case (No. 9) after and before neuropharmacological therapy.

we give some examples of the effects of neuropharmacological therapy on the progress of this type of diseases.

Neuropharmacological therapy is addressed to reducing central noradrenergic activity and to increasing DR-5HT + MR-5HT activity. To this end, we use the following neuropharmacological manipulations:

(1) Cursors of 5HT, for example 5-OH-TRP (50–100 mg).

(2) 5HT-releasing agents like the 5HT2-receptor antagonist trazodone (25–50 mg).

(3) $5HT_{1A}$-antagonist such as pindolol (2.5 mg); inhibitors of 5HT uptake including sertraline (25–50 mg) and paroxetine (20–40 mg).

(4) α_2-Agonists like clonidine (0.15 mg).

(5) Tizanidine (4 mg).

(6) Trifluoperazine (2–5 mg).

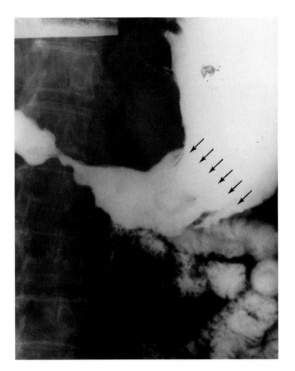

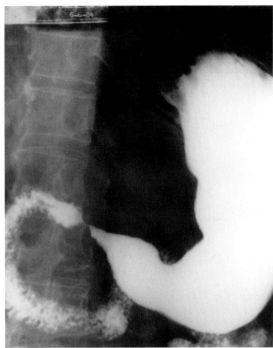

Fig. 14.10. Age 71, female. At first visit in January 1984 gastric adenocarcinoma was diagnosed in this patient who refused surgery in favor of neuropharmacological therapy. In 6 months, she showed radiological normalization of her tumor. Rejecting new endoscopic investigation, she remained free of symptoms until 1991 when she died of a cerebrovascular accident.

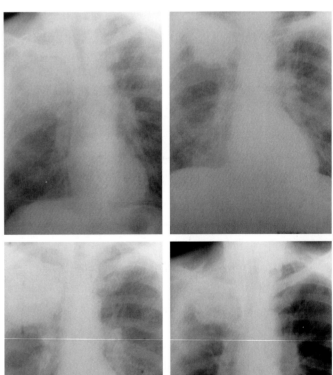

Fig. 14.11. Age 56, male. Pulmonary adenocarcinoma. Great parenchymal infiltration of the upper right lung lobe. He received neuropharmacological therapy during 3.6 years. He remained symptomless. He died following an accidental fall.

Illustrations of Some Therapeutic Results

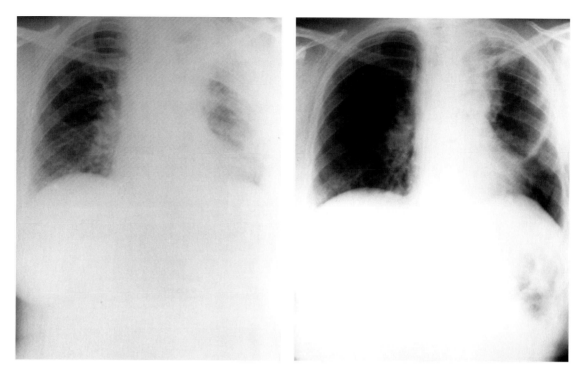

Fig. 14.12. Pleuropulmonary metastases from a previously resected mammary adenocarcinoma. Significant improvement was obtained after 3 months of neuropharmacological therapy.

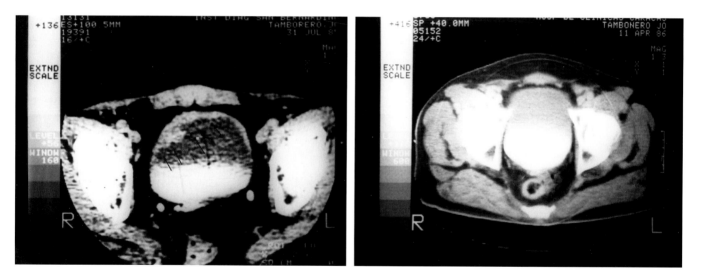

Fig. 14.13. Age 59, male. In July 1985, the patient underwent endoscopic resection of urinary bladder adenocarcinoma, followed by chemotherapy in August 1985. Bladder tumor reappeared in March 1986. Endoscopic biopsy revealed transitional cells adenocarcinoma, degree IV (Ash classification). Total disappearance was obtained after 3 months of neuropharmacological therapy. Last control in July 2000.

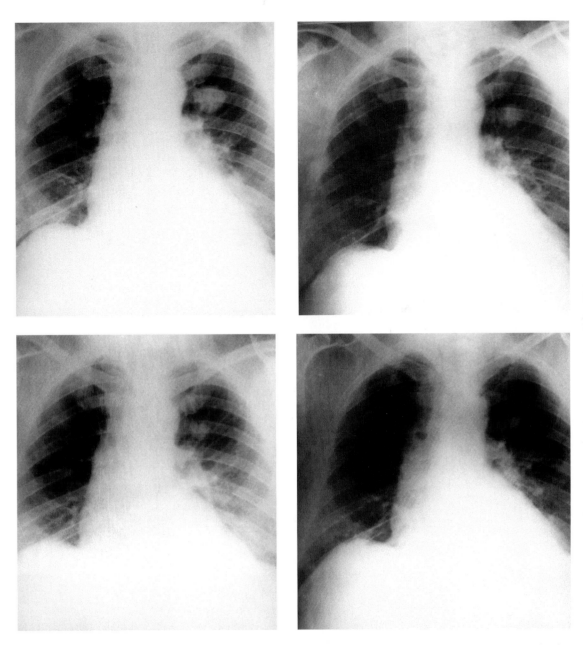

Fig. 14.14. Left pleuropulmonary metastases from a previously resected mammary adenocarcinoma. Normalization was obtained after 3 months of neuropharmacological therapy.

(7) DA antagonist that reduces NA and facilitates 5HT activity.

(8) Methotrexate (2.5–5 mg weekly).

(9) In some severe cases lithium salts are added (200 mg twice weekly).

(10) L-Tryptophan does not cross the BBB easily. We use this 5HT precursor in some cases of rheumatoid ar-

thritis looking for beneficial peripheral effects. It has been demonstrated that plasma 5HT is able to reduce macrophage activity.

We have treated many cases of multiple sclerosis with the above neuropharmacological therapy. One of these cases was an MD (ophthalmologist) who had lost his vision. He recovered his sight completely (he is now per-

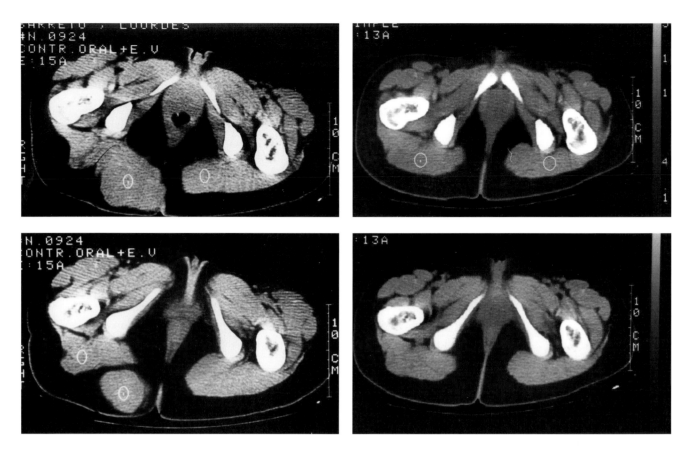

Fig. 14.15. Female, age 15. First visit in February, 1991. Surgical resection of Antoni type B schwannoma in the right gluteal region was performed in March 1989. Recidivant tumor was diagnosed in December 1990. The patient and her parents refused further surgery and visited our Institute. Neuropharmacological therapy began in March 1991. CAT scan showed complete remission after 3 months of treatment. The patient has remained symptomless. Last control in January 1995.

forming eye surgery). All types of therapy had previously failed with this patient (steroids, β-interferon, etc.). Dermatomyositis, muscular dystrophy, hemolytic anemia and other Th-1 autoimmune diseases have likewise been successfully treated with this therapy.

Summarizing, the success obtained with the neuropharmacological approach to such diverse organic (somatic), nonpsychiatric diseases is consistent with the hypothesis that the CNS circuitry, the immune system, the endocrine and the autonomic nervous system are closely interlinked, and thus all pharmacological manipulations addressed to normalizing the CNS circuitry lead to normalization of both central and peripheral physiologic disorders. In our opinion, treatment of patients should return to the hands of scientific doctors. With this aim, practitioners should receive scientific, interdisciplinary training. Medical technology is necessary but should not be the only pillar of therapy.

In the following pages, we illustrate results obtained with the above neuropharmacological approaches with some cases.

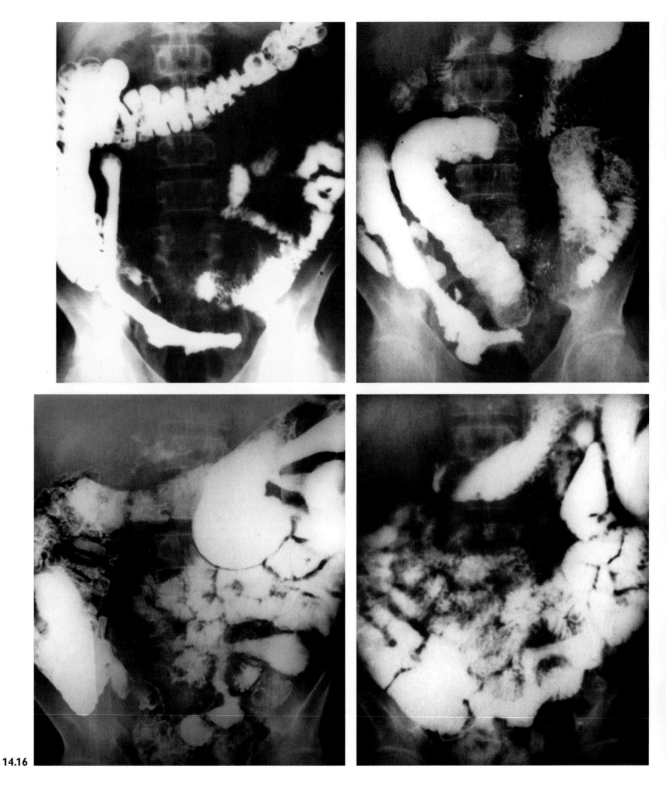

14.16

Fig. 14.16. Small bowel X-ray of a severely ill Crohn's patient. Radiological and clinical normalization occurred within 1 year of neuropharmacological treatment.

Fig. 14.17. Small bowel X-ray of a severely ill Crohn's patient. Radiological and clinical normalization occurred within 7–8 months after receiving neuropharmacological treatment.

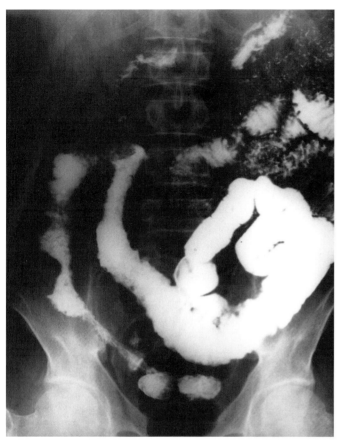

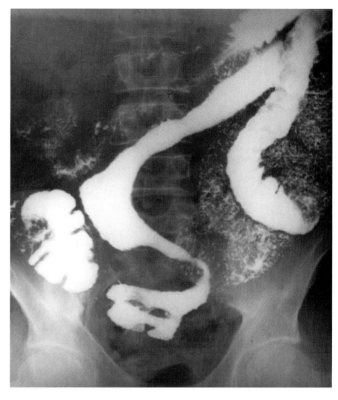

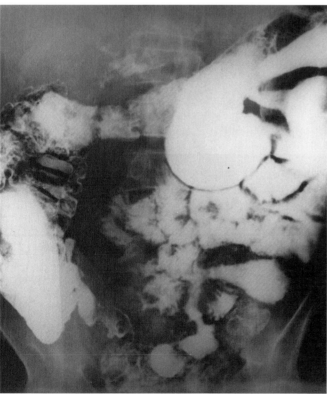

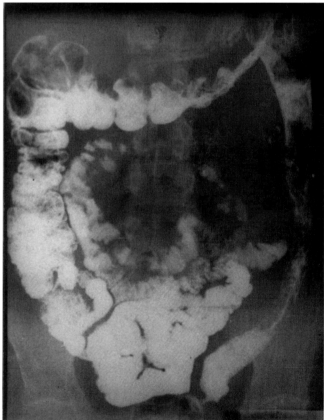

14.17

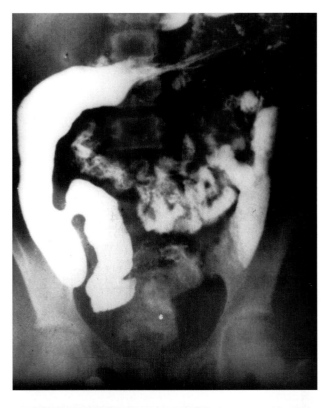
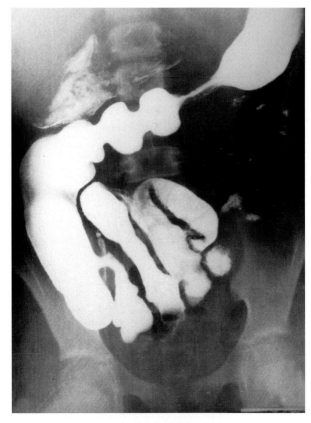
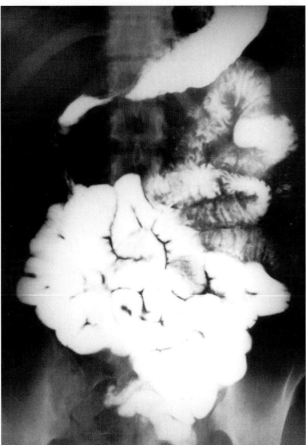
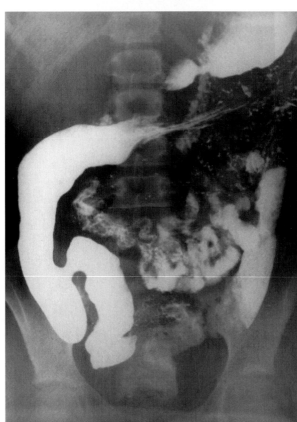

14.18

90   Illustrations of Some Therapeutic Results

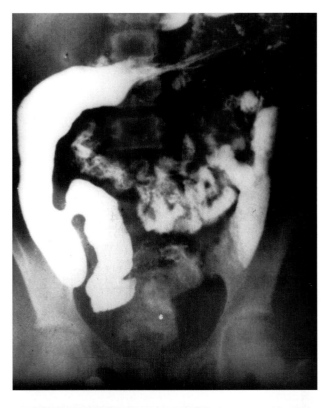
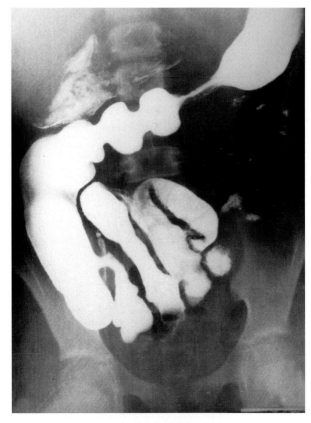
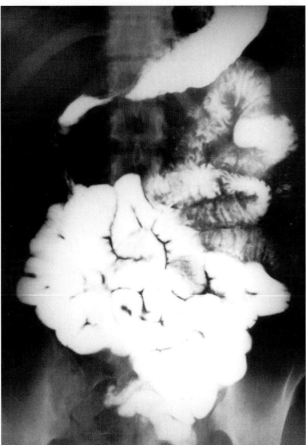
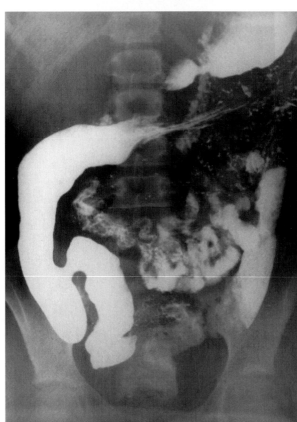

14.18

Illustrations of Some Therapeutic Results

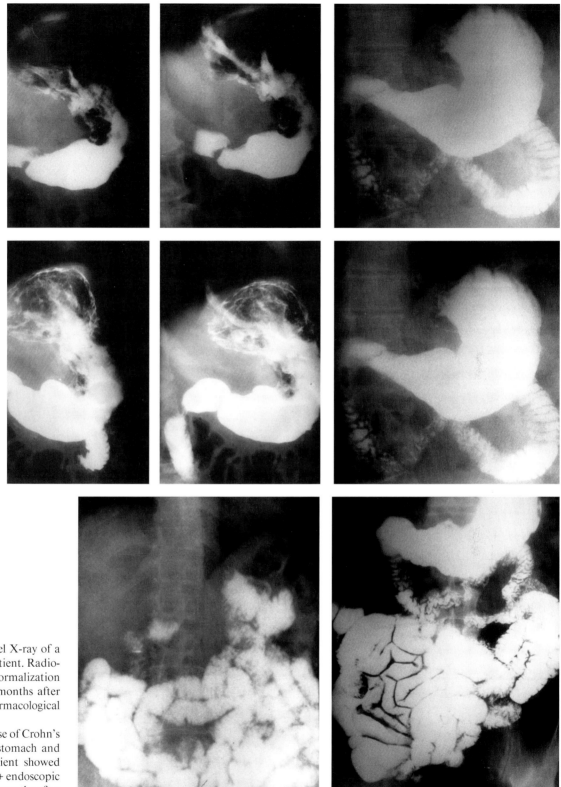

Fig. 14.18. Small bowel X-ray of a severely ill Crohn's patient. Radiological and clinical normalization occurred within 5–6 months after receiving neuropharmacological treatment.

Fig. 14.19. A severe case of Crohn's disease affecting the stomach and small bowel. The patient showed clinical + radiological + endoscopic normalization in 7–9 months after neuropharmacological therapy.

14.19

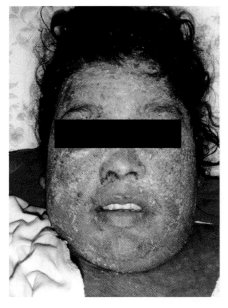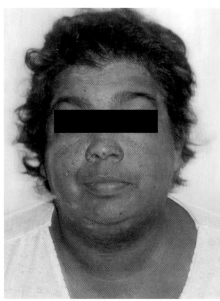

Fig. 14.20. a A severe case (No. 20) of pemphigus. Normalization of all lesions was observed after 6 weeks of neuropharmacological treatment.

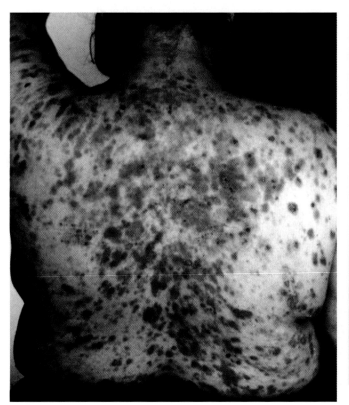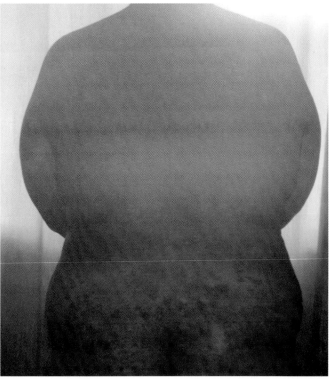

Fig. 14.20. b The same case with severe pemphigus. After and before 6 weeks of neuropharmacological treatment.

Illustrations of Some Therapeutic Results

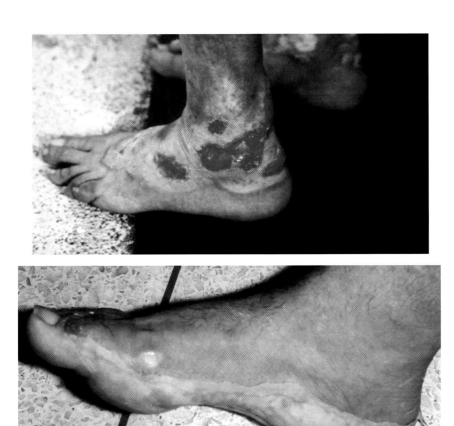

Fig. 14.20. c The same case with severe pemphigus. After and before 6 weeks of neuropharmacological treatment.

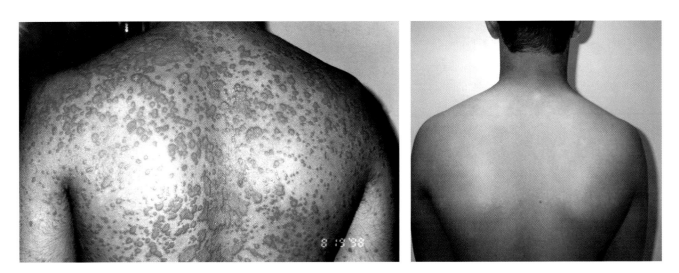

Fig. 14.21. A severe case of psoriasis was normalized after 6 months of neuropharmacological therapy.

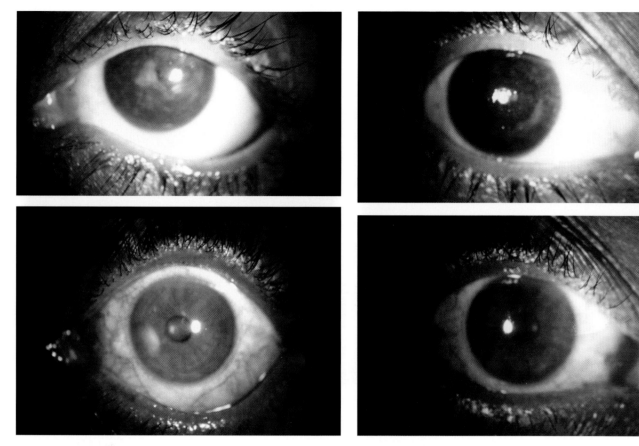

Fig. 14.22. A severe case of Sjögren was normalized after 3 months of neuropharmacological therapy. Steroid therapy had failed. The patient also presented severe rheumatoid arthritis which showed great improvement under the neuropharmacological therapy. She did not use a wheelchair anymore, after treatment.

Fig. 14.23. A severe case of Sjögren was normalized after 5 months of neuropharmacological therapy. Steroid therapy had failed. This patient had been referred to surgery for extirpation of the eye because of corneal ulceration. The patient also presented severe rheumatoid arthritis which showed great improvement under the neuropharmacological therapy. She did not use a wheelchair anymore after treatment.

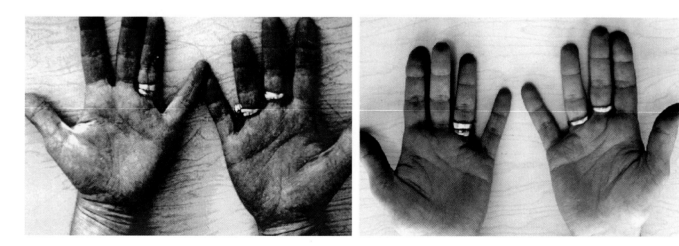

Fig. 14.24. A severe case of atopic dermatitis before and after 5 months of neuropharmacological therapy.

References

References for Introduction

Amat J, Torres A, Lechin F: Differential effect of footshock stress on humoral and cellular responses of the cat. Life Sci 1993;53:315–322.

Insausti CL, Lechin F, van der Dijs B: Severe thrombocytopenia following oral cholecystography with iodocetamic acid. Am J Haematol 1981;14:285–287.

Lechin AE, Varon J, van der Dijs B, Lechin F: Plasma catecholamines and indoleamines during attacks and remission on severe bronchial asthma: possible role of stress. Am J Respir Crit Care Med 1994;149:A778.

Lechin AE, Varon J, van der Dijs B, Lechin F: Plasma neurotransmitters, blood pressure and heart rate during rest and exercise (abstract). Am J Respir Crit Care Med 1994;149:A482.

Lechin F: The effect of secretin on serum potassium. Acta Physiol Latinoamer 1962;12:370–374.

Lechin F: Glucose disposal. Lancet 1964;ii:1122.

Lechin F: Intestinal hormones and insulin. Lancet 1966;ii:35–36.

Lechin F: Enfermedades por autoinmunidad (review). Med Cutánea 1968;1:125–132.

Lechin F: Uropepsinogen. Acta Gastroenter Latinoamer 1969;1:83–89.

Lechin F: Autoinmunidad y patologia gastroduodenal (editorial). Acta Gastroenter Latinoamer 1977;7:39–42.

Lechin F: Pimozide therapy for trigeminal neuralgia. Arch Neurol 1990;47:382.

Lechin F: Clonidine and prolactin secretion in humans. Clin Neuropharmacol 1992;15:155–156.

Lechin F: Adrenergic-serotonergic influences on gallbladder motility and irritable bowel syndrome. Am J Physiol 1992;262:G375–G376.

Lechin F: Stress, depression, neurochemistry, immunology and cancer: bases for neuropharmacological treatment (abstract). Arthur James Cancer Hospital, The Ohio State University, 1992.

Lechin F: Interaction of Stress, Immunology and Cancer (abstract). Roswell Park Cancer Institute, 1992.

Lechin F: Stress, Depression, Neurochemistry, Immunology and Cancer: Bases for Neuropharmacological Treatment (abstract). Tampa, University of South Florida, Division of Immunopharmacology, 1992.

Lechin F: Neurochemistry, Stress and the Sleep-Wake Cycle (abstract). The University of Texas Medical School, Texas Medical Center, 1992.

Lechin F: Neuropharmacological Therapy Approach to Cancer Patients (abstract). The University of Texas MD Anderson Cancer Center, 1992.

Lechin F: Neuropharmacological therapy approach to psychosomatic diseases associated with stress and depression (abstract). XXIII Congress of the International Society of Psychoneuroendocrinology, Madison, Wisconsin, 1992.

Lechin F: Letter to Eugene Renkin. News from senior physiologists. Physiologist 1999;42:102–103.

Lechin F: Central and plasma 5-HT, vagal tone and airways. Trends Pharmacol Sci 2000;21:425.

Lechin F, van der Dijs B: The relationship between gastric pepsin, uropepsin, and acidity. Acta Gastroenter Latinoamer 1969;1:91–96.

Lechin F, van der Dijs B: The effects of ADH on plasma bilirubin disappearance curves in the dog. Acta Gastroenter Latinoamer 1972;4:147–152.

Lechin F, van der Dijs B: A study of some immunological and clinical characteristics of gastritis, gastric ulcer, and duodenal ulcer in the three racial groups of the venezuelan population. Am J Phys Anthropol 1973;39:369–374.

Lechin F, van der Dijs B: The effects of ADH on hepatic blood flow in the dog. Acta Gastroenter Latinoamer 1973;5:1–18.

Lechin F, van der Dijs B: A new treatment for headache: Pathophysiological considerations. Headache 1977;16:318–21.

Lechin F, van der Dijs B: Enterohormonas, insulina y glucagon (review). Acta Gastroenter Latinoamer 1978;8:27–40.

Lechin F, van der Dijs B: The effects of dopaminergic blocking agents on distal colon motility. J Clin Pharmacol 1979;19:617–25.

Lechin F, van der Dijs B: Physiological effects of endogenous CCK on distal colon motility. Acta Gastroenter Latinoamer 1979;9:195–201.

Lechin F, van der Dijs B: Effects of diphenylhydantoin on distal colon motility. Acta Gastroenter Latinoamer 1979;9:145–152.

Lechin F, van der Dijs B: Dopamine and distal colon motility. Dig Dis Sci 1979;24:86.

Lechin F, van der Dijs B: Physiological, clinical and therapeutical basis of a new hypothesis for headache. Headache 1980;20:77–83.

Lechin F, van der Dijs B: Treatment of infertility with levodopa. Br Med J 1980;280:480.

Lechin F, van der Dijs B: Haloperidol and insulin release. Diabetologia 1981;20:78.

Lechin F, van der Dijs B: Intestinal pharmacomanometry and glucose tolerance: Evidence for two antagonistic dopaminergic mechanisms in the human. Biol Psychiatry 1981;16:969–986.

Lechin F, van der Dijs B: Colon motility and psychological traits in the irritable bowel syndrome. Dig Dis Sci 1981;26:474.

Lechin F, van der Dijs B: Glucose tolerance, nonnutrient drink and gastro-intestinal hormones. Gastroenterology 1981;80:216.

Lechin F, van der Dijs B: Noradrenergic or dopaminergic activity in chronic schizophrenia? Br J Psychiatry 1981;139:472.

Lechin F, van der Dijs B: Clonidine therapy for psychosis and tardive dyskinesia. Am J Psychiatry 1981;138:390.

Lechin F, van der Dijs B: Intestinal pharmacomanometry as a guide to psychopharmacological therapy; in Velazco M (ed): Clinical Pharmacology and Therapeutics International Congress Series No 604. Amsterdam, Excerpta Medica, 1982, p 166.

Lechin F, van der Dijs B: Opposite effects on human distal colon motility of two postulated alpha$_2$-antagonists (mianserin and chlorprothixene) and one alpha$_2$-agonist (clonidine). J Clin Pharmacol 1983;23:209–218.

Lechin F, van der Dijs B: Antimanic effect of clonazepam. Biol Psychiatry 1983;18:1511.

Lechin F, van der Dijs B: Slow wave sleep (SWS), REM sleep (REMS) and depression. Res Commun Psychol Psychiatr Behav 1984;9:227–262.

Lechin F, van der Dijs B: Remission of 23 metastatic tumors with neuropharmacological treatment. Proceedings of the Congress in Specific approaches in cancer therapy: differentiation, immunomodulation and angiogenesis. 1992 Oct 17–27; Erice, Italy.

Lechin F, Benshimol A, van der Dijs B: Histalog and secretin effects on serum electrolytes: Influence of pancreatectomy and gastrectomy. Acta Gastroenter Latinoamer 1970;2:9–18.

Lechin F, Coll-Garcia E, van der Dijs B, Peña F, Bentolila A, Rivas C: The effect of serotonin (5-HT) on insulin secretion. Acta Physiol Latinoamer 1975;25:339–346.

Lechin F, van der Dijs B, Bentolila A, Peña F: Antidiarrheal effects of dihydroergotamine. J Clin Pharmacol 1977;17:339–349.

Lechin F, van der Dijs B, Bentolila A, Peña F: The spastic colon syndrome: Therapeutic and pathophysiological considerations. J Clin Pharmacol 1977;17:431–440.

Lechin F, van der Dijs B, Lechin E, Peña F, Bentolila A: The noradrenergic and dopaminergic blockades: A new treatment for headache. Headache 1978;18:69–74.

Lechin F, van der Dijs B, Bentolila A, Peña F: The adrenergic influences on the gallbladder emptying. Am J Gastroenter 1978;69:662–667.

Lechin F, Coll-Garcia E, van der Dijs B, Bentolila A, Peña F, Rivas C: The effects of captivity on the glucose tolerance test in dogs. Experientia 1979;35:876–877.

Lechin F, Coll-Garcia E, van der Dijs B, Bentolila A, Peña F, Rivas C: The effects of dopaminergic blocking agents on the glucose tolerance test in six humans and six dogs. Experientia 1979;35:886–888.

Lechin F, van der Dijs B, Gómez F, Valls JM, Acosta E, Arocha L: Pharmacomanometric studies of colonic motility as a guide to the chemotherapy of schizophrenia. J Clin Pharmacol 1980;20:664–671.

Lechin F, Gómez F, van der Dijs B, Lechin E: Distal colon motility in schizophrenic patients. J Clin Pharmacol 1980;20:459–464.

Lechin F, van der Dijs B, Gómez F, Acosta E, Arocha L: Comparison between the effects of d-amphetamine and fenfluramine on distal colon motility in non-psychotic patients. Res Commun Psychol Psychiatr Behav 1982;7:411–430.

Lechin F, van der Dijs B, Gómez F, Arocha L, Acosta E: Effects of d-amphetamine, clonidine and clonazepam on distal colon motility in non-psychotic patients. Res Commun Psychol Psychiat Behav 1982;7:385–410.

Lechin F, van der Dijs B, Gómez F, Acosta E, Arocha L: On the use of clonidine and thioproperazine in a woman with Gilles de la Tourette's disease. Biol Psychiatry 1982;17:103–108.

Lechin F, van der Dijs B, Insausti CL, Gómez F: Treatment of ulcerative colitis with thioproperazine. J Clin Gastroenter 1982;4:445–449.

Lechin F, van der Dijs B, Gómez F, Lechin E, Oramas O, Villa S: Positive symptoms of acute psychosis: Dopaminergic or noradrenergic overactivity? Res Commun Psychol Psychiat Behav 1983;8:23–54.

Lechin F, van der Dijs B, Gómez F, Arocha L, Acosta E, Lechin E: Distal colon motility as a predictor of antidepressant response to fenfluramine, imipramine and clomipramine. J Affect Dis 1983;5:27–35.

Lechin F, van der Dijs B, Acosta E, Gómez F, Lechin E, Arocha L: Distal colon motility and clinical parameters in depression. J Affect Dis 1983;5:19–26.

Lechin F, van der Dijs B, Jakubowicz D, Camero RE, Villa S, Arocha L, Lechin A: Effects of clonidine on blood pressure, noradrenaline, cortisol, growth hormone, and prolactin plasma levels in high and low intestinal tone depressed patients. Neuroendocrinology 1985;41:156–162.

Lechin F, van der Dijs B, Jakubowicz D, Camero RE, Villa S, Lechin E, Gómez F: Effects of clonidine on blood pressure, noradrenaline, cortisol, growth hormone and prolactin plasma levels in low and high intestinal tone subjects. Neuroendocrinology 1985;40:253–261.

Lechin F, van der Dijs B, Insausti CL, Gómez F, Villa S, Lechin AE, Arocha L, Oramas O: Treatment of ulcerative colitis with clonidine. J Clin Pharmacol 1985;25:219–226.

Lechin F, van der Dijs B, Amat J, Lechin S: Central neuronal pathways involved in anxiety-like behavior syndrome: Experimental findings. Res Commun Psychol Psychiatr Behav 1986;11:113–143.

Lechin F, van der Dijs B, Amat J, Lechin M: Central neuronal pathways involved in psychotic syndromes. Res Commun Psychol Psychiatr Behav 1986;11:207–260.

Lechin F, van der Dijs B, Amat J, Lechin ME: Central neuronal pathways involved in depressive syndrome: Experimental findings. Res Commun Psychol Psychiatr Behav 1986;11:145–192:

Lechin F, van der Dijs B, Azocar J, Amat J, Vitelli-Florez G, Martinez C, Lechin S, Jimenez V, Cabrera A, Cardenas M, Villa S: Stress, immunology and cancer: Effect of psychoactive drugs. Arch Ven Farm ClinTerap 1987;6:28–43.

Lechin F, van der Dijs B, Jakubowicz D, Camero RE, Lechin S, Villa S, Reinfeld B, Lechin ME: Role of stress in the exacerbation of chronic illness: Effects of clonidine administration on blood pressure, nor-epinephrine, cortisol, growth hormone and prolactin plasma levels. Psychoneuroendocrinology 1987;12:117–129.

Lechin F, van der Dijs B, Amat J, Lechin AE: Central nervous system circuitry involved in blood pressure regulation. Arch Ven Farm Clin Terap 1987;6:79–101.

Lechin F, van der Dijs B, Amat J, Lechin A, Cabrera A, Lechin ME, Gómez F, Arocha L, Jiménez V: Definite and sustained improvement with pimozide of two patients with severe trigeminal neuralgia: Some neurochemical, neurophysiological and neuroendocrinological findings. J Med 1988;19:243–256.

Lechin F, van der Dijs B, Rada I, Jara H, Lechin M, Cabrera A, Lechin A, Gómez F, Jiménez V, Arocha L, Valderrama T: Recurrent gastroesophageal symptoms and precordial pain in a gastrectomized man improved by amytriptyline: Physiologic, metabolic, endocrine, neurochemical and psychiatric findings. J Med 1989;20:407–424.

Lechin F, van der Dijs B, Lechin ME, Amat J, Lechin AE, Cabrera A, Gómez F, Acosta E, Arocha L, Villa S, Jiménez V: Pimozide therapy for trigeminal neuralgia. Arch Neurol 1989;46:960–963.

Lechin F, van der Dijs B, Lechin S, Vitelli G, Lechin ME, Cabrera A: Neurochemical, hormonal and immunological views of stress: Clinical and therapeutic implications in Crohn's disease and cancer; in Velazco M (ed): Recent Advances in Pharmacology and Therapeutics. International Congress Series. Amsterdam, Excerpta Medica, 1989, vol 839, pp 57–70.

Lechin F, van der Dijs B, Rada I, Jara H, Lechin A, Cabrera A, Lechin M, Jiménez V, Gómez F, Villa S, Acosta E, Arocha L: Plasma neurotransmitters and cortisol in duodenal ulcer patients: role of stress. Dig Dis Sci 1990;35:1313–1319.

Lechin F, van der Dijs B, Vitelli G, Lechin-Baez S, Azócar J, Cabrera A, Lechin A, Jara H, Lechin M, Gómez F, Arocha L: Psychoneuroendocrinological and immunological parameters in cancer patients: Involvement of stress and depression. Psychoneuroendocrinology 1990;15:435–451.

Lechin F, van der Dijs B, Lechin A, Lechin M, Coll-Garcia E, Jara H, Cabrera A, Jiménez V, Gómez F, Tovar D, Rada I, Arocha A: Doxepin therapy for postprandial symptomatic hypoglycemic patients neurochemical, hormonal and metabolic disturbances. Clin Sci 1991;80:373–384.

Lechin F, van der Dijs B, Lechin M, Lechin-Báez S, Jara H, Lechin A, Orozco B, Rada I, Cabrera A, Jiménez V: Effects of an oral glucose load on plasma neurotransmitters in humans: Involvement of REM sleep? Neuropsychobiology 1992;26:4–11.

Lechin F, van der Dijs B, Lechin M, Jara H, Lechin A, Cabrera A, Rada I, Orozco B, Jimenez V, Valderrama T: Dramatic improvement with clonidine of acute pancreatitis showing raised catecholamines and cortisol plasma levels: Case report of five patients. J Med 1992;23:339–351.

Lechin F, van der Dijs B, Lechin M, Jara H, Lechin A, Lechin-Báez S, Orozco B, Rada I, Cabrera A, Arocha L, Jiménez V, León G: Plasma neurotransmitters throughout an oral glucose tolerance test in essential hypertension. Clin Exp Hypertens 1993;15:209–240.

Lechin F, van der Dijs B, Lechin AE, Orozco B, Lechin ME, Báez S, Rada I, León G, Acosta E: Plasma neurotransmitters and cortisol in chronic illness: Role of stress. J Med 1994;25:181–192.

Lechin F, van der Dijs B, Vitelli-Flores G, Báez S, Lechin ME, Lechin AE, Orozco B, Rada I, León G, Jiménez V: Peripheral blood immunological parameters in long-term benzodiazepine users. Clin Neuropharmacol 1994;17:63–72.

Lechin F, van der Dijs B, Lechin-Báez S, Lechin A, Orozco B, Lechin M, Rada I, Jara H, Gómez F, Cabrera A, Jiménez V, Arocha L, León G: Two types of irritable bowel syndrome: Differences in behavior, clinical signs, distal colon motility and hormonal, neurochemical, metabolic, physiological and pharmacological profiles. Arch Ven Farmac Terap 1994;12:105–114.

Lechin F, van der Dijs B, Orozco B, Lechin ME, Acosta E, Lechin AE, Báez S, Rada I, Arocha L, León G, García Z: Plasma neurotransmitters, blood pressure and heart rate during supine-resting, orthostasis and moderate exercise conditions in major depressed patients. Biol Psychiatry 1995;38:166–173.

Lechin F, van der Dijs B, Orozco B, Lechin AE, Báez S, Lechin ME, Rada I, Acosta E, Arocha L, Jiménez V, León G, García Z: Plasma neurotransmitters, blood pressure and heart rate during supine-resting, orthostasis and moderate exercise in dysthymic depressed patients. Biol Psychiatry 1995;37:884–891.

Lechin F, van der Dijs B, Orozco B, Báez S, Rada I, León G, García Z, Jara H, Lechin AE, Lechin ME: Plasma neurotransmitters, blood pressure and heart rate during supine-resting, orthostasis and moderate exercise stress test in healthy humans before and after parasympathetic blockade with atropine. Res Commun Biol Psychol Psychiatry 1996;21:55–72.

Lechin F, van der Dijs B, Orozco B, Lechin ME, Lechin AE: Increased levels of free serotonin in plasma of symptomatic asthmatic patients. Ann Allergy Asthma Immunol 1996;77:245–253.

Lechin F, van der Dijs B, Benaim M: Benzodiazepines: Tolerability in elderly patients (review). Psychother Psychosom 1996;65:171–182.

Lechin F, van der Dijs B, Lechin M: Plasma neurotransmitters and functional illness (review). Psychother Psychosom 1996;65:293–318.

Lechin F, van der Dijs B, Benaim M: Stress versus depression (review). Prog Neuro-Psychopharmacol Biol Psychiatry 1996;20:899–950.

Lechin F, van der Dijs B, Jara H, Baez S, Orozco B, Jahn E, Lechin ME, Jimenez V, Lechin AE: Successful neuropharmacological treatment of myasthenia gravis: Report of eight cases. Res Commun Biol Psychol Psychiatry 1997;22:81–94.

Lechin F, van der Dijs B, Jara H, Orozco B, Baez S, Jahn E, Benaim M, Lechin E, Lechin ME, Jimenez V, Lechin AE: Plasma neurotransmitter profiles of anxiety, phobia and panic disorder patients: Acute and chronic effects of buspirone. Res Commun Biol Psychol Psychiatry 1997;22:95–110.

Lechin F, van der Dijs B, Lechin ME, Orozco B, Báez S, Lechin AE, Jahn E, Jimenez V: Plasma neurotransmitters, blood pressure and heart rate during supine-resting, orthostasis, and moderate exercise conditions in two types of hypertensive patients. Res Commun Biol Psychol Psychiatry 1997;22:111–145.

Lechin F, van der Dijs B, Lechin A, Orozco B, Lechin ME, Lechin AE: The serotonin uptake-enhancing drug tianeptine suppresses asthmatic symptoms in children: A double-blind crossover placebo-controlled study. J Clin Pharmacol 1998;38:918–925.

Lechin F, van der Dijs B, Jara H, Orozco B, Baez S, Benaim M, Lechin M, Lechin A: Effects of buspirone on plasma neurotransmitters in healthy subjects. J Neural Transm 1998;105:561–573.

Lechin F, van der Dijs B, Orozco B, Jara H, Rada I, Lechin ME, Lechin AE: Neuropharmacological treatment of bronchial asthma with an antidepressant drug: tianeptine: A double-blind crossover placebo-controlled study. Clin Pharmacol Ther 1998;64:223–232.

Lechin F, van der Dijs B, Pardey-Maldonado B, Jahn E, Jiménez V, Orozco B, Baez S, Lechin ME: Enhancement of noradrenergic neural transmission: An effective therapy of myasthenia gravis. Report of 52 consecutive patients. J Med 2000;31:333–362.

Lechin F, van der Dijs B, Orozco B, Pardey-Maldonado B, Baez S, Jahn E, Naddaf R, Benaim M, Lechin ME, Lechin AE: Circulating neurotransmitter profiles throughout normal wake-sleep cycle. Part one. In press.

Lechin F, Pardey-Maldonado B, van der Dijs B, Benaim M, Baez S, Orozco B, Naddaf R, Rodriguez S, Rangel A, Lechin ME: Circulating neurotransmitter profiles throughout normal wake-sleep cycle. Part two. In press.

References for Chapter 1

Aberg-Wistedt A, Hasselmark L, Strain-Malmgren R, Apéria B, Kjellman BF, Mathé AA: Serotonergic vulnerability in affective disorder, a study of the tryptophan depletion test and relationships between peripheral and central serotonin indexes in citalopram-responders. Acta Psychiatr Scand 1998;97:374–380.

Adell A, Artigas F: Regulation of the release of 5-hydroxytryptamine in the median raphe nucleus of the rat by catecholaminergic afferents. Eur J Neurosci 1999;11:2305–2311.

Aharoni R, Teitelbaum D, Sela M, Arnon R: Bystander suppression of experimental autoimmune encephalomyelitis by T cell lines and clones of the Th2 type induced by copolymer 1. J Neuroimmunol 1998;91:135–146.

Amital H, Swissa M, Bar-Dayan Y, Buskila D, Shoenfeld Y: New therapeutic avenues in autoimmunity. Res Immunol 1996;147:361–376.

Anden NE, Grabowska M: Pharmacological evidence for a stimulation of dopamine neurons by noradrenaline neurons in the brain. Eur J Pharmacol 1976;39:275–282.

Anden NE, Strömbom JA: Adrenergic receptor blocking agents, effects on central noradrenaline and dopamine receptors and on motor activity. Psychopharmacologia (Berl) 1974;38:91–103.

Apperley GH, Drew GM, Sullivan AT: Prenalterol is an agonist at β2- as well as at β1-adrenoceptors. Eur J Pharmacol 1982;81:659–664.

Astier B, Kitahama K, Denoroy L, Berod A, Jouvet M, Renaud B: Biochemical evidence for an interaction between adrenaline and noradrenaline neurons in the rat brainstem. Brain Res 1986;397:333–340.

Aston-Jones G, Bloom FE: Norepinephine-containing locus coeruleus neurons in behaving rats exhibit pronounced responses to non-noxious environmental stimuli. J Neurosci 1981;1:887–900.

Aston-Jones G, Foote SJ, Bloom FE: Anatomy and physiology of locus coeruleus neurons, functional implications; in Zeiglen MG, Lake CR (eds): Norepinephrine, Clinical Aspects. Baltimore, Williams & Wilkins, 1984, pp 92–116.

Aston-Jones G, Hirata H, Akaoka H: Local opiate withdrawal in locus coeruleus in vivo. Brain Res 1997;765:331–336.

Aston-Jones G, Shipley MT, Chouvet G, Ennis M, van Bockstaele E, Pieribone V, Shiekhattar R, Akaoka H, Drolet G, Astier B, Charlety P, Valentino R, Williams J: Afferent regulation of locus coeruleus neurons, anatomy, physiology and pharmacology. Prog Brain Res 1991;88:47–75.

Azorin JM, Karege F, Malli M, Pringuey D, Joanny P, Tissot R: Plasma 3,4-di-hydrophenylethyleneglycol and 3-methoxy-4-hydroxy phenylethylene glycol as indicators of central noradrenergic activity: A comparative study on control subjects and depressed patients. Neuropsychobiology 1988;20:67–73.

Bamshad M, Song CK, Bartness TJ: CNS origins of the sympathetic nervous system outflow to brown adipose tissue. Am J Physiol 1999;276:R1569–R1578.

Baraban FM, Aghajanian GK: Suppression of firing activity of 5-HT neurons in the dorsal raphe by alpha-adrenoceptor antagonist. Neuropharmacology 1980;19:355–363.

Behbehani MM: Functional characteristics of the midbrain periaqueductal gray. Prog Neurobiol 1995;46:575–605.

Behbehani MM, Liu H, Jiang M, Pun RYK, Shipley MT: Activation of serotonin$_{1A}$ receptors inhibits midbrain periaqueductal gray neurons of the rat. Brain Res 1993;612:56–60.

Bhatti T, Gillin JC, Seifritz E, Moore P, Clark C, Golshan S, Stahl S, Rapaport M, Kelsoe J: Effects of a tryptophan-free amino acid drink challenge on normal human sleep electroencephalogram and mood. Biol Psychiatry 1998;43:52–59.

Björklund A, Wiklund L: Mechanisms of regrowth of the bulbospinal serotonin system following 5,6-dihydroxytryptamine induced axotomy. I. Biochemical correlates. Brain Res 1980;191:109–127.

Blier P, de Montigny C, Azzaro AJ: Effect of repeated amiflamine administration on serotonergic and noradrenergic neurotransmission: Electrophysiological studies in the rat CNS. Arch Pharmacol 1986;334:253–260.

Born GVR: Aggregation of blood platelets by adenosine diphosphate and its reversal. Nature 1962;194:927–929.

Brammer JP, Kerecsen L, Maguire MH: Effects of vinblastine on malondialdehyde formation, serotonin release and aggregation in human platelets. Eur J Pharmacol 1982;81:577–586.

Brazenor RM, Angus JA, Actions of serotonin antagonists on dog coronary artery: Eur J Pharmacol 1982;81:569–576.

Cabib S, Zocchi A, Puglisi-Allegra S: A Comparison of the behavioral effects of minaprine, amphetamine and stress. Psychopharmacology 1995;121:73–80.

Chamberlain B, Ervin FR, Pihl RO, Young SN: The effect of raising or lowering tryptophan levels on aggression in vervet monkeys. Pharmacol Biochem Behav 1987;28:503–510.

Chen S, Aston-Jones G: Anatomical evidence for inputs to ventrolateral medullary catecholaminergic neurons from the midbrain periaqueductal gray of the rat. Neurosci Lett 1995;195:140–144.

Courvoisier H, Moisan MP, Sarrieau A, Hendley ED, Mormède P: Behavioral and neuroendocrine reactivity to stress in the WKHA/WKY inbred rat strains: a multifactorial and genetic analysis. Brain Res 1996;743:77–85.

Crawley JN, Roth RH, Maas JW: Locus coeruleus stimulation increases noradrenergic metabolite levels in rat spinal cord. Brain Res 1979;166:180–184.

Curtis AL, Lechner SM, Pavcovich LA and Valentino RJ: Activation of the locus coeruleus noradrenergic system by intracoerulear microinfusion of corticotropin-releasing factor: Effects on discharge rate, cortical norepinephrine levels and cortical electroencephalographic activity. J Pharmacol Exp Ther 1997;281:163–172.

Curtis AL, Pavcovich LA, Valentino RJ: Long-term regulation of locus ceruleus sensitivity to corticotropin-releasing factor by swim stress. J Pharmacol Exp Ther 1999;289:1211–1219.

Dampney RA: The subretrofacial vasomotor nucleus, anatomical, chemical and pharmacological properties and role in cardiovascular regulation. Prog Neurobiol 1994;42:197–227.

Davies CL. Molyneux SG: Routine determination of plasma catecholamines using reversed phase ion pair high performance liquid chromatography with electrochemical detection. J Chromatogr 1982;231:41–51.

De Fanti BA, Gavel DA, Hamilton JS, Horwitz BA: Extracellular hypothalamic serotonin levels after dorsal raphe nuclei stimulation of lean (Fa/Fa) and obese (fa/fa) Zucker rats. Brain Res 2000;869:6–14.

Dehal NS, Dekaban GA, Krassioukov AV, Picard FJ, Weaver LC: Identification of renal sympathetic preganglionic neurons in hamsters using transsynaptic transport of herpes simplex type 1 virus. Neuroscience 1993;56:227–240.

Dekel B, Marcus H, Shenkman B, Shimoni A, Shechter Y, Canaan A, Berrebi A, Varon D, Reisner Y: Human/BALB radiation chimera engrafted with splenocytes from patients with idiopathic thrombocytopenic purpura produce human platelet antibodies. Immunology 1998;94:410–416.

Diana M, Muntoni AL, Pistis M, Collu M, Forgione A, Gessa GL: Chronic administration of l-sulpiride at low doses reduces A10 but not A9 somatodentritic dopamine autoreceptor sensitivity. Eur J Pharmacol 1996;312:179–181.

Dilts RP, Boadle-Biber MC: Differential activation of the 5-hydroxytryptamine-containing neurons of the midbrain raphe of the rat in response to randomly presented inescapable sound. Neurosci Lett 1995;199:78–80.

Disshon KA, Dluzen DE: Estrogen reduces acute striatal dopamine responses in vivo to the neurotoxin MPP+ in female, but not male rats. Brain Res 2000;868:95–104.

Dube S, Kumar N, Ettedgui E, Pohl R, Jones D, Sitaram N: Cholinergic REM induction response, separation of anxiety and depression. Biol Psychiatry 1985;20:408–418.

Eisenhofer G, Goldstein DS, Stull R: Simultaneous liquid chromatographic determination of 3,4-dihydroxyphenylglycol, catecholamines, and 3,4-dihydroxyphenylalanine in plasma and their responses to inhibition of monoamine oxidase. Clin Chem 1986;32:2030–2033.

Ellison GD: Behavior and the balance between norepinephrine and serotonin. Acta Neurobiol Exp 1975;35:499–515.

Elam M, Thorén P, Svensson TH: Locus coeruleus neurons and sympathetic nerves, activation by visceral afferents. Brain Res 1986;375:117–125.

Ellsworth JD, Redmond DE, Roth RH: Plasma and cerebrospinal fluid 3-methoxy-4-hydroxyphenylethylene glycol (MHPG) as indices of brain norepinephrine metabolism in primates. Brain Res 1982;235:115–124.

Farkas E, Jansen AS, Loewy AD: Periaqueductal gray matter projection to vagal preganglionic neurons and the nucleus tractus solitarius. Brain Res 1997;764:257–261.

Feldman PD: Electrophysiological effects of serotonin in the solitary tract nucleus of the rat. Arch Pharmacol 1994;349:447–454.

Fernstrom JD, Wurtman RJ: Brain serotonin content, Physiological dependence on plasma tryptophan levels. Science 1971;173:149–152.

Feng YZ, Zhang T, Rockhold RW, Ho IK: Increased locus coeruleus glutamate levels are associated with naloxone-precipitated withdrawal from butorphanol in the rat. Neurochem Res 1995;20:745–751.

Foote SL, Bloom FE, Aston-Jones G: Nucleus locus coeruleus, new evidence of anatomical and physiological specificity. Physiol Rev 1983;63:844–914:

Fozard JR: Neuronal 5-HT receptors in the periphery. Neuropharmacology 1984;23:1473–1486.

Fozard JR: Agonists and antagonists of 5-HT$_3$ receptors; in Saxena PR, Wallis DI, Wouters W, Bevan P (eds): Cardiovascular Pharmacology of 5-Hydroxytryptamine. Dordrecht, Kluwer, 1990, pp 101–115.

Gabbett T, Gass G, Gass E, Morris N, Bennett G,Thalib L: Norepinephrine and epinephrine responses during orthostatic intolerance in healthy elderly men. Jpn J Physiol 2000;50:59–66.

Gaillard JM: Brain noradrenergic activity in wakefulness and paradoxical sleep, the effect of clonidine. Neuropsychobiology 1985;13:23–25.

Gauthier P, Reader TA: 1982. Adrenomedullary secretory response to midbrain stimulation in rat: effects of depletion of brain catecholamines or serotonin. Can J Physiol Pharmacol 1982;60:1464–1474.

Gollob JA, Murphy EA, Mahajan S, Schnipper CP, Ritz J, Frank DA: Altered interleukin-12 responsiveness in Th1 and Th2 cells is associated with the differential activation of STAT5 and STAT1. Blood 1998;91:1341–1354.

Grenhoff J, Svensson H: Prazosin modulates the firing pattern of dopamine neurons in rat ventral tegmental area. Eur J Pharmacol 1993;233:79–84.

Grillner P, Berretta N, Bernardi G, Svensson TH, Mercuri NB: Muscarinic receptors depress gabaergic synaptic transmission in rat midbrain dopamine neurons. Neuroscience 2000;96:299–307:

Guyenet PG. The coeruleospinal noradrenergic neurons, anatomical and electrophysiological studies in rat. Brain Res 1980;189:121–133.

Haddad A, Bienvenu J, Miossec P: Increased production of a Th2 cytokine profile by activated whole blood cells from rheumatoid arthritis patients. J Clin Immunol 1998;18:399–405.

Haddjeri N, de Montigny C, Blier P: Modulation of the firing activity of noradrenergic neurones in the rat locus coeruleus by the 5-hydroxtryptamine system. Br J Pharmacol 1997;120:865–875.

Haft Jl, Arkel YS: Effect of emotional stress on platelet aggregation in humans. Chest 1976;70:501–506.

Harold KL, Schlinkert RT, Mann DK, Reeder CB, Noel P, Fitch TR, Braich TA, Camoriano JK: Long-term results of laparoscopic splenectomy for immune thrombocytopenic purpura. Mayo Clin Proc 1999;74:37–39.

Hay M, Bishop VS: Interactions of area postrema and solitary tract in the nucleus tractus solitarius. Am J Physiol 1991;260:H1463–H1466.

Hayes K, Weaver LC: Selective control of sympathetic pathways to the kidneys, spleen and intestine by the ventrolateral medulla in rats. J Physiol 1990;428:371–385.

Hedner J, Hedner T, Jonason J, Lundberg D: Evidence for dopamine interaction with the central respiratory control system in the rat. Eur J Pharmacol 1982;81:603–616.

Hentall ID, Kurle PJ, White TR: Correlations between serotonin level and single-cell firing in the rat's nucleus raphe magnus. Neurosci 2000;95:1081–1088.

Heym J, Steinfels GF, Jacobs BL: Medullary serotonergic neurons are insensitive to 5-MEODMT and LSD. Eur J Pharmacol 1982;81:677–680.

Horiuchi J, Potts PD, Tagawa T, Dampney RA: Effects of activation and blockade of P2x receptors in the ventrolateral medulla on arterial pressure and sympathetic activity. J Autonom Nerv Syst 1999;76:118–126.

Houzen H, Hattori Y, Kanno M, Kikuchi S, Tashiro K, Motomura M, Nakao Y, Nakamura T: Functional evaluation of inhibition of autonomic transmitter release by autoantibody from Lambert-Eaton myasthenic syndrome. Ann Neurol 1998;43:677–680.

Huang FP, Niedbala W, Wei XQ, Xu D, Feng GJ, Robinson JH, Lam Ch, Liew FY: Nitric oxide regulates Th1 cell development through the inhibition of IL-12 synthesis by macrophages. Eur J Immunol 1998;28:4062–4070.

Huang ZG, Subramanian SH, Balnave RJ, Turman AB, Chow CHM: Roles of periaqueductal gray and nucleus tractus solitarius in cardiorespiratory function in the rat brainstem. Respir Physiol 2000;120:185–195.

Ireland SJ, Tyers MB: Pharmacological characterization of 5-hydroxytryptamine-induced depolarization of the rat isolated vagus nerve. Br J Pharmacol 1987;90:229–238.

Jacobs BL, Fornal CA: Activity of brain serotonergic neurons in the behaving animal. Pharmacol Rev 1991;43:563–583.

Jansen ASP, Nguyen XV, Karpitskiy V, Mattenleiter TC, Loewy AD: Central command neurons of the sympathetic nervous system, basis of fight-or-flight response. Science 1995;270:644–646.

Jernej B, Cicin-Sain L, Kveder S: Physiological characteristics of platelet serotonin in rats. Life Sci 1989;45:485–492.

Johnson DR, Rosenheck R, Fontana A, Lubin H, Charney D, Southwick S: Outcome of intensive inpatient treatment for combat-related posttraumatic stress disorder. Am J Psychiatry 1996;153:771–777.

Jones BE, Yang TZ: The efferent projections from the reticular formation and the locus coeruleus studied by anterograde and retrograde axonal transport in the rat. J Comp Neurol 1985;242:56–92.

Joshi S, Le Vatte MA, Dekaban GA, Weaver LC: Identification of spinal interneurons antecedent to adrenal sympathetic preganglionic neurons using trans-synaptic transport of herpes simplex virus type 1. Neuroscience1995;65:893–903.

Kamiya A, Iwase S, Michikami D, Fu Q, Mano T: Head-down bed rest alters sympathetic and cardiovascular responses to mental stress. Am J Physiol 2000;279:R440–R447.

Karege F, Bovier P, Hilleret H, Gaillard JM,Tissot R: Adrenaline-induced platelet aggregation in depressed patients and control subjects. Neuropsychobiology 1993;27:21–25.

Karreman M, Moghaddam B: The prefrontal cortex regulates the basal release of dopamine in the limbic striatum: An effect mediated by ventral tegmental area. J Neurochem 1996;66:589–598.

Ke-min G, Peng L: Post-synaptic activity evoked in the rostral ventrolateral medullary neurons by stimulation of the defense areas of hypothalamus and midbrain in the rat. Neurosci Lett 1993;161:153–156.

Kennett GA, Joseph MH: Stress induced increases in 5HT release, measured in vivo, depend upon increased tryptophan availability. Neurosci Lett 1981;7:S56.

Kerry R, Scrutton MC: Platelet adrenoceptors; in Longenecker GL (ed): The Platelets, Physiology and Pharmacology. London, Academic Press, 1985, pp 113–157.

Kojima J, Yamaji Y, Matsumura M, Nambu A, Inase M, Tokuno H, Takada M, Imai H: Excitotoxic lesions of the pedunculopontine tegmental nucleus produce contralateral hemiparkinsonism in the monkey. Neurosci Lett 1997;226:111–114.

Kostowski W: Interactions between serotonergic and catecholaminergic systems in the brain. Pol J Pharmacol Pharmac 1975;27:15–24.

Kostowski W: Two noradrenergic systems in the brain and their interactions with other monoaminergic neurons. Pol J Pharmacol Pharmac 1979;31:425–436.

Kostowski W, Samanin R, Bareggi SR, Mark V, Garattini S,Valzelli L: Biochemical aspects of the interaction between midbrain raphe and locus coeruleus in the rat. Brain Res 1974;82:178–182.

Krowicki ZK, Hornby PJ: Serotonin microinjected into the nucleus raphe obscurus increases intragastric pressure in the rat via a vagally mediated pathway. J Pharmacol Exp Ther 1993;265:468–473.

Kumar AM, Kumar M, Deepika K, Fernandez JB, Eisdorfer C: A modified HPLC technique for simultaneous measurement of 5-hydroxytryptamine and 5-hydroxyindolacetic acid in cerebrospinal fluid, platelet and plasma. Life Sci 1990;47:1751–1759.

Laguzzi R, Talman WT, Reiss DJ: Serotonergic mechanisms in the nucleus tractus solitarius may regulate blood pressure and behaviour in the rat. Clin Sci 1982;63:323s–326s.

Lake CR, Pickar D, Ziegler MG, Lipper S, Slater S, Murphy DL: High plasma norepinephrine levels in patients with major affective disorder. Am J Psychiatry 1982;139:1315–1318.

Lake CR, Ziegler MG, Kopin IJ: Use of plasma norepinephrine for evaluation of sympathetic neuronal function in man. Life Sci 1976;18:1315–1321.

Lambert GW, Kaye DM, Thompson JM, Turner AG, Cox HS, Vaz M, Jennings GL, Wallin BG, Esler MD: Internal jugular venous spillover of noradrenaline and metabolites and their association with sympathetic nervous activity. Acta Physiol Scand 1998;163:155–163.

Larsen PD, Zhong S, Gebber GL, Barman SM: Differential pattern of spinal sympathetic outflow in response to stimulation of the caudal medullary raphe. Am J Physiol 2000;279:210–221.

Larsson PT, Hjemdahl P, Olsson G, Egberg N, Hornstra G: Altered platelet function during mental stress and adrenaline infusion in humans, evidence for an increased aggregability in vivo as measured by filtragometry. Clin Sci 1989;76:369–376.

Lechin AE, Varon J, van der Dijs B, Lechin F: Plasma catecholamines and indoleamines during attacks and remission on severe bronchial asthma, possible role of stress. Am J Respir Crit Care Med 1994a;149:A778.

Lechin AE, Varon J, van der Dijs B, Lechin F: Plasma neurotransmitters, blood pressure and heart rate during rest and exercise. Am J Respir Crit Care Med 1994b;149:A482.

Lechin F: Central and plasma 5-HT, vagal tone and airways. Trends Pharmacol Sci 2000;21:425.

Lechin F, van der Dijs B: Slow wave sleep (SWS), REM sleep (REMS) and depression. Res Commun Psychol Psychiat Behav 1984;9:227–262.

Lechin F, van der Dijs B, Lechin E: Experimental bases for outlining an anatomical integration model of the central autonomic nervous system; in Lechin F, van der Dijs B, Lechin E (eds): The Autonomic Nervous System: Physiological Basis of Psychosomatic Therapy. Barcelona, Editorial Cientifico-Medica, 1979a, chap II, pp 23–29.

Lechin F, van der Dijs B, Lechin E: Experimental bases for outlining a functional integration model of the central autonomic nervous system; in Lechin F, van der Dijs B, Lechin E (eds): The Autonomic Nervous System: Physiological Basis of Psychosomatic Therapy. Barcelona, Editorial Cientifico-Medica, 1979b, chap IV, pp 41–64.

Lechin F, van der Dijs B, Lechin E: Model of the functioning of the autonomic nervous system; in Lechin F, van der Dijs B, Lechin E (eds): The Autonomic Nervous System, Physiological Basis of Psychosomatic Therapy. Barcelona, Editorial Cientifico-Medica, 1979c, chap V, pp 65–72.

Lechin F, van der Dijs B, Jackubowicz D, Camero RE, Villa S, Lechin E, Gomez F: Effects of clonidine on blood pressure, noradrenaline, cortisol, growth hormone, and prolactin plasma levels in high and low intestinal tone subjects. Neuroendocrinology 1985a;40:253–261.

Lechin F, van der Dijs B, Jackubowicz D, Camero RE, Villa S, Arocha L, Lechin AE: Effects of clonidine on blood pressure, noradrenaline, cortisol, growth hormone, and prolactin plasma levels in high and low intestinal tone depressed patients. Neuroendocrinology 1985b;41:156–162.

Lechin F, van der Dijs B, Amat J, Lechin M: Neuroanatomical basis; in Lechin F, van der Dijs B (eds): Neurochemistry and Clinical Disorders, Circuitry of Some Psychiatric and Psychosomatic Syndromes. Boca Raton, CRC Press, 1989a, pp 1–48.

Lechin F, van der Dijs B, Gomez F, Lechin E, Acosta E, Arocha L: Biological markers in the assessment of central autonomic nervous functioning, an approach to the diagnosis of some psychiatric and psychosomatic syndromes; in Lechin F, van der Dijs B (eds): Neurochemistry and Clinical Disorders, Circuitry of Some Psychiatric and Psychosomatic Syndromes. Boca Raton, CRC Press, 1989b, pp 151–226.

Lechin F, van der Dijs B, Lechin ME, Amat J, Lechin AE, Cabrera A, Gomez F, Acosta E, Arocha L, Villa S, Jimenez V: Pimozide therapy for trigeminal neuralgia. Arch Neurol 1989c;46:960–963.

Lechin F, van der Dijs B, Rada I, Jara H, Lechin AE, Cabrera A, Lechin ME, Jimenez V, Gomez F, Villa S, Acosta E, Arocha L: Plasma neurotransmitters and cortisol in duodenal ulcer patients: Role of stress. Dig Dis Sci 1990a;35:1313–1319.

Lechin F, van der Dijs B, Vitelli-Florez G, Lechin-Baez S, Azocar J, Cabrera A, Lechin AE, Jara H, Lechin ME, Gomez F, Arocha L: Psychoneuroendocrinological and immunological parameters in cancer patients: Involvement of stress and depression. Psychoneuroendocrinology 1990b;15:435–451.

Lechin F, van der Dijs B, Lechin AE, Lechin ME, Coll-Garcia E, Jara H, Cabrera A, Jimenez V, Gomez F, Tovar D, Rada I, Arocha L: Doxepin therapy for postprandial symptomatic hypoglycemic patients: Neurochemical, hormonal and metabolic disturbances. Clin Sci 1991;80:373–384.

Lechin F, van der Dijs B, Lechin ME, Baez S, Jara H, Lechin A, Orozco B, Rada I, Cabrera A, Jimenez V, Leon G: Effects of an oral glucose load on plasma neurotransmitters in humans: Involvement of REM sleep? Neuropsychobiology 1992;26:4–11.

Lechin F, van der Dijs B, Lechin ME, Jara H, Lechin A, Baez S, Orozco B, Rada I, Cabrera A, Arocha L, Jimenez V, Leon G: Plasma neurotransmitters throughout oral glucose tolerance test in non-depressed essential hypertension patients. Clin Exp Hypertens 1993;15:209–240.

Lechin F, van der Dijs B, Lechin AE, Orozco B, Lechin ME, Baez S, Rada I, Leon G, Acosta E: Plasma neurotransmitters and cortisol in chronic illness: Role of stress. J Med 1994;25:181–192.

Lechin F, van der Dijs B, Orozco B, Lechin AE, Baez S, Lechin ME, Rada I, Acosta E, Arocha L, Jimenez V, Leon G, Garcia Z: Plasma neurotransmitters, blood pressure and heart rate during supine-resting, orthostasis and moderate exercise in dysthymic depressed patients. Biol Psychiatry 1995a;37:884–891.

Lechin F, van der Dijs B, Orozco B, Lechin ME, Baez S, Lechin AE, Rada I, Acosta E, Arocha L, Jimenez V, Leon G, Garcia Z: Plasmaneurotransmitters, blood pressure, and heart rate during supine-resting, orthostasis, and moderate exercise conditions in major depressed patients. Biol Psychiatry 1995b;38:166–173.

Lechin F, van der Dijs B, Benaim M: Stress vs depression. Prog Neuro-Psychopharmacol Biol Psychiatry 1996a;20:899–950.

Lechin F, van der Dijs B, Lechin AE, Orozco B, Lechin ME, Baez-Lechin S, Rada I, Leon G, Garcia Z, Jimenez V: Plasma neurotransmitters, blood pressure and heart rate during supine-resting, orthostasis and moderate exercise stress test in healthy humans before and after the parasympathetic blockade with atropine. Res Commun Biol Psychol Psychiat 1996b;21:55–72.

Lechin F, van der Dijs B, Orozco B, Lechin AE, Baez S, Lechin ME, Benaim M, Acosta E, Arocha L, Jimenez V, Leon G, Garcia Z: Plasma neurotransmitters, blood pressure and heart rate during supine resting, orthostasis and moderate exercise in severely ill patients: A model of failing to cope with stress. Psychother Psychosom 1996c;65:129–136.

Lechin F, van der Dijs B, Orozco B, Lechin ME, Lechin AE: Increased free serotonin plasma levels in symptomatic asthmatic patients. Ann Allergy Asthma Immunol 1996d;77:245–253.

Lechin F, van der Dijs B, Jara H, Orozco B, Baez S, Jahn E, Benaim M, Lechin E, Lechin ME, Jimenez V, Lechin AE: Plasma neurotransmitter profiles of anxiety, phobia and panic disorder patients: Acute and chronic effects of buspirone. Res Commun Biol Psychol Psychiatry 1997;22:113–156.

Lechin F, van der Dijs B, Jara H, Orozco B, Baez S, Benaim M, Lechin M, Lechin A: Effects of buspirone on plasma neurotransmitters in healthy subjects. J Neural Transm 1998;105:561–573.

Lechin F, Pardey-Maldonado B, van der Dijs B, Benaim M, Baez S, Orozco B, Naddaf R, Rodriguez S, Rangel A, Lechin ME: Circulating neurotransmitter profiles throughout normal wake-sleep cycle. Part two. In press.

Levine SP, Towell BL, Suarez AM, Knieriem LK, Harris MM, George JN: Platelet activation and secretion associated with emotional stress. Circulation 1985;71:1129–1134.

Li Q, Murakami I, Stall S, Levy AD, Brownfield MS, Nichols DE, van de Kar LD: Neuroendocrine pharmacology of three serotonin releasers: 1-(1,3-benzodioxol-5-yl)-2-(methylamino)butane (MBDB), 5-methoxy-6-methyl-2-aminoindan (MMAI) and p-methylthioamphetamine (MTA). J Pharmacol Exp Ther 1996; 279:1261–1267.

Li YW, Ding ZQ, Wesseling SL, Blessin WW: Renal sympathetic preganglionic neurons demonstrated by herpes simplex virus transneuronal labelling in the rabbit, close apposition of neuropeptide Y-immunoreactive terminals. Neuroscience 1993;53:1143–1152.

Luppi PH, Charlety PJ, Fort P, Akaoka H, Chouvet G, Jouvet M: Anatomical and electrophysiological evidence for a glycinergic inhibitory innervation of the rat locus coeruleus. Neurosci Lett 1991;128:33–36.

Luppi PH, Aston-Jones G, Akaoka H, Chouvet G, Jouvet M: Afferent projections of the rat locus coeruleus demonstrated by retrograde and anterograde tracing with cholera-toxin B subunit and Phaseolus vulgaris leucoagglutinin. Neuroscience 1995;65:119–116.

MacCarley RW: REM sleep and depression, common neurobiological control mechanisms. Am J Psychiatry 1982;139:5–13.

Maes M, Scharpé S, Verkerk R, D'Hondt P, Peeters D, Cosyns P, Thompson P, De Meyer F, Wauters A, Neels H: Seasonal variation in plasma l-tryptophan availability in healthy volunteers. Arch Gen Psychiatry 1995;52:937–946.

Maling TJB, Dollery CT, Hamilton CA: Clonidine and sympathetic activity during sleep. Clin Sci 1979;57:509–514.

McCall RB, Harris LT: 5-HT2 receptor agonists increase spontaneous sympathetic nerve-discharge. Eur J Pharmacol 1988;151:113–116.

McCann MJ, Hermann GE, Rogers RC: Nucleus raphe obscurus (nRO) influences vagal control of gastric motility in rats. Brain Res 1989;486:181–184.

McGinty DJ, Harper RM: Dorsal raphe neurons, depression of firing during sleep in cats. Brain Res 1976;101:569–875.

McKitrick DJ, Calaresu FR: Nucleus ambiguus inhibits activity of cardiovascular units in RVLM. Brain Res 1996;742:203–210.

Merahi N, Orer HS, Laguzzi R: 5-HT2 receptors in the nucleus tractus solitarius, characterization and role in cardiovascular regulation in the rat. Brain Res 1992;575:74–78.

Mileykovskiy BY, Kiyaschenko LI, Kodama T, Lai Y-Y, Siegel JM: Activation of pontine and medullary motor inhibitory regions reduces discharge in neurons located in the locus coeruleus and the anatomical equivalent of the midbrain locomotor region. J Neurosci 2000;20:8551–8558.

Minabe Y, Emori K, Ashby CHR: The depletion of brain serotonin levels by para-chlorophenylalanine administration significantly alters the activity of midbrain dopamine cells in rats: An extracellular single cell recording study. Synapse 1996;22:46–53.

Mohammed JR, Saska TA, Chi J, Stephens RL: Stimulation of the nucleus raphe obscurus produces market serotonin release into the dorsal medulla of fed but not fasted rats-glutamatergic dependence. Brain Res 1995;695:100–103.

Morgan WW, Saldana JJ, Yndo CA, Morgan JF: Correlations between circadian changes in serum aminoacids or brain tryptophan and the contents of serotonin and 5-hydroxy-indoleacetic acid in regions of the rat brain. Brain Res 1975;84:75–86.

Moroni F: Tryptophan metabolism and brain function, focus on kynurenine and other indole metabolites. Eur J Pharmacol 1999;375:87–100.

Muramatsu M, Tamari-Ohashi J, Usuki C, Araki H, Aihara H: Serotonin-2 receptor-mediated regulation of release of acetylcholine by minaprine in cholinergic nerve terminal of hippocampus of rat. Neuropharmacology 1988;27:603–609.

Nishiike S, Takeda N, Kubo T, Nakamura S: Neurons in rostral ventrolateral medulla mediate vestibular inhibition of locus coeruleus in rats. Neuroscience 1997;77:219–232.

Page ME, Valentino RJ: Locus coeruleus activation by physiological challenges. Brain Res Bull 1994;35:557–560.

Park SB, Coull JT, McShane RH, Young AH, Sahakian BJ, Robins TW, Cowen PJ: Tryptophan depletion in normal volunteers produces selective impairments in learning and memory. Neuropharmacology 1994;33:575–588.

Pickworth WB, Sharpe LG, Gupta VN: Morphine-like effects of clonidine on the EEG, slow wave sleep and behavior in the dog. Eur J Pharmacol 1982;81:551–558.

Piguet P, Stoeckel ME, Schlichter R: Synaptically released 5-HT modulates the activity of tonically discharging neuronal populations in the rostral ventral medulla (RVM). Eur J Neurosci 2000;12:2662–2675.

Plaznik A, Danysz W, Kostowski W, Bidzinski A, Hauptmann M: Interaction between noradrenergic and serotonergic brain systems as evidenced by behavioral and biochemical effects of microinjections of adrenergic agonists and antagonists into the median raphe nucleus. Pharmacol.Biochem Behav 1983;19:27–32.

Pratt GD, Bowery NG: The 5-HT$_3$ receptor ligand (^{3}H)BRL43694, binds to presynaptic sites in the nucleus tractus solitarius of the rat. Neuropharmacology 1989;28:1367–1376.

Przegalinski E, Tatarczynska E, Deren-Wesolek A, Chojnacka-Wójcik E: Anticonflict effects of a competitive NMDA receptor antagonist and a partial agonist at strychnine-insensitive glycine receptors. Pharmacol Biochem Behav 1996;54: 73.

Pyner S, Coote JH: Rostroventrolateral medulla neurons preferentially project to target-specified sympathetic preganglionic neurons. Neuroscience 1998;83:617–631.

Rahman S, Neuman RS: Action of 5-hydroxytryptamine in facilitating N-methyl-D-aspartate depolarization of cortical neurones mimicked by calcimycin, cyclopiazonic acid and thapsigargin. Br J Pharmacol 1996:119:877–884.

Rausch JL, Janowsky SC, Risch SC, Huey LY: Physostigmine effects on serotonin uptake in human blood platelets. Eur J Pharmacol 1985; 109:91–96.

Reese NB, Garcia-Rill E, Skinner RD: The pedunculopontine nucleus-auditory input, arousal and pathophysiology. Prog Neurobiol 1995;42: 105–133.

Reynolds DJM, Leslie RA, Grahame-Smith DG, Harvey JM: Localization of 5HT₃ receptor binding sites in human dorsal vagal complex. Eur J Pharmacol 1989;174:127–130.

Ricci A, Bronzetti E, Mannino F, Mignini F, Morosetti C, Tayebati SK, Amenta F: Dopamine receptors in human platelets. Arch Pharmacol 2001;363:376–382.

Robertson D, Garland AJ, Robertson RM, Nies AS, Shand DG, Oates JA: Comparative assessment of stimuli that release neuronal and adrenomedullary catecholamines in man. Circulation 1979;59:637–643.

Robinson SE: Effect of specific serotonergic lesions on cholinergic neurons in the hippocampus cortex and striatum. Life Sci 1982;32:345–353.

Sawchenko PE: Central connections of the sensory and motor nuclei of the vagus nerve. J Autonom Nerv Syst 1981;9:13–26.

Schaechter JD, Wurtman RJ: Serotonin release varies with brain tryptophan levels. Brain Res 1990;532:203–210.

Scheurink AJW, Steffens AB, Gaykema RP: Hypothalamic adrenoceptors mediate sympathoadrenal activity in exercising rats. Am J Physiol 1990;259:R470–R477.

Shafton AD, Ryan A, Badoer E: Neurons in the hypothalamic paraventricular nucleus send collaterals to the spinal cord and to the rostral ventrolateral medulla in the rat. Brain Res 1998;801:239–243.

Shepperson NB, Duval N, Langer SZ: Dopamine decreases mesenteric blood flow in the anaesthetised dog through the stimulation of postsynaptic α₂-adrenoceptors. Eur J Pharmacol 1982;81:627–636.

Sheu YS, Nelson JP, Bloom FE: Discharge patterns of cat raphe neurons during sleep and waking. Brain Res 1974;73:263–276.

Shopsin B, Wilk S, Gershon S: Cerebrospinal fluid MHPG, an assessment of norepinephrine metabolism in affective disorders. Arch Gen Psychiatry 1973;28:230–233.

Sim LJ, Joseph SA: Efferent projections of the nucleus raphe magnus. Brain Res Bull 1992;28: 679–682.

Soares-Da Silva P: Evidence for a non-precursor dopamine pool in noradrenergic neurons of the dog mesenteric artery. Arch Pharmacol 1986; 333:219–223.

Soares-Da Silva P: A comparison between the pattern of dopamine and noradrenaline release from sympathetic neurons of the dog mesenteric artery. Br J Pharmacol 1987;90:91–98.

Sourkes TL: Neurotransmitters and central regulation of adrenal functions. Biol Psychiatry 1985; 20:182–191.

Sporton SCE, Shepeard SL, Jordan D, Ramage AG: Microinjections of 5-HT₁A agonists into the dorsal motor vagal nucleus produce a bradycardia in the atenolol-pretreated anaesthetized rat. Br J Pharmacol 1991;104:466–470.

Sprouse J, Braselton J, Reynolds L: 5-HT₁A agonist potential of pindolol electrophysiologic studies in the dorsal raphe nucleus and hippocampus. Biol Psychiatry 2000;47:1050–1055.

Stamford JA, Muscat R, O'Connor JJ, Patel J, Trout SJ, Wieczorek WJ, Kruk ZL, Willner P: Voltammetric evidence that subsensitivity to reward following chronic mild stress is associated with increased release of mesolimbic dopamine. Psychopharmacology 1991;105:275–282.

Strack AM, Sawyer WB, Marubio LM, Loewy AD: Spinal origin of sympathetic preganglionic neurons in the rat. Brain Res 1988;455:187–191.

Swerdlow NR, Bakshi V, Geyer MA: Seroquel restores sensorimotor gating in phencyclidine-treated rats. J Pharmacol Exp Ther 1996;279: 1290–1299.

Ter-Horst GJ, Toes GJ, Van Willigen JD: Locus coeruleus projections to the dorsal motor vagus nucleus in the rat. Neuroscience 1991;45:153–160.

Thurston-Stanfield CL, Ranieri JT, Vallabhapurapu R, Barnes-Noble D: Role of vagal afferents and the rostral ventral medulla in intravenous serotonin-induced changes in nociception and arterial blood pressure. Physiol Behav 1999;67: 753–767.

Trulson ME, Jacobs BL: Raphe unit activity in freely moving cats, correlation with level of behavioral arousal. Brain Res 1979,163:135–142.

Trulson ME, Jacobs BL: Activity of serotonin-containing neurons in freely moving cats; in Jacobs BL, Gelperin A (eds): Serotonin Neurotransmission and Behavior. Cambridge, MIT Press, 1981, pp 339–402.

Trulson ME, Crisp T: Role of norepinephrine in regulating the activity of serotonin-containing dorsal raphe neurons. Life Sci 1984;35:511–515.

Trulson ME, Jacobs BL, Morrison AR: Raphe unit activity across the sleep-waking cycle in normal cats and in pontine lesioned cats displaying REM sleep without atonia. Brain Res 1981; 226:75–91.

Trulson ME, Crisp T, Howell GA: Raphe unit activity in freely moving cats, effects of quipazine. Neuropharmacology 1982a;21:681–686.

Trulson ME, Preussler DW, Howell GA, Frederickson CJ: Raphe unit activity in freely moving cats, effects of benzodiazepines. Neuropharmacology 1982b;21:1045–1050.

Tsukamoto K, Sved AF, Ito S, Komatsu K, Kanmatsuse K: Enhanced serotonin-mediated responses in the nucleus tractus solitarius of spontaneously hypertensive rats. Brain Res 2000;863:1–8.

Van Gaalen M, Kawahara H, Kawahara Y, Westerink BH: The locus coeruleus noradrenergic system in the rat studied by dual-probe microdialysis. Brain Res 1997;763:56–62.

van der Maelen CP, Aghajanian GK: Noradrenergic activation of serotonergic dorsal raphe neurons recorded in vitro. Soc Neurosci Abstr 1982;8:482.

Vertes RP, Fortin, Crane AM: Projections of the raphe nucleus in the rat. J Comp Neurol 1999; 407:555–582.

Wang QP, Ochiai H, Nakai Y: GABAergic innervation of serotonergic neurons in the dorsal raphe nucleus of the rat studied by electron microscopy double immunostaining. Brain Res Bull 1992;29:943–948.

Watkins LL, Grossman P, Krishnan R, Sherwood A: Anxiety and vagal control of heart rate. Psychosom Med 1998;60:498–502.

Whalen EJ, Johnson AK, Lewis SJ: Functional evidence for the rapid desensitization of 5-HT₃ receptors on vagal afferents mediating the Bezold-Jarisch reflex. Brain Res 2000;873:302–305.

Wilffert B, Smitt G, de Jonge A, Thoolen MJ, Timmermans PB, van Zwieten PA: Inhibitory dopamine receptors on sympathetic neurons innervating the cardiovascular system of the pithed rat: Characterization and role in relation to presynaptic alpha-2-adrenoceptors. Arch Pharmacol 1984;326:91–98.

Wilkinson LO, Abercrombie ED, Rasmussen K, Jacobs BL: Effect of buspirone on single unit activity in locus coeruleus and dorsal raphe nucleus in behaving cats. Eur J Pharmacol 1987;136:123–127.

Yates BJ, Goto T, Kerman I, Bolton PS: Responses of caudal medullary raphe neurons to natural vestibular stimulation. J Neurophysiol 1993; 70:938–945.

Yildiz O, Tuncer M: 5-HT₁-like and 5-HT₂A receptors mediate 5-hydroxytryptamine-induced contraction of rabbit isolated mesenteric artery. Arch Pharmacol 1995;352:127–131.

Yusof APM, Coote JH: Patterns of activity in sympathetic postganglionic nerves to skeletal muscle, skin and kidney during stimulation of the medullary raphe area of the rat. J Autonom Nerv Syst 1988;24:71–79.

Zagon A: Internal connections in the rostral ventromedial medulla of the rat. J Autonom Nerv Syst 1995;53:43–56.

Zheng Y, Riche D, Rekling JC, Foutz AS, Denavit-Saubié M: Brainstem neurons projecting to the rostral ventral respiratory group (VRG) in the medulla oblongata of the rat revealed by co-application of NMDA and biocytin. Brain Res 1998;782:113–125.

Ziegler MG, Lake CR, Wood JH: Relationship between norepinephrine in blood and cerebrospinal fluid in the presence of a blood cerebrospinal fluid barrier for NE. J Neurochem 1977; 28:677–679.

References for Chapter 2

Bodnar R, Paul D, Pasternak GW: Synergistic analgesic interactions between the periaqueductal gray and the locus coeruleus. Brain Res 1991;558:224–230.

Callera JC, Bonagamba LG, Sévoz C, Laguzzi R, Machado BH: Cardiovascular effects of microinjection of low doses of serotonin into the NTS of unanesthetized rats. Am J Physiol 1997;272:1135–1142.

Chen S, Aston-Jones G: Anatomical evidence for inputs to ventrolateral medullary catecholaminergic neurons from the midbrain periaqueductal gray of the rat. Neurosci Lett 1995;195:140–144.

Chitravanshi VC, Calaresu FR: Dopamine microinjected into the nucleus ambiguus elicits vagal bradycardia in spinal rats. Brain Res 1992;583:308–311.

Clement HW, Gemsa D, Wesemann W: Serotonin-norepinephrine interactions: A voltametric study on the effect of serotonin receptor stimulation followed in the n. raphe dorsalis and the locus coeruleus of the rat. J Neur Transm 1992;88:11–23.

Farkas E, Jansen AS, Loewy AD: Periaqueductal gray matter projection to vagal preganglionic neurons and the nucleus tractus solitarius. Brain Res 1997;764:257–261.

Feuerstein TJ, Mutschler A, Lupp A, Van Velthoven V, Schlicker E, Göthert M: Endogenous noradrenaline activates α_2-adrenoceptors on serotonergic nerve endings in human and rat neocortex. J Neurochem 1993;61:474–480.

Gauthier P, Reader T: Adrenomedullary secretory response to midbrain stimulation in rat: Effects of depletion of brain catecholamines or serotonin. Can J Physiol Pharmacol 1982;60:1464–1474.

Haddjeri N, de Montigny C, Blier P: Modulation of the firing activity of noradrenergic neurones in the rat locus coeruleus by the 5-hydroxtryptamine system. Br J Pharmacol 1997;120:865–875.

Hermann GE, Bresnahan JC, Holmes GM, Rogers RC, Beattie MS: Descending projections from the nucleus raphe obscurus to pudendal motoneurons in the male rat. J Comp Neurol 1998;397:458–474.

Heym J, Steinfels GF, Jacobs BL: Activity of serotonin-containing neurons in the nucleus raphe pallidus of freely moving cats. Brain Res 1982;251:259–276

Hillegaart V, Hjorth S. Median raphe, but not dorsal raphe, application of the 5-HT1A agonist 8-OH-DPAT stimulates rat motor activity. Eur J Pharmacol 1989;160:303–307.

Kawano S, Osaka T, Kannan H, Yamashita H: Excitation of hypothalamic paraventricular neurons by stimulation of the raphe nuclei. Brain Res Bull 1992;28:573–579.

Kirby LG, Rice KC, Valentino RJ: Effects of corticotropin-releasing factor on neuronal activity in the serotonergic dorsal raphe nucleus. Neuropsychopharmacology 1999;22:148–162.

Llewelyn MB, Azami J, Roberts MH: Effects of 5-hydroxytryptamine applied into nucleus raphe magnus on nociceptive thresholds and neuronal firing rate. Brain Res 1983;258:59–68.

Meyer-Bernstein EL, Blanchard JH, Morin LP: The serotonergic projection from the median raphe nucleus to the suprachiasmatic nucleus modulates activity phase onset, but not other circadian rhythm parameters. Brain Res 1997;755:112–120.

Morrison SF, Sved AF, Passerin AM: GABA-mediated inhibition of raphe pallidus neurons regulates sympathetic outflow to brown adipose tissue. Am J Physiol 1999;276:R290–R297.

Sotgiu ML: The effects of periaqueductal gray and nucleus raphe magnus stimulation on the spontaneous and noxious-evoked activity of lateral reticular nucleus neurons in rabbits. Brain Res 1987;414:219–227.

Starkey SJ, Skingle M: 5-HTID as well as 5-HTIA autoreceptors modulate 5-HT release in the guinea-pig dorsal raphe nucleus. Neuropharmacology 1994;33:393–402.

Ter Horst GJ, Toes GJ, Van Willigen JD: Locus coeruleus projections to the dorsal motor vagus nucleus in the rat. Neuroscience1991;45:153–160.

Thurston-Stanfield CL, Ranieri JT, Vallabhapurapu R, Barnes-Noble D: Role of vagal afferents and the rostral ventral medulla in intravenous serotonin-induced changes in nociception and arterial blood pressure. Physiol Behav 1999;67:753–767.

References for Chapter 3

Adell A, Artigas F: Regulation of the release of 5-hydroxytryptamine in the median raphe nucleus of the rat by catecholaminergic afferents. Eur J Neurosci 1999;11:2305–2311.

Amat J, Torres AR, Lechin F: Differential effect of footshock stress on humoral and cellular immune responses of the rat. Life Sci 1993;53:315–322.

Apperley GH, Drew GM, Sullivan AT: Prenalterol is an agonist at β_2- as well as β1-adrenoceptors. Eur J Pharmacol 1982;81:659–664.

Armario A, Garcia-Marquez C, Jolin T: The effects of chronic stress on corticosterone, GH and TSH response to morphine administration. Brain Res 1987;401:200–203.

Armario A, Marti O, Gavalda A, Lopez-Calderón A: Evidence for the involvement of serotonin in acute stress-induced release of luteinizing hormone in the male rat. Brain Res Bull 1993;31:29–31.

Astier B, Kitahama K, Denoroy L, Berod A, Jouvet M, Renaud B: Biochemical evidence for an interaction between adrenaline and noradrenaline neurons in the rat brainstem. Brain Res 1986;397:333–340.

Aston-Jones G, Bloom FE: Norepinephine-containing locus coeruleus neurons in behaving rats exhibit pronounced responses to non-noxious environmental stimuli. J Neurosci 1981;1:887–900.

Aston-Jones G, Hirata H, Akaoka H: Local opiate withdrawal in locus coeruleus in vivo. Brain Res 1997;765:331–336.

Aston-Jones G, Shipley MT, Chouvet G, Ennis M, van Bockstaele E, Pieribone V, Shiekhattar R, Akaoka H, Drolet G, Astier B, Charlety P, Valentino R, Williams J: Afferent regulation of locus coeruleus neurons: Anatomy, physiology and pharmacology. Prog Brain Res 1991;88:47–75.

Bamshad M, Song CK, Bartness TJ: CNS origins of the sympathetic nervous system outflow to brown adipose tissue. Am J Physiol 1999;45:1569–1578.

Behbehani MM, Liu H, Jiang M, Pun RYK, Shipley MT: Activation of serotonin1A receptors inhibit midbrain periaqueductal gray neurons of the rat. Brain Res 1993;612:56–60.

Behbehani MM: Functional characteristics of the midbrain periaqueductal gray. Prog Neurobiol 1995;46:575–605.

Blizard DA, Freedman LS, Liang B: Genetic variation, chronic stress, and the central and peripheral noradrenergic systems. Am J Physiol 1983;245:600–605.

Brady LS: Stress, antidepressant drugs, and the locus coeruleus. Brain Res Bull 1994;35:545–556,

Brammer JP, Kerecsen L, Maguire MH: Effects of vinblastine on malondialdehyde formation, serotonin release and aggregation in human platelets. Eur J Pharmacol 1982;81:577–586.

Brazenor RM, Angus JA: Actions of serotonin antagonists on dog coronary artery. Eur J Pharmacol 1982;81:569–576.

Brennan Jr. FX, Cobb CL, Silbert LH, Watkins LR, Maier SF: Peripheral β-adrenoceptors and stress-induced hypercholesterolemia in rats. Physiol Behav 1996;60:1307–1310.

Casanovas JM, Lèsourd M, Artigas F: The effect of the selective 5-HT1A agonists alnespirone (S-20499) and 8-OH-DPAT on extracellular 5-hydroxytryptamine in different regions of rat brain. Br J Pharmacol 1997;122:733–741.

Coenen AML, Van Luijtelaar ELJM: Stress induced by three procedures of deprivation of parodoxical sleep. Physiol Behav 1985;35:501–504.

Conti LH, Foote SL: Effects of pretreatment with corticotropin-releasing factor on the electrophysiological responsivity of the locus coeruleus to subsequent corticotropin-releasing factor challenge. Neuroscience 1995;69:209–219.

Conti LH, Youngblood KL, Printz MP, Foote SL: Locus coeruleus electrophysiological activity and responsivity to corticotropin-releasing factor in inbred hypertensive and normotensive rats. Brain Res 1997;774:27–34:

Crawley JN, Roth RH, Maas JW: Locus coeruleus stimulation increases noradrenergic metabolite levels in rat spinal cord. Brain Res 1979;166: 180–184.

Cunnick JE, Lysle DT, Kucinski BJ, Rabin BS: Evidence that shock-induced immune suppression is mediated by adrenal hormones and peripheral α-adrenergic receptors. Biochem Behav 1990;36:645–651.

Curtis AL, Drolet G, Valentino RJ: Hemodynamic stress activates locus coeruleus neurons of anesthetized rats. Brain Res Bull 1993;31:737–744.

Curtis AL, Lechner SM, Pavcovich LA, Valentino RJ: Activation of the locus coeruleus noradrenergic system by intracoerulear microinfusion of corticotropin-releasing factor: Effects on discharge rate, cortical norepinephrine levels and cortical electroencephalographic activity. J Pharmacol Exp Ther 1997;281:163–172.

Curtis AL, Pavcovich LA, Valentino RJ: Long-term regulation of locus coeruleus sensitivity to corticotropin-releasing factor by swim stress. J Pharmacol Exp Ther 1999;289:1211–1219.

Dampney RA: The subretrofacial vasomotor nucleus: Anatomical, chemical and pharmacological properties and role in cardiovascular regulation. Prog Neurobiol 1994;42:197–227.

Dantagostino G, Amoretti G, Frattini P, Zerbi F, Cucchi ML, Preda S, Corona GL: Catecholaminergic, neuroendocrine and anxiety responses to acute psychological stress in healthy subjects: Influence of alprazolam administration. Neuropsychobiology 1996;34:36–43.

De Fanti BA, Gavel DA, Hamilton JS, Horwitz BA: Extracellular hypothalamic serotonin levels after dorsal raphe nuclei stimulation of lean (Fa/Fa) and obese (fa/fa) Zucker rats. Brain Res 2000;869:6–14.

De Souza E: Corticotropin-releasing factor receptors in the rat central nervous system: characterization and regional distribution. J Neurosci 1987;7:88–100.

Elam M, Thorén P, Svensson TH: Locus coeruleus neurons and sympathetic nerves: activation by visceral afferents. Brain Res 1986;375:117–125.

Elam M, Yao T, Svensson TH, Thorn P: Regulation of locus coeruleus neurons and splanchnic, sympathetic nerves by cardiovascular afferents. Brain Res 1984;290:281–287.

Ennis M, Aston-Jones G, Shiekhattar R: Activation of locus coeruleus neurons by nucleus paragigantocellularis or noxious sensory stimulation is mediated by intracoerulear excitatory amino acid neurotransmission. Brain Res 1992;598: 185–195.

Ennis M, Aston-Jones G: Activation of locus coeruleus from nucleus paragigantocellularis: A new excitatory amino acid pathway in the brain. J Neurosci 1988;8:3644–3657:

Feenstra MGP, Botterblom MHA: Rapid stimulation of extracellular dopamine in the rat prefrontal cortex during food consumption, handling and exposure to novelty. Brain Res 1996; 742:17–24.

Feldman PD: Electrophysiological effects of serotonin in the solitary tract nucleus of the rat. Arch Pharmacol 1994;349:447–454.

Feng YZ, Zhang T, Rockhold RW, Ho IK: Increased locus coeruleus glutamate levels are associated with naloxone-precipitated withdrawal from butorphanol in the rat. Neurochem Res 1995;20:745–751:

Ferretti C, Blengio M, Ricci Gamalero S, Ghi P: Biochemical and behavioural changes induced by acute stress in a chronic variate stress model of depression: the effect of amitriptyline. Eur J Pharmacol 1995;280:19–26.

File SE: Recent developments in anxiety, stress, and depression. Phamacol Biochem Behav 1996;54:3–12.

Fontana DJ, McMiller LV, Commissaris RL: Depletion of brain norepinephrine: Differential influence on anxiolyic treatment effects. Psychopharmacol 1999;143:197–208.

Foote SL, Aston-Jones G, Bloom FE: Impulse activity of locus coeruleus neurons in awake rats and monkeys is a function of sensory stimulation and arousal. Proc Natl Acad Sci USA 1980;77:3033–3037.

Foote SL, Berridge C, Adams L, Pineda J: Electrophysiological evidence for involvement of the locus coeruleus in alerting, orienting and attention. Prog Brain Res 1991;88:521–532.

Fuchs E, Kramer M, Hermes B, Netter P, Hiemke C: Psychosocial stress in three shrews: Clomipramine counteracts behavioral and endocrine changes. Pharmacol Biochem Behav 1996;54: 219–228.

Funk D, Stewart J: Role of catecholamines in the frontal cortex in the modulation of basal and stress-induced autonomic output in rats. Brain Res 1996;741:220–229.

Gauthier P: Pressor responses and adrenomedullary catecholamine release during brain stimulation in the rat. Can J Physiol Pharmacol 1981; 59:485–492.

Gorka Z, Moryl E, Papp M: Effect of chronic mild stress on circadian rhythms in the locomotor activity in the rats. Pharmacol Biochem Behav 1996;54:229–234.

Graeff FG, Guimaraes FS, De Andrade TGCS, Deakin JFW: Role of 5HT in stress, anxiety, and depression. Pharmacol Biochem Behav 1996;54:129–141.

Graeff FG, Viana MB, Mora PO: Dual Role of 5-HT in defense and anxiety. Neurosci Biobehav Rev 1997;21:791–799.

Grillner P, Berretta N, Bernardi G, Svensson TH, Mercuri NB: Muscarinic receptors depress GABAergic synaptic transmission in rat midbrain dopamine neurons. Neuroscience 2000; 96:299–307.

Guillaume V, Conte-Devolx B, Szafarcczyk A, Malaval F, Pares-Herbute N, Grino M, Alonso G, Assenmacher I, Oliver Ch: The corticotropin-releasing factor release in rat hypophysial portal blood is mediated by brain catecholamines. Neuroendocrinology 1987;46:143–146.

Haas DA, George SR: Single or repeated mild stress increases synthesis and release of hypothalamic corticotropin-releasing factor. Brain Res 1988; 461:230–237.

Hedner J, Hedner T, Jonason J, Lundberg D: Evidence for dopamine interaction with the central respiratory control system in the rat. Eur J Pharmacol 1982;81:603–616.

Hentall ID, Kurle PJ, White TR: Correlations between serotonin level and single-cell firing in the rat's nucleus raphe magnus. Neuroscience 2000;95:1081–1088.

Heym J, Steinfels GF, Jacobs BL: Medullary serotonergic neurons are insensitive to 5-MEODMT and LSD. Eur J Pharmacol 1982; 81:677–680.

Holtman Jr. JR, Dick TE, Berger AJ: Serotonin-mediated excitation of recurrent laryngeal and phrenic motoneurons evoked by stimulation of the raphe obscurus. Brain Res 1987;417:12–20.

Ireland SJ, Tyers MB: Pharmacological characterization of 5-hydroxytryptamine-induced depolarization of the rat isolated vagus nerve. Br J Pharmac 1987;90:229–238.

Jacobs BL, Fornal CA: Activity of brain serotonergic neurons in the behaving animal. Pharmacol Rev 1991;43:563–583.

Jacobs EH, Yamatodani A, Timmerman H: Is histamine the final neurotransmitter in the entrainment of circadian rhythms in mammals? Trends Pharmacol Sci 2000;21:293–294.

Jernej B, Cicin-Sain L, Kveder S: Physiological characteristics of platelet serotonin in rats. Life Sci 1989;45:485–492.

Jones BE, Harper ST, Halaris AE: Effects of locus coeruleus lesions upon cerebral monoamine content, sleep-wakefulness states and the response to amphetamine in the cat. Brain Res 1977;124:473–496.

Kant GJ, Pastel RH, Bauman RA, Meininger GR, Maughan KR, Robinson TN, Wright WL, Covington PS: Effects of chronic stress on sleep in rats. Physiol Behav 1995;57:359–365.

Karreman M, Moghaddam B: The prefrontal cortex regulates the basal release of dopamine in the limbic striatum: An effect mediated by ventral tegmental area. J Neurochem 1996;66: 589–598.

Kaur S, Saxena RN, Mallick BN: GABA in locus coeruleus regulates spontaneous rapid eye movement sleep by acting GABAA receptors in freely moving rats. Neurosci Lett 1997;223: 105–108.

Kawahara Y, Kawahara H, Westerink BHC: Comparison of effects of hypotension and handling stress on the release of noradrenaline and dopamine in the locus coeruleus and medial prefrontal cortex of the rat. Arch Pharmacol 1999; 360:42–49.

King D, Zigmond MJ, Finaly JM: Effects of dopamine depletion in the medial prefrontal cortex on the stress-induced increase in extracellular dopamine in the nucleus accumbens core and shell. Neuroscience 1997;77:141–153.

Knigge U, Matzen S, Warberg J: Histaminergic mediation of the stress-induced release of prolactin in male rats. Neuroendocrinology 1988; 47:68–74.

Korf J, Aghajanian GK, Roth RH: Increased turnover of norepinephrine in the rat cerebral cortex during stress: Role of the locus coeruleus. Neuropharmacology 1973;12:933–938.

Krowicki ZK, Hornby PJ. Serotonin microinjected into the nucleus raphe obscurus increases intragastric pressure in the rat via a vagally mediated pathway. J Pharmacol Exp Ther 1993; 265:468–475.

Laaris N, Le Poul E, Hamon M, Lanfumey L: Stress-induced alterations of somatodendritic 5-HT1A autoreceptor sensitivity in the rat dorsal raphe nucleus: In vitro electrophysiological evidence. Fundam Clin Pharmacol 1997;11: 206–214.

Laguzzi R, Talman WT, Reiss DJ: Serotonergic mechanisms in the nucleus tractus solitarius may regulate blood pressure and behaviour in the rat. Clin Sci 1982;63:323s–326s.

Lambert GW, Kaye DM, Thompson JM, Turner AG, Cox HS, Vaz M, Jennings GL, Wallin BG, Esler MD: Internal jugular venous spillover of noradrenaline and metabolites and their association with sympathetic nervous activity. Acta Physiol Scand 1998;163:155–163.

Larsen PD, Zhong S, Gebber GL, Barman SM: Differential pattern of spinal sympathetic outflow in response to stimulation of the caudal medullary raphe. Am J Physiol Regulatory Integrative Comp Physiol 2000;279:R210–R221.

Lechin AE, Varon J, van der Dijs B, Lechin F: Plasma catecholamines and indoleamines during attacks and remission on severe bronchial asthma: possible role of stress. Am J Respir Crit Care Med 1994;149:A778.

Lechin AE, Varon J, van der Dijs B, Lechin F: Plasma neurotransmitters, blood pressure and heart rate during rest and exercise. Am J Respir Crit Care Med 1994;149:A482.

Lechin F, van der Dijs B, Azocar J, Amat J, Vitelli-Florez G, Martinez C, Lechin-Baez S, Jimenez V, Cabrera A, Cardenas M, Villa S: Stress, immunology and cancer: Effect of psychoactive drugs. Arch Ven Farmac Terap 1987;6:28–43.

Lechin F, van der Dijs B, Azocar J, Vitelli-Florez G, Lechin S, Villa S, Jara H, Cabrera A: Neurochemical and immunological profiles of three clinical stages in 50 advanced cancer patients. III Interamerican Congress of Clinical Pharmacology and Therapeutics. Arch Ven Farm Terap 1988;7(suppl 1):abstr 39.

Lechin F, van der Dijs B, Jackubowicz D, Camero RE, Lechin S, Villa S, Reinfeld B, Lechin ME: Role of stress in the exacerbation of chronic illness: Effects of clonidine administration on blood pressure and plasma norepinephrine, cortisol, growth hormone and prolactin concentrations. Psychoneuroendocrinology 1987; 12:117–129.

Lechin F, van der Dijs B, Jara H, Orozco B, Baez S, Benaim M, Lechin M, Lechin A: Effects of buspirone on plasma neurotransmitters in healthy subjects. J Neural Transm 1998;105:561–573.

Lechin F, van der Dijs B, Lechin AE, Lechin ME, Coll-Garcia- E, Jara H, Cabrera A, Jimenez V, Gomez F, Tovar D, Rada I, Arocha L: Doxepin therapy for postprandial symptomatic hypoglycemic patients: Neurochemical, hormonal and metabolic disturbances. Clin Sci 1991;80:373–384.

Lechin F, van der Dijs B, Lechin AE, Orozco B, Lechin ME, Baez S, Rada I, Leon G, Acosta E: Plasma neurotransmitters and cortisol in chronic illness: Role of stress. J Med 1994;25: 181–192.

Lechin F, van der Dijs B, Lechin AE, Orozco B, Lechin ME, Baez-Lechin S, Rada I, Leon G, Garcia Z, Jimenez V: Plasma neurotransmitters, blood pressure and heart rate during supine-resting, orthostasis and moderate exercise stress test in healthy humans before and after the parasympathetic blockade with atropine. Res Commun Biol Psychol Psychiat 1996;21: 55–72.

Lechin F, van der Dijs B, Lechin ME, Jara H, Lechin A, Baez S, Orozco B, Rada I, Cabrera A, Arocha L, Jimenez V, Leon G: Plasma neurotransmitters throughout oral glucose tolerance test in non-depressed essential hypertension patients. Clin Exp Hypertens 1993;15:209–240.

Lechin F, van der Dijs B, Lechin ME, Baez S, Jara H, Lechin A, Orozco B, Rada I, Cabrera A, Jimenez V, Leon G: Effects of an oral glucose load on plasma neurotransmitters in humans: Involvement of REM sleep? Neuropsychobiology 1992;26:4–11.

Lechin F, van der Dijs B, Lechin ME: Plasma neurotransmitters and functional illness. Psychother Psychosom 1996;65:293–318.

Lechin F, van der Dijs B, Lechin-Baez S, Vitelli G, Lechin M, Cabrera A: Neurochemical, hormonal and immunological views of stress: Clinical and therapeutic implications in Crohn's disease and cancer; in Velazco M (ed): Recent Advances in Pharmacology and Therapeutics. Amsterdam, Elsevier, 1989, pp 57–70.

Lechin F, van der Dijs B, Orozco B, Lechin AE, Baez S, Lechin ME, Benaim M, Acosta E, Arocha L, Jimenez V, Leon G, Garcia Z: Plasma neurotransmitters, blood pressure and heart rate during supine-resting, orthostasis, and moderate exercise in severely ill patients: A model of failing to cope with stress. Psychother Psychosom 1996;65:129–136.

Lechin F, van der Dijs B, Orozco B, Lechin ME, Lechin AE: Increased free serotonin plasma levels in symptomatic asthmatic patients. Ann Allergy Asthma Immunol 1996;77:245–253.

Lechin F, van der Dijs B, Rada I, Jara H, Lechin AE, Cabrera A, Lechin ME, Jimenez V, Gomez F, Villa S, Acosta E, Arocha L: Plasma neurotransmitters and cortisol in duodenal ulcer patients: Role of stress. Dig Dis Sci 1990;35: 1313–1319.

Lechin F, van der Dijs B, Vitelli-Florez G, Lechin-Baez S, Azocar J, Cabrera A, Lechin AE, Jara H, Lechin ME, Gomez F, Arocha L: Psychoneuroendocrinological and immunological parameters in cancer patients: Involvement of stress and depression. Psychoneuroendocrinology 1990;15:435–451.

Lechin F, van der Dijs B: Stress vs. depression. Prog Neuro-Psychopharmacol Biol Psychiatry 1996;20:899–950.

Lee EHY, Lin HH, Yin HM: Differential influences of different stressors upon midbrain raphe neurons in rats. Neurosci Lett 1987;80: 115–119.

Levine ES, Litto WJ, Jacobs BL: Activity of cat locus coeruleus noradrenergic neurons during the defense reaction. Brain Res 1990;531:189–195.

Lindsey BG, Arata A, Morris KF, Hernandez YM, Shannon R: Medullary raphe neurons and baroreceptor modulation of the respiratory motor pattern in the cat. J Physiol 1998;512:863–882.

Linton EA, Tilders FJH, Hodgkinson S, Berkenbosch F, Vermes I, Lowry PJ: Stress-induced secretion of adrenocorticotropin in rats is inhibited by administration of antisera to ovine corticotropin-releasing factor and vasopressin. Endocrinology 1985;116:966–970.

Luppi PH, Charlety PJ, Fort P, Akaoka H, Chouvet G, Jouvet M: Anatomical and electrophysiological evidence for a glycinergic inhibitory innervation of the rat locus coeruleus. Neurosci Lett 1991;128:33–36.

Matsuno K, Kobayashi T, Tanaka MK, Mita S: δ_1-Receptor subtype is involved in the relief of 'behavioral despair' in the mouse forced swimming test. Eur J Pharmacol 1996;312:267–271.

McCann MJ, Hermann GE, Rogers RC: Nucleus raphe obscurus (nRO) influences vagal control of gastric motility in rats. Brain Res 1989;486: 181–184.

McKitrick DJ, Calaresu FR: Nucleus ambiguus inhibits activity of cardiovascular units in RVLM. Brain Res 1996;742:203–210.

Melia KR, Duman RS: Involvement of corticotropin-releasing factor in chronic stress regulation of the brain noradrenergic system. Proc Natl Acad Sci USA 1991;88:8382–8386.

Merahi N, Orer HS, Laguzzi R: 5-HT2 receptors in the nucleus tractus solitarius: Characterization and role in cardiovascular regulation in the rat. Brain Res 1992;575:74–78.

Merchenthaler I: Corticotropin-releasing factor (CRF)-like immunoreactivity in the rat central nervous system: Extrahypothalamic distribution. Peptides 1984;5:53–69.

Minabe Y, Emori K, Ashby CR Jr: The depletion of brain serotonin levels by para-chlorophenylalanine administration significantly alters the activity of midbrain dopamine cells in rats: An extracellular single cell recording study. Synapse 1996;22:46–53.

Mohammed JR, Saska TA, Chi J, Stephens RL Jr: Stimulation of the nucleus raphe obscurus marked serotonin release into dorsal medulla of fed but not fasted rats-glutamatergic dependence. Brain Res 1995;695:100–103.

Morrison AP: Brain stem regulation of behavior during sleep and waking. Prog Psychobiol Psychophysiol 1979;8:91–131.

Mosko SS, Haubrich D, Jacobs BL: Serotonergic afferents to the dorsal raphe nucleus: evidence from HRP and synaptosomal uptake studies. Brain Res 1977;119:291–303.

Muramatsu M, Tamaki-Ohashi J, Usuki C, Araki H, Aihara H: Serotonin-2 receptor-mediated regulation of release of acetylcholine by minaprine in cholinergic nerve terminal of hippocampus of rat. Neuropharmacology 1988;27:603–609.

Murburg MM, McFall ME, Lewis N, Veith RC: Plasma norepinephrine kinetics in patients with posttraumatic stress disorder. Biol Psychiatry 1995;38:819–825.

Natelson BH, Creighton D, McCarty R, Tapp WN, Pitman D, Ottenweller JE: Adrenal hormonal indices of stress in laboratory rats. Physiol Behav 1987;39:117–125.

Natelson BH, Ottenweller JE, Cook JA, Pitman D, McCarty R, Tapp WN: Effect of stressor intensity on habituation of the adrenocortical stress response. Physiol Behav 1988;43:41–48.

Nishiike S, Takeda N, Kubo T, Nakamura S: Neurons in rostral ventrolateral medulla mediate vestibular inhibition of locus coeruleus in rats. Neuroscience 1997;77:219–232.

Nitz D, Siegel JM: GABA release in the locus coeruleus as a function of sleep/wake state. Neuroscience 1997;78:795–801.

Nörenberg W, Schöffel E, Szabo B, Starke K: Subtype determination of soma-dendritic 2-autoreceptors in slices of rat locus coeruleus. Arch Pharmacol 1997;356:159–165.

Ogasahara S, Taguchi Y, Wada H: Changes in serotonin in rat brain during slow-wave sleep and paradoxical sleep: Application of the microwave fixation method to sleep research. Brain Res 1980;189:570–575.

Olpe HR, Berecek K, Jones RSG, Steinman MW, Sonnenburg C, Hofbauer KG: Reduced activity of locus coeruleus neurons in hypertensive rats. Neurosci Lett 1985;61:25–29.

Olpe HR: The cortical projection of the dorsal raphe nucleus: Some electrophysiological and pharmacological properties. Brain Res 1981:216:61–71.

Ottenweller JR, Natelson BH, Pitman DL, Drastal SD: Adrenocortical and behavioral responses to repeated stressors: Toward an animal model of chronic stress and stress-related mental illness. Biol Psychiatry 1989;26:829–841.

Page ME, Abercrombie ED: Afferent regulation of locus coeruleus responsivity: An hypothesis of variable dominance of excitatory inputs; in Kvetnansky R, McCart R (eds): Stress, Molecular and Genetic Neurobiological Advances. New York, Gordon & Breach Science, 1996, pp 63–87.

Page ME, Valentino RJ: Locus coeruleus activation by physiological challenges. Brain Res Bull 1994;35:557–560.

Pavcovich LA, Cancela LM, Volosin M, Molina VA, Ramirez OA: Chronic stress-induced changes in locus coeruleus neuronal activity. Brain Res Bull 1990;24:293–296.

Pickworth WB, Sharpe LG, Gupta VN: Morphine-like effects of clonidine on the EEG slow wave sleep and behavior in the dog. Eur J Pharmacol 1982;81:551–558.

Piñeyro G, Blier P: Autoregulation of serotonin neurons: Role in antidepressant drug action. Pharmacol Rev 1999;51:533–538.

Plaznik A, Danysz W, Kostowski W, Bidzinski A, Hauptmann M: Interaction between noradrenergic and serotonergic brain systems as evidenced by behavioral and biochemical effects of microinjections of adrenergic agonists and antagonists into the median raphe nucleus. Pharmacol Biochem Behav 1983;19:27–32.

Pol O, Campmany LL, Armario A: Inhibition of catecholamine synthesis with α-methyl-p-tyrosine apparently increases brain serotoninergic activity in the rat: No influence of previous chronic immobilization stress. Pharmacol Biochem Behav 1995;52:107–112.

Privitera PJ, Granata AR, Underwood MD, Gaffney TE, Reis DJ: C1 area of the rostral ventrolateral medulla as a site for the central hypertensive action of propranolol. J Pharmacol Exp Ther 1988;246:529–535.

Puglisi-Allegra S, Imperato A, Angelucci L, Cabib S: Acute stress induces time-dependent responses in dopamine mesolimbic system. Brain Res 1991;554:217–222.

Rabkin SW: Effect of D-ALA-2-Me-Phe-4-Gly-ol-5 enkephalin on epinephrine-induced arrhythmias in the rat and the interrelationship to the parasympathetic nervous system. Life Sci 1989;45:1039–1047.

Rausch JL, Janowsky SC, Risch SC, Huey LY: Physostigmine effects on serotonin uptake in human blood platelets. Eur J Pharmacol 1985;109:91–96.

Reese NB, Garcia-Rill E, Skinner RD: The pedunculopontine nucleus-auditory input, arousal and pathophysiology. Prog Neurobiol 1995;42:105–133.

Richard ChA, Stremel RW: Involvement of the raphe in the respiratory effects of gigantocellular area activation. Brain Res Bull 1990;25:19–23.

Rivier C, Vale W: Modulation of stress-induced ACTH release by corticotropin-releasing factor, catecholamines and vasopressin. Nature 1983;305:325–333.

Robinson SE: Effect of specific serotonergic lesions on cholinergic neurons in the hippocampus cortex and striatum. Life Sci 1982;32:345–353.

Roth KA, Mefford IM, Barchas JD: Epinephrine, norepinephrine, dopamine, and serotonin: Differential effects of acute and chronic stress on regional brain amines. Brain Res 1982;239:417–424.

Sauerbier I, von Mayersbach H: Circadian variations of serotonin levels in human blood. Horm Metab Res 1976;8:157–158.

Sawchenko PE: Central connections of the sensory and motor nuclei of the vagus nerve. J Autonom Nervous System 1983;9:13–26.

Scheurink AJW, Steffens AB, Gaykema RPA: Hypothalamic adrenoceptors mediate sympathoadrenal activity in exercising rats. Physiol 1990;28:470–477.

Schreihofer AM, Guyenet PG: Sympathetic reflexes after depletion of bulbospinal catecholaminergic neurons with anti-DβH-saporin. Am J Physiol 2000;279:R729–R742.

Schworer H, Kuyyumi AA, Brush JE, Epstein SE: Cholinergic modulation of the release of 5-hydroxytryptamine from the guinea pig ileum. Arch Pharmacol 1987;336:127–132.

Seals DR: Sympathetic neural adjustments to stress in physically trained and untrained humans. Hypertension 1991;17:36–43.

Shepperson NB, Duval N, Langer SZ: Dopamine decreases mesenteric blood flow in the anesthetised dog through the stimulation of postsynaptic α_2-adrenoceptors. Eur J Pharmacol 1982;81:627–636.

Shibasaki T, Yamauchi N, Hotta M, Imaki T, Oda T, Ling N, Demura H: Brain corticotropin-releasing hormone increases arousal in stress. Brain Res 1991;554:352–354.

Sim LJ, Joseph SA: Efferent projections of the nucleus raphe magnus. Brain Res Bull 1992;28:679–682.

Smolen A, Smolen TN, van de Kamp JL: Alterations in brain catecholamines during pregnancy. Pharmacol Biochem Behav 1987;26:613–618.

Sporton SCE, Shepeard SL, Jordan D, Ramage AG: Microinjections of 5-HT$_{1A}$ agonists into the dorsal motor vagal nucleus produce a bradycardia in the atenolol-pretreated anaesthetized rat. Br J Pharmacol 1991;104:466–470.

Sprouse J, Braselton J, Reynolds L: 5-HT$_{1A}$ agonist potential of pindolol: Electrophysiologic studies in the dorsal raphe nucleus and hippocampus. Biol Psychiatry 2000;47:1050–1055.

Stanford SC: Stress: A major variable in the psychopharmacologic response. Pharmacol Biochem Behav 1996;54:211–217.

Svensson TH: Peripheral autonomic regulation of locus coeruleus noradrenergic neurons in brain: Putative implications of psychiatry and psychopharmacology. Psychopharmacology 1987;92:1–7.

Swenson RM, Vogel WH: Plasma catecholamine and costicosterone as well as brain catecholamine changes during coping in rats exposed to stressful footshock. Pharmacol Biochem Behav 1983;18:689–693.

Tobe T, Izumikawa F, Sano M, Tanaka C: Release mechanisms of 5HT in mammalian gastrointestinal tract-especially vagal release of 5HT; in Fujita T (ed): Endocrine Gut-Pancreas. Amsterdam, Elsevier, 1976, pp 371–380.

Tsopanakis A, Stalikas A, Sgouraki E, Tsopanakis C: Stress adaptation in athletes: Relation of lipoprotein levels to hormonal response. Pharmacol Biochem Behav 1994;48:377–382.

Tsukamoto K, Sved AF, Ito S, Komatsu K, Kanmatsuse K: Enhanced serotonin-mediated responses in the nucleus tractus solitarius of spontaneously hypertensive rats. Brain Res 2000;863:1–8.

Tung CS, Ugedo L, Grenhoff J, Engberg G, Svensson TH: Peripheral induction of burst firing in locus coeruleus neurons by nicotine mediated via excitatory amino acids. Synapse 1989;4:313–318.

Valentino RJ, Foote SL: Corticotropin-releasing hormone increases tonic but not sensory-evoked activity of noradrenergic locus coeruleus neurons in unanesthetized rats. J Neurosci 1988;8:1016–1025.

Valentino RJ, Page M, van Bockstaele E, Aston-Jones G: Corticotropin-releasing factor innervation of the locus coeruleus region: Distribution of fibers and sources of input. Neuroscience 1992;48:689–705.

Valentino RJ, Page ME, Curtis AL: Activation of noradrenergic locus coeruleus neurons by hemodynamic stress is due to local release of corticotropin-releasing factor. Brain Res1991;555: 25–34.

Van Gaalen M, Kawahara H, Kawahara Y, Westerink BHC: The locus coeruleus noradrenergic system in the rat brain studied by dual-probe microdialysis. Brain Res 1997;763:56–62.

Vertes RP, Fortin WJ, Crane AM: Projections of the median raphe nucleus in the rat. J Comp Neurol 1999;407:555–582.

Vesifeld IL, Vasilijiev VN, Iljicheva RF: Relationship of catecholamines, histamine and serotonin in men under different kind of stress; in Usdin E, Kvetnansky R, Kopin IJ (eds): Catecholamines and Stress. Oxford, Pergamon Press, 1976, pp 527–534.

Vollmayr B, Keck S, Henn FA, Schloss P: Acute stress decreases serotonin transporter mRNA in the raphe pontis but not in other raphe nuclei of the rat. Neurosci Lett 2000;290:109–112.

Weiss JM, Stout JC, Aaron MF, Quan N, Owens MJ, Butler PD, Nemeroff CB: Depression and anxiety: Role of the locus coeruleus and corticotropin-releasing factor. Brain Res Bull 1994; 35:561–572.

Wilkinson LO, Abercrombie ED, Rasmussen K, Jacobs BL: Effect of buspirone on single unit activity in locus coeruleus and dorsal raphe nucleus in behaving cats. Eur J Pharmacol 1987;136:123–127.

Willette RN, Punnen S, Krieger AJ, Sapru HN: Interdependence of rostral and caudal ventrolateral medullary areas in the control of blood pressure. Brain Res 1984;321:169–174.

Williamson DE, Birmaher B, Dahl RE, Al-Shabbout M, Ryan ND: Stressful life events influence nocturnal growth hormone secretion in depressed children. Biol Psychiatry 1996;40: 1176–1180.

Yang Z, Coote JH: Influence of the hypothalamic paraventricular nucleus on cardiovascular neurones in the rostral ventrolateral medulla of the rat. J Physiol 1998;513:521–530.

Yehuda R, Teicher MH, Trestman RL, Levengood RA, Siever LJ: Cortisol regulation in posttraumatic stress disorder and major depression: A chronobiological analysis. Biol Psychiatry 1996;40:79–88.

Zebrowska-Lupina I, Ossowska G, Klenk-Majewska B: Chronic stress reduces fighting behavior of rats: The effects of antidepressants. Pharmacol Biochem Behav 1991;39:293–296.

References for Chapter 4

Åberg-Wistedt A, Hasselmark L, Strain-Malmgren R, Apéria B, Kjellman BF, Mathé AA: Serotonergic vulnerability in affective disorder: A study of the tryptophan depletion test and relationships between peripheral and central serotonin indexes in citalopram-responders. Acta Psychiatr Scand 1998;97:374–380.

Ackerman KD, Martino M, Heyman R, Moyna NM, Rabin BS: Stressor-induced alteration of cytokine production in multiple sclerosis patients and controls. Psychosom Med 1998;60: 484–491.

Aghajanian GK, Haigler HJ: Studies on the physiological activity of 5-HT neurons; in Acheson G (ed): Pharmacology and the Future of Man. Basel, Karger, 1973, pp 269–285.

Aghajanian GK, Wang RY: Physiology and pharmacology of central serotonergic neurons; in: Psychopharmacology: A Generation of Progress. New York, Raven Press, 1978, pp 171–183.

Ågmo A, Belzung C, Rodriguez C: A rat model of distractibility: Effects of drugs modifying dopaminergic, noradrenergic and GABAergic neurotransmission. J Neural Transm 1997;104: 11–29.

Agren H: Symptom patterns in unipolar and bipolar depression correlating with monoamine metabolites in the cerebrospinal fluid. I. General patterns. Psychiatr Res 1980;3:211–223.

Agren H: Symptom patterns in unipolar and bipolar depression correlating with monoamine metabolites in the cerebrospinal fluid. II. Suicide. Psychiatr Res 1980;3:225–236.

Alojz, Tepes B, Gubina M: Diminished Th1-type cytokine production in gastric mucosa T-lymphocytes after *H. pylori* eradication in duodenal ulcer patients. Eur J Physiol 2000;440: R89–R90.

Anden NE, Grabowska M: Pharmacological evidence for a stimulation of dopamine neurons by noradrenaline neurons in the brain. Eur J Pharmacol 1976;39:275–282.

Anden NE, Strömbom JA: Adrenergic receptor blocking agents: Effects on central noradrenaline and dopamine receptors and on motor activity. Psychopharmacologia (Berl) 1974;38: 91–103.

Anden NE, Atack CV, Svensson TH: Release of dopamine from central noradrenaline and dopamine nerves induced by a dopamine-beta-hydroxylase inhibitor. J Neural Transm 1973; 34:93–100.

Anderson C, Pasquier D, Forbes W, Morgane P: Locus coeruleus-to-dorsal raphe input examined by electrophysiological and morphological methods. Brain Res Bull 1977;2:209–221.

Anisman H, Sklar LS: Catecholamine depletion in mice upon reesposure to stress: Mediation of the escape deficits produced by inescapable shock. J Comp Physiol 1979;93:610–625.

Anisman H, Irwin J, Sklar LS: Deficits of escape performance following catecholamnie depletion: Implications for behavioral deficits induced by uncontrollable stress. Psychopharmacology 1979;64:163–170.

Anisman H, Ritch M, Sklar LS: Noradrenergic and dopaminergic interactions in escape behavior: Analysis of uncontrollable stress effects. Psychopharmacology 1981;74:263–268.

Anisman H, Suissa A, Sklar LS: Escape deficits produced by uncontrollable stress: Antagonism by dopamine and norepinephrine agonists. Behav Neurol Biol 1980;28:34–47.

Antelman SM, Caggiula AR: Norepinphrine-dopamine interactions and behavior. Science 1977; 195:646–652.

Aprison MH, Hingtgen JN: Hypersensitive serotonergic receptors: a new hypothesis for one subgroup of unipolar depression derived from an animal model; in Haber B, Gabay S, Issidorides MR, Alivisatos SGA (eds): Serotonin: Current Aspects of Neurochemistry and Function. New York, Plenum Press, 1981, pp 627–656.

Arranz B, Blennow K, Eriksson A, Månsson JE, Marcusson J: Serotonergic, noradrenergic and dopaminergic measures in suicide brains. Biol Psychiatry 1997;41:1000–1009.

Asberg M, Thoren P, Traskman L, Bertilsson L, Ringberger V: Serotonin depression: A biochemical subgroup within the affective disorders? Science 1976;191:478–483.

Askenazy F, Candito M, Caci H, Myquel M, Chambon P, Darcourt, Pucch AJ: Whole blood serotonin content, tryptophan concentrations, and impulsivity in anorexia nervosa. Biol Psychiatry 1998;43:188–195.

Assaf SY, Miller JJ: The role of a raphe serotonin system in the control of septal unit activity and hippocampal desynchoronization. Neuroscience 1978;3:539–550.

Aulakh CS, Mazzola-Pomietto P, Murphy DL: Long-term antidpressant treatment restores clonidine's effect on growth hormone secretion in a genetic animal model of depression. Pharmacol Biochem Behav 1996;55:265–268.

Azmitia EC, Segal M: An autoradiographic analysis of the differential ascending projections of the dorsal and medial raphe nuclei of the rat. J Comp Neurol 1978;179:641–668.

Azorin JM, Raucoules D, Valli M, Levy C, Lancon C, Luccioni JM, Tissot R: Plasma levels of 3-methoxy-4-hydroxyphenylglycol in depressed patients compared with normal controls. Neuropsychobiology 1990;23:18–24.

Bamshad M, Song CK, Bartness TJ: CNS origins of the sympathetic nervous system outflow to brown adipose tissue. Am J Physiol 1999;276: R1569–R1578.

Bannon MJ, Roth RH: Pharmacology of mesocortical dopamine neurons. Pharmacol Rev 1983; 35:53–68.

Bannon MJ, Wolf ME, Roth RH: Pharmacology of dopamine neurons innervating the prefrontal, cingulated and piriform cortices. Eur J Pharmacol 1983;92:119–125.

Baraban JM, Aghajanian GK: Suppresion of firing activity of 5HT neurons in the dorsal raphe by alpha-adrenoceptor antagonists. Neuropharmacology 1980;19:335–341.

Baraban JM, Aghajanian GK: Suppresion of serotonergic neuronal firing by alpha-adrenoceptor antagonists: Evidence against GABA mediation. Eur J Pharmacol 1980;66:287–294.

Bateman A, Singh A, Kral T, Solomon S: The immune-hypothalamic-pytuitary-adrenal axis. Endocrinol Rev 1989;10:92–112.

Benarroch EE, Balda MS, Finkielman S, Nahmod VE: Neurogenic hypertension after depletion of norepinephrine in anterior hypothalamus induced by 6-hydroxydopamine administration into the ventral pons: role of serotonin. Neuropharmacology 1983;22:29–34.

Benson KL, Faull KF, Zarcone VP: The effects of age and serotonergic activity on slow-wave sleep in depressive illness. Biol Psychiatry 1993;33:842–844.

Berger B, Tassin JP, Blanc G, Moyne MA, Thierry AM: Histochemical confirmation for dopaminergic innervation of the rat cerebral cortex after destruction of the noradrenergic ascending pathways. Brain Res 1974;81:332–337.

Berger B, Thierry AM, Tassin JP, Moyne MA: Dopaminergic innervation of the rat prefrontal cortex: a fluorescence histochemical study. Brain Res 1976;106:133–145:

Berger M, Doerr P, Lund R, Bronisch T, von Zerssen D: Neuroendocrinological and neurophysiological studies in major depressive disorders: Are there biological markers for the endogenous subtype? Biol Psychiatry 1982;17:1217–1242.

Berger PA, Faull KF, Kilkowski J, Anderson PJ, Kraemer H, Davis KL, Barchas JD: CSF monoamine metabolites in depression and schiozophrenia. Am J Psychiatry 1980;137: 174–180.

Berman RM, Narasimhan M, Miller HL, Anand A, Cappiello A, Oren DA, Heninger GR, Charney DS: Transient depressive relapse induced by catecholamine depletion. Arch Gen Psychiatry 1999;56:395–403.

Berridge KC, Robinson TE: What is the role of dopamine in reward: Hedonic impact, reward learning, or incentive salience? Brain Res Rev 1998;28:309–369.

Bhatti T, Gillin JC, Seifritz E, Moore P, Clark C, Golshan S, Stahl S, Rapaport M, Kelsoe J: Effects of a tryptophan-free amino acid drink challenge on normal human sleep electroencephalogram and mood. Biol Psychiatry 1998;43: 52–59.

Blanc G, Herve D, Simon H, Lisoprawski A, Glowinski J, Tassin JP: Response to stress of mesocortico-frontal dopaminergic neurons in rats after long-term isolation. Nature 1980;284: 265–267.

Blier P, de Montigny C, Azzaro AJ: Effect or repeated amiflamine adminstration on serotonergic and noradrenergic neurotransmission: Electrophysiological studies in the rat CNS. Arch Pharmacol 1986;334:253–260.

Bobillier P, Petitjean F, Salvert D, Lighier M, Seguin S: Differential prejections of the nucleus raphe dorsalis and nucleus raphe centralis as revealed by autoradiography. Brain Res 1975; 85:205–210.

Bobillier P, Sequin S, Petitjean F, Salvert D, Touret M, Jouvet M: The raphe nuclei of the cat brain stem: A topographical atlas of their efferent projections as revealed by autoradiography. Brain Res 1976;113:449–486.

Bondolfi G, Chautems C, Rochat B, Bertschy G, Baumann P: Non-response to citalopram in depressive patients: Pharmacokinetic and clinical consequences of a fluvoxamine augmentation. Psychopharmacology 1996;128:421–425.

Breier A, Albus M, Pickar D, Zahn TP, Wolkowitz OM, Paul SM: Controllable and uncontrollable stress in humans: Alterations in mood and neuroendocrine and psychophysiological function. Am J Psychiatry 1987;144:1419–1425.

Brown AS, Gershon S: Dopamine and depression. J Neural Transm 1993;91:75–109.

Brown GL, Ballenger JC, Minichiello MD, Goodwin FK: Human aggression and its relationship to cerebrospinal fluid 5-hydroxy-indoleacetic acid, 3-methoxy-4-hydroxyphenylglycol, and homovanillic acid; in Sandler M (ed): Psychopharmacology of Aggression. New York, Raven Press, 1979.

Brown GL, Ebert MH, Goyer PF, Jimerson DC, Klein WJ, Bunney WE, Goodwin FK: Agression, suicide and serotonin: Relationship to CSF amine metabolites. Am J Psychiatry 1982; 139:741–746.

Brown GL, Goodwin FK, Ballenger JC, Goyer PF, Major LF: Agression in humans correlates with cerebrospinal fluid amine metabolites. Psychiatr Res 1979;1:131–140.

Brown GL, Goodwin FK, Bunney WJ: Human aggression and suicide: Their relationship to neuropsychiatric diagnoses and serotonin metabolism; in Ho BT (ed): Serotonin in Biological Psychiatry. New York, Raven Press, 1982.

Brown L, Rosellini RA, Samuels OB, Riley EP: Evidence for a serotonergic mechanism of the learned helplessness phenomenon. Pharmacol Biochem Behav 1982;17:877–883.

Bunney BS, Aghajanian GK: Mesolimbic and mesocortical dopaminergic systems: Physiology and pharmacology; in Lipton MA, DiMascio A, Killam KF (eds): Psychopharmacology: A Generation of Progress. New York, Raven Press, 1978, pp 221–234.

Bunney BS: The electrophysiological pharmacology of midbrain dopaminergic systems; in Horn AS, Korf J, Westerink BHC (eds): The Neurobiology of Dopamine. New York, Academic Press, 1979, pp 417–452.

Bunney WE, Davis JM: Norepinephrine in depressive reactions. Arch Gen Psychiatry 1965;13: 483–487.

Carter CJ, Pycock CJ: Behavioural and biochemical effects of dopamine and noradrenaline depletion within the medial prefrontal cortex of the rat. Brain Res 1980;192:163–176.

Casanovas JM, Lésourd M, Artigas F: The effect of the selective 5-HT1A agonists alnespirone (S-20499) and 8-OH-DPAT on extracellular 5-hydroxytryptamine in different regions of rat brain. Brit J Pharmacol 1997;122:733–741.

Catalán R, Gallart JM, Castellanos JM, Galard R: Plasma corticotropin-releasing factor in depressive disorders. Biol Psychiatry 1998;44: 15–20.

Charney DS, Price LH, Heninger GR: Desipramine-yohimbine combination treatment of refractory depression. Arch Gen Psychiatry 1986;43:1155–1161.

Checkley SA, Slade PA, Shur E: Growth hormone and other responses to clonidine in patients with endogenous depression. Br J Psychiatry 1981;138:51–55.

Clemente CD, Chase MH: Neurological substrates of aggresive behaviour. Ann Rev Physiol 1973; 35:329–356.

Cochran E, Robins E, Grote S: Regional serotonin levels in brain: A comparison of depressive suicides and alcoholic suicides with controls. Biol Psychiatry 1976;11:283–294.

Conrad ICA, Leonard CM, Pfaff DW: Connections of the median and dorsal raphe nuclei in the rat: An autoradiographic an degeneration study. J Comp Neurol 1974;107:513–525.

Costall B, Naylor RJ, Marsden CB, Pycock CJ: Serotonergic modulation of the dopamine response form the nucleus accumbens. J Pharm Pharmacol 1976;28:523–526.

Cowan WM, Raisman G, Powell TPS: The connections of the amygdala. J Neurol Neurosurg Psychiatry 1965;28:137–151.

Delgado PL, Charney DS, Price LH, Aghajanian GK, Landis H, Heninger GR: Serotonin function and the mechanism of antidepressant action. Arch Gen Psychiatry 1990;47:411–418.

Descarries L, Beaudet A: The serotonin innervation of adult rat hypothalamus; in Vincent JD, Kordon C (eds): Cell Biology of Hypothalamic Neurosecretion. Paris, CNRS, 1978.

Dey S: Physical exercise as a novel antidepressant agent: Possible role of serotonin receptor subtypes. Physiol Behav 1992;55:323–329.

Diamant M, de Wied D: Autonomic and behavioral effects of centrally administered corticotropin-releasing factor in rats. Endocrinology 1991;129:446–454.

Dichiara G, Camb R, Spano PF: Evidence for inhibition by brain serotonin of mouse killing behavior in rats. Nature 1971;233:272–273.

Dilts RP, Boadle-Biber MC: Differential activation of the 5-hydroxytryptamine-containing neurons of the midbrain raphe of the rat in response to randomly presented inescapable sound. Neurosci Lett 1995;199:78–80.

Dube S, Kumar N, Ettedgui E, Pohl R, Jones D, Sitaram N: Cholinergic REM induction response: separation of anxiety and depression. Biol Psychiatry 1985;20:408–418.

Dyr W, Kostowski W, Zacharski B, Bidzinski A: Differential clonidine effects on EEG following lesions of the dorsal and median raphe nuclei in rats. Pharmacol Biochem Behav 1983;19: 177–185.

Dziedzicka-Wasylewska M, Mackowiak M, Fijar K, Wedzony S: Adaptive changes in the rat dopaminergic transmission following repeated lithium administration. J Neural Transm 1996; 103:765–776.

Earley CJ, Yaffee JB, Allen RP: Randomized, double-blind, placebo-controlled trial of pergolide in restless legs syndrome. Neurology 1998;51: 1599–1602.

Elam M, Thorén P, Svensson TH: Locus coeruleus neurons and sympathetic nerves: Activation by visceral afferents. Brain Res 1986;375:117–125.

Elkind-Hirsch K, King JC, Gerall AA, Leeman SE: Neonatal estrogen affects preoptic/anterior hypothalamic LHRH differently in adult male and female rats. Neuroendocrinology 1984;38: 68–74.

Ellenbroek B, Cools AR: The neurodevelopment hypothesis of schizopharenia: Clinical evidence and animal models. Neurosci Res Commun 1998;22:127–133.

Ellison G: Behavioral and the balance norepinephrine and serotonin. Acta Neurobiol Exp 1975; 35:499–515.

Eriksson E, Eden S, Modigh K: Up-and down-regulation of central postsynaptic alpha$_2$-receptors reflected in the growth hormone response to clonidine in reserpine-pretreated rats. Psychopharmacology 1982;77:327–335.

Evans DL, Leserman J, Pedersen CA, Golden R, Lewis MH, Folds JA, Ozer H: Immune correlates of stress and depression. Psychopharm Bull 1989;25:319–323.

Evans DL, Pedersen CA, Folds JD: Major depression and immunity: Preliminary evidence of decreased natural killer cell populations. Neuro-Psychopharmacol Biol Psychiatry 1988;12: 739–748.

Fadda F, Argiolas A, Melin ME, Tissari AM, Onali PL, Gesssa GL: Stress induced increase in 3,4-dihydroxyphenylacetic acid (DOPAC) levels in the cerebral cortex and in n. accumbens: Reversal by diazepam. Life Sci 1978;23:2219–2224.

File SE, Hyde JRG, MacLeod NK: 5,7-Dihydroxytryptamine lesions of dorsal and median raphe nuclei and performance in the social interaction test of anxiety and in a home cage aggression test. J Affect Dis 1979;1:155–122.

File SE: Clinical lesions of both dorsal and median raphe nulei and changes in social and aggressive behaviour in rats. Pharmacol Biochem Behav 1980;12:855–859.

Fishman RH, Feigenbaum JJ, Yanai J, Klawans HL: The relative importance of dopamine and norepinephrine in mediating locomotor activity. Prog Neurobiol 1983;20:55–88.

Fletcher PJ, Davies M: Dorsal raphe microinjection of 5-HT and indirect 5-HT agonists induces feeding in rats. Eur J Pharmacol 1990; 184:265–271.

Foote SL, Aston-Jones G, Bloom FE: Impulse activity of locus coeruleus neurons in awake rats and monkeys is a function of sensory stimulation an arousal. Proc Natl Acad Sci USA 1980; 77:3033–3039.

Frankhuyzen AL, Mulder AH: Noradrenaline inhibits ^{3}H-serotonin release from slices of rat hippocampus. Eur J Pharmacol 1980;63:179–187.

Fride E, McIntyre T, Skolnick P, Arora PK: Immunocompetence in the long sleep and short sleep mouse lines: Baseline versus primed responses. Brain Behav Immun 1993;7:231–242.

Friedman Y, Bacchus R, Raymond R, Joffe RT, Nobrega JN: Acute stress increases thyroid hormone levels in rat brain. Biol Psychiatry 1999; 45:234–237.

Funakoshi K, Kadota T, Atobe Y, Nakano M, Goris RC, Kishida R: Serotonin-immunoreactive axons in the cell column of sympathetic preganglionic neurons in the spinal cord of the filefish Stephanolepis cirrhifer. Neurosci Lett 2000;280:115–118.

Fuxe K, Hokfelt T, Agnati L, Johansson D, Ljangdahl A, Perez de la Mora M: Regulation of the mesocortical dopamine neurons; in Costa E, Gessa GL (eds): Nonstriatal Dopaminergic Neurons. Adv Biochem Psychopharmacol. New York, Raven Press, 1977, pp 47–55.

Fykse EM, Fonnum F: Amino acid neurotransmission: Dynamics of vesicular uptake. Neurochem Res 1996;21:1053–1060.

Gabbett T, Gass G, Gass E, Morris N, Bennett G, Thalib L: Norepinephrine and epinephrine responses during orthostatic intolerance in healthy elderly men. Jpn J Physiol 2000;50:59–66.

Gaillard JM: Brain noradrenergic activity in wakefulness and paradoxical sleep: The effect of clonidine. Neuropsychobiology 1985;13:23–25.

Galey S, LeMoal M: Behavioural effects of lesions in the A10 dopaminergic area of the rat. Brain Res 1977;124;83–97.

Gann DS, Ward DE, Carlson DE: Neural pathways controlling release of corticotropin (ACTH); in Jones MT, Gillham B, Dallman MF, Chattopadhyay S (eds): Interaction within the Brain-Pituitary-Adrenocortical System. London, Academic Press, 1979, pp 75–86.

Goodwin FK, Post RM: 5-Hydroxytryptamine and depression: A model for the interaction of normal variance with pathology. Br J Clin Pharmacol 1983;15:3935–4055.

Goodwin FK, Rubovits R, Jimerson DC, Post RM: Serotonin and norepinephrine 'subgroups' in depression: Metabolite findings and clinical-pharmacological correlations. Sci Proc Am Psychiat Assoc 1977;130:108–115.

Granat AR, Kumada M, Reis DJ: Sympathoinhibition by A1-noradrenergic neurons is mediated by neurons in the C1 area of the rostral medulla. J Auton Nerv System 1985;14:387–395.

Green JD, Arduini AA: Hippocampal electrical activity in arousal. J Neurophysiol 1954;17: 533–557.

Grenhoff J, Svensson H: Prazosin modulates the firing pattern of dopamine neurons in rat ventral tegmental area. Eur J Pharmacol 1993;233: 79–84.

Gudelsky GA, Meltzer HY: Function of tuberoinfundibular dopamine neurons in pargyline-and reserpine-treated rats. Neuroendocrinology 1984;38:51–55.

Guillaume V, Conte-Devolx B, Szafarczyk A, Malaval F, Pares-Herbute N, Grino M, Alonso G, Assenmacher I, Oliver C: The corticotropin-releasing factor release in rat hypophysial portal blood is mediated by brain catecholamines. Neuroendocrinology 1987;46:143–146.

Gumulka W, Samanin R, Valzelli L, Consolo S: Behavioural and biochemical effects following the stimulatin of the nucleus raphe dorsalis in rats. J Neurochem 1971;18:533–535.

Gupta S: Molecular steps of cell suicide: An insight into immune senescence. J Clin Immunol 2000;20:229–236.

Hahn YS, Kim Y, Jo SO, Han HS: Reduced frequencies of peripheral interferon-y-producing CD4+ and CD4– cells during acute Kawasaki disease. Int Arch Allergy Immunol 2000;122: 293–298.

Halper JP, Brown RP, Sweeney JA, Kocsis JH, Peters A, Mann JJ: Blunted α-adrenergic responsivity of peripheral blood mononuclear cells in endogenous depression. Arch Gen Psychiatry 1988;45:241–244.

Hashimoto K, Ohno N, Yunoki S, Kageyama J, Takahara AY, Ofuji T: Characterization of corticotropin-releasing factor (CRF) and arginine vasopress in median eminence extracts on sephadex gel-filtration. Endocr Jpn 1981;28:1–7.

Hellhammer DH, Rea MA, Bell M, Belkien L, Ludwig M: Learned helplessness: Effects on brain monoamines and the pituitary-gonada axis. Pharmacol Biochem Behav 1984;21:481–485.

Hengeveld MW: Serotonin in attempted suicide. J Psychosom Res 1994;38:639–641.

Herman JP, Guillonneau D, Dantzer R, Scatton B, Semerdjian-Rouquier L, LeMoal M: Differential effects of inescapable foot-shocks and of stimuli previously paired with inescapable foot-shocks on dopamine turnover in cortical and limbic areas of the rat. Life Sci 1982;30: 2207–2214.

Hernandez F, Blanquer A, Linares M, López A, Tarin F, Cerveró A: Autoimmune thrombocytopenia associated with hepatitis C virus infection. Acta Haematol 1998;99:217–220.

Herve D, Simon H, Blanc G, LeMoal M, Glowinski J, Tassin JP: Opposite changes in dopamine utilization in the nucleus accumbens and the frontal cortex after electrolytic lesion of the median raphe in the rat. Brain Res 1981;3: 152–165.

Herve D, Simon H, Blanc G, Lisoprawski A, LeMoal M, Glowinski J, Tassin JP: Increased utilization of dopamine in the nucleus accumbens but not in the cerebral cortex after dorsal raphe lesion in the rat. Neurosci Lett 1979;15:127–134.

Hirata-Hibi M, Higashi S, Tachibana T, Watanabe N: Stimulated lymphocytes in schizophrenia. Arch Gen Psychiatry 1982;39:82–87.

Hodge GK, Butcher LL: Catecholamine correlates of isolation-induced aggression in mice. Eur J Pharmacol 1973;31:81–93.

Huang ZG, Subramanian H, Balnave RJ, Turman AB, Chow CM: Roles of periaqueductal gray and nucleus tractus solitarius in cardiorespiratory function in the rat brainstem. Respir Physiol 2000;12:185–195.

Huyse Frits J, Zwaan W A, Kupka R: The applicability of antidepressants in the depressed medically ill: An open clinical trial with fluoxetine. J Psychosom Res 1994;38:695–703.

Invernizzi R, Bramante M, Samanin R: Role of 5-HT1A receptors in the effects of acute and chronic fluoxetine on extracellular serotonin in the frontal cortex. Pharmac Biochem Behav 1996;54:143–147.

Irwin M, Smith TL, Gillin JC: Low natural killer cytotoxicity in major depression. Life Sci 1987;41:2127–2133.

Jacobs BL, Cohen A: Differential behavioral effects of lesions of the median or dorsal raphe nuclei in rats: Open field and pain elicited aggression. J Comp Physiol Psychol 1976;46:102–112.

Jacobs BL, Asher R, Dement WC: Electrophysiological and behavioral effect of electrical stimulation of raphe nuclei in cats. Physiol Behav 1973;11:489–495.

Jacobs BL, Foote SL, Bloom FE: Differential projections of neurons within the dorsal raphe nucleus of the rat: A horseradish peroxidase (HRP) study. Brain Res 1978;147:149–153.

Jakovljevik M, Mück-Šeler D, Pivac M, Ljubijij D, Bujas M, Dogig G: Seasonal influence on platelet 5-HT levels in patients with recurrent major depression and schizophrenia. Biol Psychiatry 1997;41:1028–1034.

Jimerson DC, Post RM, Stoddard FJ, Gillin JC, Bunney WE: Preliminary trial of the noredrenergic agonist clonidine in psychiatric patients. Biol Psychiatry 1980;139:1315–1319.

Jones MT, Hillhouse EW, Burden J: Effect of various putative neurotransmitters on the secretion of corticotrophin releasing hormone from the rat hypothalamus in vitro. J Endocrinol 1976;69:1–20.

Jones MT: Control of corticotropin (ACTH) secretion; in Jeffcoate SL, Hutchinson JSM (eds): The Endocrine Hypothalamus. New York, Academic Press, 1978, pp 385–419.

Joseph MH, Kennett GA: Corticosteroid response to stress depends upon increased tryptophan availability. Psychopharmacology 1983;79:79–81.

Kaneko M, Honda K, Kanno T, Horikoshi R, Manome T, Watanabe A, Kumashiro H: Plasma free 3-methoxy-4-hydroxyphenylglycol in acute schizophrenics before and after treatment. Neuropsychobiology 1992;25:126–129.

Karege F, Bovier P, Hilleret H, Gaillard JM, Tissot R: Adrenaline-induced platelet aggregation in depressed patients and control subjects. Neuropsychobiology 1993;27:21–25.

Kawahara Y, Kawahara H, Westerink BH: Tonic regulation of the activity of noradrenergic neurons in the locus coeruleus of the conscious rat studied by dual-probe microdialysis. Brain Res 1999;823:42–48.

Keell SD, Chambers JS, Francis DP, Edwards DF, Stables RH: Shuttle-walk test to assess chronic heart failure. Lancet 1998;352:705.

Kellner M, Yassouridis A, Manz B, Steiger A, Holsboer F, Wiedemann K: Corticotropin-releasing hormone inhibits melatonin secretion in healthy volunteers: A pontential link to low-melatonin syndrome in depression? Neuroendocrinology 1997;65:284–290.

Kennett GA, Joseph MH: Stress induced increases in 5HT release, measured in vivo, depend upon increased tryptophan availability. Neurosci Lett 1981;7:S56.

Key B, Krzywosinski L: Electrocortical changes induce by the perfusion of noradrenaline, acetylcholine and their antagonists directly into the dorsal raphe nucleus of the cat. Br J Pharmacol 1977;61:297–305.

Kiianmaa K, Fuxe K: The effects of 5,7-DHT-induced lesions of the ascending 5-HT pathways on the sleep wakefulness cycle. Brain Res 1977;131:287–301.

Kinney GG, Vogel GW, Feng P: Decreased dorsal raphe nucleus neuronal activity in adult chloral hydrate anesthetized rats following neonatal clomipramine treatment: Implications for endogenous depression. Brain Res 1997;756:68–75.

Ko GN, Elsworth JD, Roth RH, Rifkin BG, Leigh H, Redmond DE: Panic-induced elevation of plasma MHPG in phobic-anxious patients: Effects of clonidine or imipramine. Arch Gen Psychiatry 1983;40:425–430.

Ko HC, LU RB, Shiah IS, Hwang CC: Plasma free 3-methoxy-4-hydroxyphenylglycol predicts response to fluoxetine. Biol Psychiatry 1997;41:774–781.

Koek RJ, Yerevanian BI, Tachiki KH, Smith JC, Alcock J, Kopelowicz A: Hemispheric asymmetry in depression and mania: A longitudinal QEEG study in bipolar disorder. J Affect Dis 1999;53:109–122.

Koh KB, Lee BK: Reduced lymphocyte proliferation and interleukin-2 production in anxiety disorders. Psychosom Med 1998;60:479–483.

Košnik M, Wraber B: Shift from Th2 to Th1 response in immunotheraphy with venoms. Eur J Physiol 2000;440:R71–R72.

Kostowski W, Jerlicz M, Bidzinski A, Hauptmann M: Evidence for existence of two opposite noradrenergic brain systems controlling behavior. Psychopharmacology 1978;59:311–312.

Kostowski W, Samanin R, Bareggi SR, Mark V, Garanttini S, Valzelli L Biochemical aspects of the interaction between midbrain raphe and locus coeruleus in the rat. Brain Res 1974;82:178–182.

Kostowski W: Interactions between Serotonergic and catecholaminergic systems in the brain. Pol J Pharmacol Pharmac 1975;27:15–24.

Kostowski W: Two noradrenergic systems in the brain and their interactions with other monoaminergic neurons. Pol J Pharmacol Pharma 1979;31:425–436.

Kraemer GW, Ebert MH, Lake CR, McKinney WT: Cerebrospinal fluid measures of neurotransmitter changes associated with pharmacological alteration of the despair response to social separation in rhesus monkeys. Psychiatr Res 1984:11:303–315.

Kulkarni A, Jan Ravi MD T, Brodmerkel GJ, Agrawal R: Inflammatory myositis in association with inflammatory bowel disease. Dig Dis Sci 1997;42:1142–1145.

Lai YY, Clements JR, Wu XY, Shalita T, Wu JP, Kuo JS, Siegel JM: Brainstem projections to the ventromedial medulla in cat: Retrograde transport horseradish peroxidase and immunohistochemical studies. J Comp Neurol 1999;408:419–436.

Lake CR, Pickar D, Ziegler MG, Lipper S, Slater S, Murphy DL: High plasma norepinephrine levels in patients with major affective disorders. Am J Psychiatry 1982;139:1315–1319.

Lake CR, Ziegler MG, Kopin IJ: Use of plasma norepinephrine for evaluation of sympathetic neuronal function in man. Life Sci 1976;18:1315–1321.

Lambert GW, Kaye DM, Thompson JM, Turner AG, Cox HS, Vaz M, Jennings GL, Walling BG, Esler MD: Internal jugular venous spillover of noradrenaline and metabolites and their association with sympathetic nervous activity. Acta Physiol Scand 1998;163:155–163.

Larsson PT, Hjemdahl P, Olsson G, Egberg N, Hornstra G: Altered platelet function during mental stress and adrenaline infusion in humans: Evidence for an increase aggregability in vivo as measured by filtragometry. Clin Sci 1989;76:369–376.

Lavielle S, Tassin JP, Thiery AM, Blanc G, Herve D, Barthelemy C, Glowinski J: Blockade by benzodiazepines of the selective high increase in dopamine turnover induced by stress in mesocortical dopaminergic neurons of the rat. Brain Res 1979;168:585–594.

Lechin AE, Varon J, van der Dijs B, Lechin F: Plasma cathecholamines and indoleamines during attacks and remission on severe bronchial asthma: possible role of stress. Am J Respir Crit Care Med 1994;149:A778.

Lechin F, van der Dijs B: Clonidine therapy for psychosis and tardive dyskinesia. Am J Psychiatry 1981;138:390.

Lechin F, van der Dijs B, Benaim M: Benzodiazepines: Tolerability in elderly patients. Psychother Psychosom 1996;65:171–182.

Lechin F, van der Dijs B, Amat J, Lechin M: Central neuronal pathways involved in psychotic syndromes; in Lechin F, van der Dijs B (eds): Neurochemistry and Clinical Disorders of Some Psychiatric and Psychosomatic Syndromes. Boca Raton, CRC Press, 1989, pp 91–120.

Lechin F, van der Dijs B, Cabrera A, Jimenez V, Guerrero H, Lechin AE: Plasma neurotransmitters profile in depressive syndromes. Arch Ven Farm Clin Terap 1988;7(suppl 1):abstr 7.

Lechin F, van der Dijs B, Orozco B, Lechin AE, Baez S, Lechin ME, Rada I, Acosta E, Arocha L, Jimenez V, Leon G, Garcia Z: Plasma neurotransmitters, blood pressure, and heart rate during supine resting, orthostasis, and moderate exercise in dysthymic depressed patients. Biol Psychiatry 1995;37:884–891.

Lechin F, van der Dijs B, Orozco B, Lechin ME, Baez S, Lechin AE, Rada I, Acosta E, Arocha L, Jimenez V, Leon G, Garcia Z: Plasma neurotransmitters, blood pressure, and heart rate during supine-resting, orthostasis, and moderate exercise conditions in major depressed patients. Biol Psychiatry 1995;38:166–173.

Lechin F, van der Dijs B: Noradrenergic or dopaminergic activity in chronic schizophrenia? Br J Psychiatry 1981;139:472–473.

Leger L, McRae-Deguerce A, Pujol JE: Origine de l'innervation serotoninergique du locus coeruleus chez le rat. CR Acad Sci 1980;290:807–810.

Lindbrink P: The effect of lesions of ascending noradrenaline pathways on sleep and waking in the rat. Brain Res 1974;74:19–40.

Lindvall O, Bjorklund A: Organization of catecholamine neurons in the rat central nervous systems. Chemical pathways in the brain; in Iversen LL, Iversen SD, Snyder SH (eds): Handbook of Psychopharmacology. New York, Plenum Press, 1978, pp 139–122.

Lipowski ZJ: Somatization and depression. Psychosomatics 1990;31:13–20.

Lloyd KG, Farley IJ, Deck JHN, Hornykiewicz O: Serotonin and 5-hydroxyindoleacetic acid in discrete areas of the brainstem of suicide victims and control patients; in Costa E, Gessa GL, Sandler M (eds): Advances in Biochemical Pharmacology. New York, Raven Press, 1974, pp 387–397.

Maas JW, Dekirmenjian H, DeLeon JF: The identification of depressed patients who have a disorder of norepinephrine metabolism and/or disposition; in Usdin E, Snyder SH (eds): Frontiers in Catecholamine Research. New York, Pergamon Press, 1974, pp 1091–1096.

Maas JW: Biogenic amines and depression: Biochemical and pharmacological separation of two types of depression. Arch Gen Psychiatry 1975;32:1357–1361.

Maccarley RW: REM sleep and depression: common neurobiological control mechanisms. Am J Psychiatry 1982;139:5–13.

Madden KS, Felten SY, Felten DY, Sundaresan RL, Liunat S: Sympathetic neural modulation of the immune system. I. Depression of T-cell immunity in vivo and in vitro following chemical sympathectomy. Brain Behav Immun 1989;3:72–89.

Maes M, Scharpé S, Verkerk R, D'Hondt P, Peeters D, Cosyns P, Thompson P, De Meyer F, Wauters A, Neels H: Seasonal variation in plasma l-tryptophan availability in healthy volunteers. Arch Gen Psychiatry 1995;52:937–946.

Maes M, Vandoolaeghe E, Ranjan R, Bosmans E, Van Gastel A, Bergmans R, Desnyder R: Increased serum soluble CD8 or suppressor/cytotoxic antigen concentrations in depression: Suppressive effects of glucocorticoids. Biol Psychiatry 1996;40:1273–1281.

Maran JW, Carlson DE, Grizzlw WE, Ward GE, Gann DS: Organization of the medial hypothalamus for control of adrenocorticotropin in the cat. Endocrinology 1978;103:957–970.

Marazziti D, Ambrogi F, Venacore R, Mignani V, Savino M, Palego L, Cassano GB, Akiskal HS: Immune cell imbalance in major depressive and panic disorders. Neuropsychobiology 1992;26:23–26.

Martí O, Martí J, Armario A: Effects of chronic stress on food intake in rats: influence of stressor intensity and duration of daily exposure. Physiol Behav 1994;55:747–753.

Martinez V, Rivier J, Wang L, Taché Y: Central injection of a new corticotropin-releasing factor (CFR) antagonist, astressin, blocks CRF- and stress-related alterations of gastric and colonic motor function. J Pharmacol Exp Ther 1997;280:754–760.

Mason ST: Noradrenaline and selective attention: A review of the model and the evidence. Life Sci 1980;27:617–631.

Mathé JM, Nomikos GG, Hildebrand BE, Hertel P, Svensson TH: Prazosin inhibits MK-801-induced hyperlocomotion and dopamine release in the nucleus accumbens. Eur J Pharmacol 1996;309:1–11.

Matthews J, Akil H, Greden J, Charney D, Weinberg V, Rosenbaum A, Watson SJ: β-Endorphin/β-lipotropin immunoreactivity in endogenous depression. Arch Gen Psychiatry 1986;43:374–381.

McCall RB, Harris LT: 5-HT$_2$ receptor agonists increase spontaneous sympathetic nerve discharge. Eur J Pharmacol 1988;151:113–116.

McGinty DJ, Harper RM: Dorsal raphe neurons: Depression of firing during sleep in cats. Brain Res 1976;101:569–875.

McRae-Deguerce A, Milton H: Serotonin and dopamine afferents to the rat locus coeruleus: A biochemical study after lesioning of the ventral mesencephalic tegmental A10 region and the raphe dorsalis. Brain Res 1983;263:344–347.

Meeusen R, Thorré K, Chaouloff F, Sarre S, De Meirleir K, Ebinger G, Michotte Y: Effects of tryptophan and/or acute running on extracellular 5-HT and 5-HIAA levels in the hippocampus of food-deprived rats. Brain Res 1996;740:245–252.

Mendlovic S, Mozes E, Eilat E, Doron A, Lereya J, Zakuth V, Spirer Z: Immune activation in nontreated suicidal major depression. Immunol Lett 1999;67:105–108.

Milon H, McRae-Degueurce A: Pharmacological investigation on the role of dopamine in the rat locus coeruleus. Neurosci Lett 1982;30:297–301.

Mongeau R, Blier P, de Montigny C: The serotonergic and noradrenergic systems of the hippocampus: Their interactions and the effects of antidepressant treatments. Brain Res Rev 1997;23:145–195.

Moore H, West AR, Grace AA: The regulation of forebrain dopamine transmission: Relevance to the pathophysiology and psychopathology of schizophrenia. Biol Psychiatry 1999;46:40–55.

Moore KE, Kelly PH: Biochemical pharmacology of mesolimbic and mesocortical dopaminergic neurons; in Lipton MA, DiMascio A, Killam KF (eds): Psychopharmacology: A Generation of Progress. New York, Raven Press, 1978, pp 221–234.

Moore RY, Halaris AE, Jones BE: Serotonin neurons of the midbrain raphe: ascending projections. J Comp Neurol 1978;180:417–438.

Morley JE, Raleigh MJ, Brammer GL, Yuwiler A, Geller E, Flannery J, Hershman JM: Serotonergic and catecholaminergic influence on thyroid function in the vervet monkey. Eur J Pharmacol 1980;67:283–288.

Moroni F: Tryptophan metabolism and brain function: Focus on kynurenine and other indole metabolites. Eur J Pharmacol 1999;375:87–100.

Mosko SS, Haubrich K, Jacobs BL: Serotonergic afferents to the dorsal raphe nucleus: Evidence from HRP and synaptosomal uptake studies. Brain Res 1977;119:269–290.

Müller N, Ackenheil M, Hofschuster E, Mempel W, Eckstein R: Cellular immunity in schizophrenic patients before and during neuroleptic treatment. Psychiatr Res 1991;37:147–160.

Murphy DL, Campbell IC, Costa JL: The brain serotonergic system in the effective disorders. Prog Neuropsychopharmacol 1978;2:1–31.

Musselman DL, Tomer A, Manatunga AK, Knight BT, Porter MR, Kasey S, Marzec U, Harker LA, Nemeroff CB: Exaggerated platelet reactivity in major depression. Am J Psychiatry 1996;153:1313–1317.

Nagata T, Kiriike N, Tobitani W, Kawarada Y, Matsunaga H, Yamagami S: Lymphocyte subset, lymphocyte proliferative response, and soluble interleukin-2 receptor in anorexic patients. Biol Psychiatry 1999;45:471–474.

Natelson BH, Denny T, Zhou X-D, LaManca JJ, Ottenweller JE, Tiersky L, DeLuca J, Gause WC: Is depression associated with immune activation? J Affect Disord 1999;53:179–186.

Nishijima K, Kashiwa A, Nishikawa T: Preferential stimulation of extracellular release of dopamine in rat frontal cortex to striatum following competitive inhibition of the N-methyl-d-aspartate receptor. J Neurochem 1994;63:375–378.

Nishikawa T, Scatton B: Inhibitory influence of GABA on central serotonergic transmission: Raphe nuclei as the neuroanatomical site of the GABAergic inhibition of cerebral serotonergic neurons. Brain Res 1985;331:91–103.

Nörenberg W, Schöffel E, Szabo B, Starke K: Subtype determination of soma-dendritc α$_2$-autoreceptors in slices of rat locus coeruleus. Arch Pharmacol 1997;356:159–165.

Obál F Jr, Kacsóh B, Bredow S, Guha-Thakurta N, Krueger JM: Sleep in rats rendered chronically hyperprolactinemic with anterior pituitary grafts. Brain Res 1997;755:130–136.

Ogren SO, Fuxe K, Agnati LF, Gustafsson JA, Johansson G, Holm AC: Reevaluation of the indoleamine hypothesis of depression: Evidence for a reduction of functional activity of central 5HT systems by antidepressant drugs. J Neural Transm 1979;46:85–103.

Okamoto S, Ibaraki K, Hayashi S, Saito M: Ventromedial hypothalamus suppresses splenic lymphocyte activity through sympathetic innervation. Brain Res 1996;739:308–313.

Ortiz J, Mocaër E, Artigas F: Effects of the antidepressant drug tianeptine on plasma and platelet serotonin concentrations in the rat. J Pharmacol 1991;199:335–339.

Ost RM, Ballenger JC, Goodwin FK: Cerebrospinal fluid studies on neurotransmitter function in manic and depressive illness; in Wood JH (ed): The Neurobiology of Cerebrospinal Fluid. New York, Plenum Press, 1980, pp 685–717.

Overton PG, Clark D: Burst firing in midbrain dopaminergic neurons. Brain Res Rev 1997; 25:312–334.

Palkovits M, Zaborsky L, Brownstein MJ, Fekete MIK, Herman JP, Kanycska B: Distribution of norepinephrine and dopamine in cerebral cortical areas of the rat. Brain Res Bull 1979;4: 593–601.

Pandey SC, Kim SW, Davis JM, Pandey GN: Platelet serotonin-2 receptors in obsessive-compulsive disorder. Biol Psychiatry 1993;33: 367–372.

Pare CM, Yeung DP, Price K, Stacey RS: 5-Hydroxytryptamine, noradrenaline and dopamine in brainstem, hypothalamus and caudate nucleus of controls and of patients commiting suicide by coal gas poisoning. Lancet 1969; ii:133–135.

Pasquier DA, Kemper TL, Forbes WB, Morgane PJ: Dorsal raphe, substantia nigra and locus coeruleus: Interconnections with each other and the neostriatum. Brain Res Bull 1977;2: 323–329.

Penit-Soria J, Eudinat E, Crepel F: Excitation of rat prefrontal cortical neurons by dopamine: An in vitro electrophysiological study. Brain Res 1987;425:263–274.

Petty F, Sherman AD: A neurochemical differentiation between exposure to stress and the development of learned helplessness. Drug Dev Res 1982;2:43–45.

Petty F, Sherman AD: Learned helplessness induction decreases in vivo cortical serotonin release. Pharmacol Biochem Behav 1983;18: 649–650.

Piñeyro G, Blier P: Autoregulation of serotonin neurons: Role in antidepressant drug action. Pharmacol Rev 1999;51:533–578.

Plaznik A, Danysz W, Kostowski W, Bidzinski A, Hauptmann M: Interaction between noradrenergic and serotonergic brain systems as evidenced by behavioral and biochemical effects of microinjections of adrenergic agonists and antagonists into the median raphe nucleus. Pharmacol Biochem Behav 1983;19:27–32.

Pop VJ, Maartens LH, Leusink G, Van Son MJ, Knottnerus AA, Ward AM, Metcalfe R, Weetman: Are autoimmune thyroid dysfunction and depression related? J Clin Endocrinol Metab 1998;83:3194–3197.

Post RM, Gordon EK, Goodwin FK: Central norepinephrine metabolism in affective illness: MHPG in the cerebrospinal fluid. Science 1973;179:1002–1003.

Pradalier A, Launay JM: Immunological aspects of migraine. Biomed Pharmacother 1996;50:64–70.

Printz DJ, Strauss DH, Goetz R, Sadiq S, Malaspina D, Krolewski J, Gorman JM: Elevation of CD5+B lymphocytes in schizophrenia. Biol Psychiatry 1999;46:110–118.

Przewlocka B, Kukulka L, Tarczynska E: The effect of lesions of dorsal or median raphe nucleus on rat behavior. Pol J Pharmac Pharm 1977;29: 573–579.

Pujol JF, Stein D, Blondaux Ch, Petitijean F, Frament JL, Jouvet M: Biochemical evidence for interation phenomena between noradrenergic and serotonergic system in the cat brain; in Usdin E, Snyder SH (eds): Frontiers in Catecholamine Research. New York, Pergamon Press, 1973, pp 771–772.

Pycock CJ, Carter CJ, Kerwin RW: Effect of 6-hydroxydopamine lesions of the medial prefrontal cortex on neurotransmitters systems in subcortical sites in the rat. J Neurochem 1980; 34:91–99.

Reinhard JF, Nannon MJ, Roth RH: Acceleration by stress of dopamine synthesis and metabolism in prefrontal cortex. Arch Pharmacol 1982;318:374–377.

Richter DW, Schmidt-Garcon P, Pierrefiche O, Bischoff AM, Lalley PM: Neurotransmitters and neuromodulators controlling the hypoxic respiratory response in anaesthetized cats. J Physiol 1999;514:567–578.

Romero L, Hervás I, Artigas F: The 5-HT1A antagonist WAY-100635 selectively potentiates the presynaptic effects of serotonergic antidepressants in rat brain. Neurosci Lett 1996;219:123–126.

Rosenbaum AH, Schatzberg AF, Maruta T, Orsualak PJ, Cole JO, Grab EL, Shildkraut JJ: MHPG as a predicter of antidepressant response to imipramine and maprotiline. Am J Psychiatry 1980;137:1090–1097.

Rothermundt M, Arolt V, Weitzsch C, Eckhoff D, Kirchner H: Immunological dysfunction in schizophrenia: A systematic approach. Neuropsychobiology 1998;37:186–193.

Roy A, Guthrie S, Pickar D, Linnoila M: Plasma norepinephrine responses to cold challenge in depressed patients and normal controls. Psychiatry Res 1987;21:161–168.

Roy A, Pickard D, Linnoila M, Doran AR, Paul SM: Cerebrospinal fluid monoamine and monoamine metabolite levels and the dexamethasone suppression test in depression. Arch Gen Psychiatry 1986;43:356–360.

Roy A: Suicidal behavior in depression: Relationship to platelet serotonin transporter. Neuropsychobiology 1999;39:71–75.

Rudorfer MV, Scheinin M, Karou F, Ross RJ, Potter WZ, Linnoila M: Reduction of norepinephrine turnover by serotonergic drug in man. Biol Psychiatry 1984;19:179–185.

Samanin R, Quattrone A, Consolo S, Ladinsky H, Algeri S: Biochemical and pharmacological evidence of the interaction of serotonin with other aminergic systems in the brain; in Garattini S, Pujol JF, Samanin R (eds): Interactions between Putative Neurotransmitters. New York, Raven Press, 1978, pp 355–368.

Schatzberg AF, Orsulak PJ, Rosenbaum AH, Maruta T, Kruger ER, Cole JO, Schildkraut JJ: Toward a biochemical classification of depressive disorders. V. Heterogeneity of unipolar depressions. Am J Psychiatry 1982;139:4–10.

Schatzberg AF: Classification of depressive disorders; in Cole JO, Schatzberg AF, Frazier SH (eds): Depression, Biology, Psychodynamics and Treatment. New York, Plenum Press, 1978, pp 13–40.

Schedlowsky M, Jacobs R, Alker J, Pröhl F, Stratmann G, Richter S, Hädicke A, Wagner TOF, Schmidt RE, Tewes U: Psychophysiological, neuroendocrine and cellular immune reactions under psychological stress. Neuropsychobiology 1993;28:87–90.

Scheel-Kruger J, Randrup A: Stereotyped hyperactive behavior produced by dopamine in the absence of noradrenaline. Life Sci 1967;6: 1389–1398.

Schildkraut JJ, Keeler BA, Papusek M: MHPG excretion in depressive disorders: Relation to clinical subtypes and desynchronized sleep. Science 1973;181:762–764.

Schildkraut JJ: Catecholamine metabolism and affective disorders; in Usdin E, Snyder SH (eds): Frontiers in Catecholamine Research. New York, Pergamon Press, 1974, pp 1165–1171.

Schildkraut JJ: Norepinephrine metabolites as biochemical criteria for classifying depressive disorders and predicting responses to treatment. Am J Psychiatry 1973;130:695–698.

Schildkraut JJ: The catecholamine hypothesis of affective disorders: A review of supporting evidence. Am J Psychiatry 1965;122:508–522.

Schmidt RH, Bjorklund A, Lindvall O, Loren I: Prefrontal cortex: dense dopaminergic input in the newborn rat. Dev Brain Res 1982;5:222–228.

Schutz MTB, Aguiar JC, Graeff FG: Anti-aversive role of serotonin in the dorsal periaqueductal gray matter. Psychopharmacology 1985;85: 340–345.

Shaw DM, O'Keefe R, MacSweeney DA: 3-Methoxy-4-hydroxyphenylglycol in depression. Psychol Med 1973;3:333–336.

Sherman AD, Petty F: Neurochemical basis of the action of antidepressants on learned helplessness. Behav Neural Biol 1980;30:119–134.

Sheu YS, Nelson JP, Bloom FE: Discharge patterns of cat raphe neurons during sleep and waking. Brain Res 1974;73:263–276.

Shopsin B, Wilk S, Gershon S: Cerebrospinal fluid MHPG: An assessment of norepinephrine metabolism in affective disorders. Arch Gen Psychiatry 1973;28:230–233.

Sim LJ, Joseph SA: Efferent projections of the nucleus raphe magnus. Brain Res Bull 1992;28: 679–682.

Simon H, LeMoal M, Stinus L, Calas A: Anatomical relationships between the ventral mesencephalic tegmentum-A10 region and the locus coeruleus as demostrated by anterograde and retrograde tracing techniques. J Neural Transm 1979;44:77–86.

Simon H, Scatton B, LeMoal M: Dopaminergic A10 neurons are involved in cognitive functions. Nature 1980;286:150–151.

Sinha AK, Henticksen S, Dement WC, Barchas JD: Cat brain amine content during sleep. Am J Physiol 1973;224:381–383.

Sladek J, Walker P: Serotonin-containing neuronal perikarya in the primate locus coeruleus and subcoeruleus nuclei. Brain Res 1977;134:359–366.

Slopsema JS, Van der Gugten J, Bruin JPC: Regional concentrations of noradrenaline and dopamine in the frontal cortex of the rat: Dopaminergic innervation of the prefrontal subareas and lateralization of prefrontal dopamine. Brain Res 1982;250:197–200.

Smee ML, Weston PF, Kinner DS, Day T: Dose-related effects of central noradrenaline stimulation of behavioural arousal in rats. Psychopharmacol Commun 1975;1:123–130.

Souêtre E, Candito M, Salvati E, Pringuey D, Chambon P, Darcourt G: 24-Hour profile of plasma norepinephrine in affective disorders. Neuropsychobiology 1986;16:1–8.

Sourkes TL: Neurotransmitters and central regulation of adrenal functions. Biol Psychiatry 1985;20:182–191.

Stamford JA, Mucat R, O'Connor JJ, Patel J, Trout SP, Wieczorek WJ, Kruk ZL, Willner P: Voltammetric evidence that subsensitivity to reward following chronic mild stress is associated with increased release of mesolimbic dopamine. Psychopharmacology 1991;105:275–282.

Steiger A, Guldner J, Colla-Müller M, Friess E, Sonntag A, Schier T: Growth hormone-releasing hormone (GHRH)-induced effects on sleep EEG and nocturnal secretion of growth hormone, cortisol and ACTH in patients with major depression. J Psychiatr Res 1994;28:225–238.

Stein L, Wise DC: Serotonin and behavioral inhibition; in Costa E, Gessa GL, Sandler M (eds): Serotonin – New Vistas. New York, Raven Press, 1974, pp 281–292.

Stein L, Wise DC, Belluzi JD: Effects of benzodiazepines on central serotonergic mechanisms; in Costa E, Greengard P (eds): Mechanism of Action of Benzodiazepines. New York, Raven Press, 1975, pp 29–44.

Steplewski Z, Vogel WH, Ehya H, Poropatich C, McDonald-Smith J: Effects of restraint stress or inoculated tumor growth and immune response in rats. Cancer Res 1985;45:5128–5133.

Storm-Mathisen J, Goldberg HC: 5-hydroxytryptamine and noradrenaline in the hippocampal region: Effect of transection of afferent pathways on endogenous levels, high affinity uptake and some transmitter-related enzymes. J Neurochem 1974;22:793–803.

Swanson LW: The projections of the ventral tegmental area and adjacent regions: A combined fluorescent retrograde and immuno-fluorescense study in the rat. Brain Res Bull 1982;9:321–354.

Syvalahti E, Eskola J, Ruuskanen O, Laine T: Non-suppression of cortisol in depression and immune function. Prog Neuro-Psychopharmacol Biol Psychiatry 1985;9:413–422.

Takahata R, Moghaddam B: Target-specific glutamatergic regulation of dopamine neurons in the ventral tegmental area. J Neurochem 2000; 75:1775–1778.

Tassin JP, Stinus J, Simon H, Blanc G, Thierry AM, LeMoal H Cardo B, Glowinski J: Relationship between the locomotor activity induced by A10 lesions and the destruction of the fronto-cortico dopaminergic innervation in the rat. Brain Res 1978;141:267–281.

Thase ME, Kupfer DJ, Fasiczka AJ, Buysse DJ, Simons AD, Frank E: Identifying an abnormal electroencephalographic sleep profile to characterize major depressive disorder. Biol Psychiatry 1997;41:964–973.

Thiel A, Dressler D, Reimer A, Rother E: Effects of clozapine on CSF homovanillic acid in spasmodic torticollis. J Neural Transm (Gen Sect) 1994;97:245–251.

Thierry AM, Tassin JP, Blanc G, Glowinski J: Selective activation of the mesocortical dopaminergic system by stress. Nature 1976;263:242–244.

Toner BB, Stuckless N, Ali A, Downe F, Emmott S, Akman D: The development of a cognitive scale for functional bowel disorders. Psychosom Med 1998;60:492–497.

Traskman L, Asberg M, Bertilsson L, Sjostrand L: Monoamine metabolites in CSF and suicidal behaviour. Arch Gen Psychiatry 1981;38:631–636.

Trimbach C: Hippocampal modulation of behavioral arousal: Mediation by serotonin; Dissertation, Princeton University, 1972.

Trulson ME, Crisp T: Role of norepinephrine in regulating the activity of serotonin-containing dorsal raphe neurons. Life Sci 1984;35:511–515.

Trulson ME, Jacobs BL: Activity of serotonin-containing neurons in freely moving cats; in Jacobs BL, Gelperin A (eds): Serotonin Neurotransmission and Behavior. Cambridge, MIT Press, 1981, pp 339–402.

Trulson ME, Jacobs BL: Raphe unit activity in freely moving cats: correlation with level of behavioral arousal. Brain Res 1979;163:135–142.

Trulson ME, Crisp T, Howell GA: Raphe unit activity in freely moving cats: Effects of quipazine. Neuropharmacology 1982;21:681–686.

Trulson ME, Jacobs BL, Morrison AR: Raphe unit activity across the sleep-waking cycle in normal cats and in pontine lesioned cats diplaying REM sleep without atonia. Brain Res 1981; 226:75–91.

Trulson ME, Preussler DW, Howell GA, Frederickson CJ: Raphe unit activity in freely moving cats: Effects of benzodiazepines. Neuropharmacology 1982;21:1045–1050.

Van Dogen P: Locus coeruleus region: effects on behavior of cholinergic, noradrenergic, and opiate drugs injected intracerebrally into freely moving cats. Exp Neurol 1980;67:52–78.

Van Loon GR, Shum A, Sole MJ: Decreased brain serotonin turnover after short-term (two-hour) adrenalectomy in rats: A comparison of four hour turnover methods. Endocrinology 1981; 108:1392–1402.

Van Praag HM: Central monoamine metabolism in depression. Compreh Psychiatry 1980;21:30–43.

Vandermaelen CP, Aghajanian GK: Noradrenergic activation of serotonergic dorsal raphe neurons recorded in vitro. Soc Neurosci Abstr 1982;8:482.

Vertes RP, Fortin WJ, Crane AM: Projections of the raphe nucleus in the rat. J Comp Neurol 1999;407:555–582.

Vestergaard P, Sorensen T, Hoppe E, Rafaelsen OJ, Yates CM, Nicolaou N: Biogenic amine metabolites in cerebrospinal fluid of patients with affective disorders. Acta Psychiatr Scand 1978; 58:88–96.

Waldbilig RJ: The role of the dorsal raphe and median raphe in the inhibition of muricide. Brain Res 1979;160:341–346.

Waldmeier PC: Serotonergic modulation of mesolimbic and frontal cortical dopamine neurons. Experientia 1980;36:1092–1094.

Wang QP, Ochiai H, Nakai Y: GABAergic innervation of serotonergic neurons in the dorsal raphe nucleus of the rat studied by electron microscopy double immunostaining. Brain Res Bull 1992;29:943–948.

Wang RY: Dopaminergic neurons in the rat ventral tegmental area. Brain Res Rev 1981;3:152–165.

Watkins LL, Grossman P, Krishnan R, Sherwood A: Anxiety and vagal control of heart rate. Psychosom Med 1998;60:498–502.

Weiss JM, Goodman PA, Losito PG, Corrigan S, Charry JM, Bailey WH: Behavioral depression produced by an uncontrollable stressor relationship to norepinephrine, dopamine and serotonin levels in various region of rat brain. Brain Res Rev 1981;3:167–205.

Weiss JM, Stout JC, Aaron MF, Quan N, Owens MJ, Butler PD, Nemeroff CB: Depression and axiety: Role of the locus coeruleus and corticotropin-releasing factor. Brain Res Bull 1994;35:561–572.

Whitnall MH, Regulation of the hypothalamic corticotropin-releasing hormone neurosecretrory system: Prog Neurobiol 1993;40:573–629.

Wiklund L: Studies on anatomical, functional, and plastic properties of central serotonergic neurons; Diss, Department of Histology, Lund, 1980.

Wilde MI, Benfield P: Tianeptine: A review of its pharmacodynamic and pharmacokinetic properties, and therapeutic efficacy in depression and coexisting anxiety and depression. Drugs 1995;49:411–439.

Yadid G, Nakash R, Dery Ilana, Tamar G, Kinor N, Gispan I, Zangen A: Elucidation of the neurobiology of depression: Insights from a novel genetic animal model. Prog Neurobiol 2000; 62:353–378.

Yamamoto T, Watanabe T, Shibata S, Ueki S: The effect of locus coeruleus and midbrain raphe stimulation on muricide in rats. Jpn J Pharmacol 1979;29:41–50.

Yavari P, Vogel GW, Neill DB: Decreased raphe unit activity in a rat model of endogenous depression. Brain Res 1993;611:31–36.

Yeragani V, Balon R, Pohl R, Ramesh C: Depression and heart rate variability. Biol Psychiatry 1995;38:768–770.

Young LT, Robb JC, Levitt AJ, Cooke RG, Joffe RT: Serum Mg^{2+} and Ca^{2+}/Mg^{2+} ratio in major depressive disorder. Neuropsychobiology 1996;34:26–28.

Yusof APM, Coote J: Patterns of activity in sympathetic postganglionic nerves to skeletal muscle, skin and kidney during stimulation of the medullary raphe area of the rat. J Autonom Nerv Syst 1988;24:71–79.

Zheng Y, Riche D, Rekling JC, Foutz AS, Denavit-Saubié M: Brainstem neurons projecting to the rostral ventral respiratory group (VRG) in the medulla oblongata of the rat revealed by co-application of NMDA and biocytin. Brain Res 1998;782:113–125.

Ziegler MG, Lake CR, Wood JH, Ebert MH: Norepinephrine in cerebro-spinal fluid: basic studies, effects of drugs and diseases; in Wood JH (ed): Neurobiology of Cerebrospinal Fluid. New York, Plenum Press, 1979, pp 141–156.

References for Chapter 5

Aberg-Wisted A, Ross SB, Jostell KG, Sjoquist B: A double-blind study of zimelidine, a serotonin uptake inhibitor, and desipramine, a noradrenaline uptake inhibitor, in endogenous depression. II. Biochemical findings. Acta Psychiatr Scand 1982;66:66–82.

Andreoli A, Keller SE, Rabaeus M, Zaugg L, Garrone G, Taban C: Immunity, major depression, and panic disorder comorbidity. Biol Psychiatry 1992;31:896–908.

Anisman H: Neurochemical changes elicited by stress; in Anisman H, Bignami G (eds): Psychopharmacology of Aversively Motivated Behavior. New York, Plenum Press, 1978, pp 19–172.

Anisman H, Irwin J, Sklar LS: Deficits of escape performance following catecholamine depletion: Implications or behavior deficits induced by uncontrollable stress. Psychopharmacology 1979;64:163–170.

Anisman H, Pizzino A, Sklar LS: Coping with stress, norepinephrine depletion and escape performance. Brain Res 1980;191:583–588.

Anisman H, Ritch M, Sklar LS: Noradrenergic and dopaminergic interactions in escape behavior: Analysis of uncontrollable stress effects. Psychopharmacology 1981;64:263–268.

Anisman H, Sklar LS: Catecholamine depletion in mice upon re-exposure to stress: Mediation of the escape deficits produced by inescapable shock. J Comp Physiol 1979;93:610–625.

Anisman H, Suissa A, Sklar LS: Escape deficits produced by uncontrollable stress: antagonism by dopamine and norepinephrine agonists. Behav Neurol Biol 1980;28:34–47.

Anisman H, Zacharko RM: Depression: The predisposing influence of stress. Behav Brain Sci 1982;5:89–137.

Aprison MH, Hingtgen JN: Hypersensitive serotonergic receptors: A new hypothesis for one subgroup of unipolar depression derived from an animal model; in Haber B, Gabay S, Issidorides MR, Alivisatos SGA (eds): Serotonin: Current Aspects of Neurochemistry and Function. New York, Plenum Press, 1981, pp 627–656.

Aprison MH, Hingtgen JN, Nagayama M: Testing a new theory of depression with an animal model: Neurochemical-behavioural evidence for postsynaptic serotonergic receptor involvement; in Langer S, Takahashi R, Segawa T, Briley M (eds): New Vistas in Depression. New York, Pergamon Press, 1982, pp 171–178.

Ardlie NG, Cameron HA, Garreu J: Platelet activation by circulating levels of hormones: A possible link in coronary heart disease. Thromb Res 1984;36:315–321.

Azorin JM, Karege F, Malli M, Pringuey D, Joanny P, Tissot R: Plasma 3,4-di-hydrophenylethyleneglycol and 3-methoxy-4-hydroxy phenylethylene glycol as indicators of central noradrenergic activity: A comparative study on control subjects and depressed patients. Neuropsychobiology 1988;20:67–73.

Banki CM, Molnar G, Vojnik M: Cerebrospinal fluid amine metabolites, tryptophan and clinical parameters in depression: Psychopathological symptoms. J Affect Dis 1991;3:91–109.

Baldessarini RJ: Treatment of depression by altering monoamine metabolism: Precursors and metabolic inhibitors. Psychopharmacol Bull 1984;20:224–239.

Baraban FM, Aghajanian GK: Suppression of firing activity of 5-HT neurons in the dorsal raphe by alpha-adrenoceptor antagonist. Neuropharmacology 1980;19:355–363.

Benarroch EE, Balda MS, Finkelman S, Nahmod E: Neurogenic hypertension after depletion of norepinephrine in anterior hypothalamus induced by 6-hydroxydopamine administration into the ventral pons: Role of serotonin. Neuropharmacology 1983;22:29–34.

Benfield P, Heel RC, Lewis SP: Fluoxetine: A review of its pharmacodynamic and pharmacokinetic properties, and therapeutic effects during depressive illness. Drugs 1986;32:481–508.

Berger M, Doerr P, Lund R, Bronisch T, Von Zerssen D: Neuroendocrinological and neurophysiological studies in major depressive disorders: Are there biological markers for the endogenous subtype? Biol Psychiatry 1982;17:1217–1242.

Blackard W, Heidingsfelder S: Adrenergic receptor control mechanism for growth hormone secretion. J Clin Invest 1968;47:1407–1414.

Bower MB: Cerebrospinal fluid 5-hydroxyindoleacetic acid (5-HIAA) and homovanillic acid (HVA) following probenecid in unipolar depressives treated with amitriptyline. Psychopharmacology 1972;23:26–33.

Breier A, Albus M, Pickar D, Zahn TP, Wolkowitz OM, Paul SM: Controllable and uncontrollable stress in humans: Alterations in mood and neuroendocrine and psychophysiological function. Am J Psychiatry 1987;144:1419–1425.

Burchfield SR: The stress response: A new perspective. Psychosom Med 1979;41:661–672.

Cabib S, Kempf E, Schleef C, Oliveiro A, Puglisi-Allegra S: Effects of immobilization stress on dopamine and its metabolites in different brain areas of the mouse: Role of genotype and stress duration. Brain Res 1988;441:153–160.

Cabrera A, van der Dijs B, Jimenez V, Guerrero H, Lechin F: Plasma neurotransmitters profile in normal subjects. III Interamerican Congress of Clinical Pharmacology and Therapeutics. Arch Ven Farm Terap 1988;7(suppl 1):abstr 107.

Caramona MM, Soares Da Silva P: The effects of chemical sympathectomy on dopamine, noradrenaline and adrenaline content in some peripheral tissues. Br J Pharmacol 1985;86:351–356.

Carrol BJ: Neuroendocrine diagnosis of depression: the dexamethasone suppression test; in Clayton PJ, Barret J (eds): Treatment of Depression: Old Controversies and New Approaches. New York, Raven Press, 1982.

Charney DS, Heninger GR, Sternberg DE, Hafstad KM, Giddings S, Lancis DH: Adrenergic receptor sensitivity in depression: Effects of clonidine in depressed patients and healthy subjects. Arch Gen Psychiatry 1982;39:290–294.

Checkley SA, Slade AP, Shur E: Growth hormone and other responses to clonidine in patients with endogenous depression. Br J Psychiatry 1981;138:51–55.

Civeira J, Cervera S, Giner J: Moclobemide versus clomipramine in the treatment of depression: A multicentre trial in Spain. Acta Psychiatr Scand 1990;82(suppl 360):48–49.

Clement-Jewery S: The development of cortical beta-adrenoceptor subsensitivity in the rat by chronic treatment with trazodone, doxepin and mianserine. Neuropharmacology 1978;17: 779–781.

Croiset G, Heijnen CJ, Veldhuis HD, De Wied D, Ballieux RE: Modulation of the immune response by emotional stress. Life Sci 1987;40: 775–782.

Cross RJ, Roszman TL: Central catecholamine depletion impairs in vivo immunity but not in vitro lymphocyte activation. J Neuroimmunol 1988;19:33–45.

Dantzer R, Kelley KW: Stress and immunity: An integrated view of relationships between the brain and the immune system. Life Sci 1989; 44:1995–2008.

Darko DF, Lucas AH, Gillin JC, Risch SC, Golshan S., Hamburger RN, Silverman MB, Janowsky DS: Age, cellular immunity and the HP axis in major depression. Prog Neuro-Psychopharmacol Biol Psychiatry 1988;12:713–720.

Davies KL, Hollister LE, Mathe AA, Davis BM, Rothpearl AB, Faull K, Hsieh JYK, Barchas JD, Berger PA: Neuroendocrine and neurochemical measurements in depression. Am J Psychiatry 1981;38:1555–1562.

Day TA, Willoughby JO: Noradrenergic afferent to median eminence: Inhibitory role in the rhythmic growth hormone secretion. Brain Res 1980;202:335–345.

De Boer SF, Koopmans SJ, Slangen JL, van der Gugten J: Plasma catecholamines, corticosterone and glucose responses to repeated stress in rats: effects of interstressor interval length. Physiol Behav 1990;47:1117–1124.

Delbende C, Contesse V, Mocaer E, Kamoun A, Vaudry H: The novel antidepressant, tianeptine, reduces stress-evoked stimulation of the hypothalamo-pituitary-adrenal axis. Eur J Pharmacol 1991;202:391–396.

DeMontigny C, Blier P: Effects of antidepressant treatments on 5HT neurotransmission: Electrophysiological and clinical studies. Adv Biol Psychiatry 1984;39:223–239.

Dilsaver SC, Coffman JA: Cholinergic hypothesis of depression: A reappraisal. J Clin Pharmacol 1989;9:173–179.

Dimsdale JE, Moss J: Plasma catecholamines in stress and exercise. JAMA 1980;243:340–345.

Dunn AJ: Stress-related changes in cerebral catecholamine and indoleamine metabolism: Lack of effect of adrenalectomy and corticosterone. J Neurochem 1988a;51:406–412.

Dunn AJ: Changes in plasma and brain tryptophan, and brain serotonin and 5-hydroxyindoleacetic acid after footshock stress. Life Sci 1988b;42:1847–1853.

Eden S, Bolle P, Modigh K: Monoaminergic control of episodic growth hormone secretion in the rat: Effects of reserpine, alpha-methyl-p-tyrosine, p-chlorophenylalanine and haloperidol. Endocrinology 1979;105:523–529.

Ellsworth JD, Redmond DE, Roth RH: Plasma and cerebrospinal fluid 3-methoxy-4-hydroxyphenylethylene glycol (MHPG) as indices of brain norepinephrine metabolism in primates. Brain Res 1982;235:115–124.

Eriksson E, Eden B, Modigh K: Up- and down-regulation of central postsynaptic alpha$_2$-receptors reflected in the growth hormone response to clonidine in reserpine pretreated rats. Psychopharmacology 1982;77:327–331.

Fuxe K, Anderson K, Eneroth P, Siegel R, Agnati LF: Immobilization stress-induced changes in discrete catecholamine levels and turnover, their modulation by nicotine and relationship to neuroendocrine function. Acta Physiol Scand 1983;117:421–426.

Fuxe K, Ogren SO, Agnati LF, Calza L: Evidence for stabilization of cortical 5HT neurotransmission by chronic treatment with antidepressant drugs: Induction of a high and low affinity component in 3H-5HT binding sites. Acta Physiol Scand 1982;114:477–480.

Fuxe K, Ogren SO, Agnati LF, Eneroth P, Holm AC, Andersson K: Long-term treatment with zimelidine leads to a reduction in 5-hydroxytryptamine neurotransmission within central nervous system of the mouse and rat. Neurosci Lett 1981;21:57–62.

Fuxe K, Ogren SO, Agnati L, Gustafsson JA, Jonsson G: On the mechanisms of action of the antidepressant drugs amitriptyline and nortriptyline: Evidence for 5-hydroxytryptamine receptor blocking activity. Neurosci Lett 1977;6: 339–343.

Gamallo A, Villanua A, Trancho G, Fraile A: Stress adaptation and adrenal activity in isolated and crowded rats. Physiol Behav 1986;36:217–221.

Geerts S, Bruynooghe F, De Cuyper H: Moclobemide versus fluoxetine for major depressive episodes. Clin Neuropharmacol 1994;17(suppl 1):14.

Gibbons RD, Davis JM: Consistent evidence for a biological subtype of depression characterized by low CSF-5-HIAA monoamine levels. Acta Psychiatr Scand 1986;74:8–12.

Gomez F, Lechin AE, Jara H, Jimenez V, Cabrera A, Guerrero H, van der Dijs B, Lechin F: Plasma neurotransmitters in anxiety patients. Proceedings of the III Interamerican Congress of Clinical Pharmacological and Therapeutics. Arch Ven Farm Terap 1988;7(suppl 1):abstr 4.

Glavin GB: Selective noradrenaline depletion markedly alters stress responses in rats. Life Sci 1985;37:461–465.

Guelfi JD, Payan C, Fermanian J: Moclobemide versus clomipramine in endogenous depression: A double-blind randomized clinical trial. Br J Psychiatry 1992;160:519–524.

Haft Jl, Arkel YS: Effect of emotional stress on platelet aggregation in humans. Chest 1976;70: 501–506.

Heinsbroek RPW, Van Haaren F, Feenstra MGP, Boon P, van de Poll NE: Controllable and uncontrollable footshock and monoaminergic activity in the frontal cortex of male and female rats. Brain Res 1991;551:247–255.

Hellhammer DH: Learned helplessness: An animal model revisited; in Agnst J (ed): The Origins of Depression. Berlin, Springer, 1983, pp 147–161.

Hendley ED, Cierpial MA, McCarty R: Sympathetic-adrenal medullary response to stress in hyperactive and hypertensive rats. Physiol Behav 1988;44:47–51.

Heninger GR, Charney DS, Sternberg DE: Serotonergic function in depression. Arch Gen Psychiatry 1984;41:398–402.

Herman JP, Guillonneau D, Dantzer R, Scatton B, Smerdjian-Rouquier L, Le Moal M: Differential effects of inescapable foot-shocks and of stimuli previously paired with inescapable foot-shocks on dopamine turnover in cortical and limbic areas of the rat. Life Sci 1982;30: 2207–2214.

Hsu CY, Knapp DR, Halushka PV: The effects of alpha adrenergic agents on human blood platelet aggregation. J Pharmacol Exp Ther 1979; 208:366–372.

Huang YH: Net effect of acute administration of desipramine on the locus coeruleus-hippocampal system. Life Sci 1979;25:739–746.

Imperato A, Puglisi-Allegra S, Casolini P, Zocchi A, Angelucci L: Stress-induced enhancement of dopamine and acetylcholine release in limbic structures: role of corticosterone. Eur J Pharmacol 1989;165:337–338.

Irwin J, Ahluwalia P, Zacharko RM, Anisman H: Central norepinephrine and plasma corticosterone following acute and chronic stressors: Influence of social isolation and handling. Pharmacol Biochem Behav 1986;24:1151–1154.

Jara H, Lechin AE, Rada I, Villa S, Cabrera A, Guerrero H, van der Dijs B, Lechin F: Plasma neurotransmitters profile in duodenal ulcer patients. Proceedings of the III Interamerican Congress of Clinical Pharmacology and Therapeutics. Arch Ven Farm Terap 1988;7(suppl 1):abstr 86.

Kahn RS, Wetzler S, Asnis GM, Papolos D, van Praag HM: Serotonin receptor sensitivity in major depression. Biol Psychiatry 1990;28: 358–362.

Khansari DN, Murgo AJ, Faith RE: Effects of stress on the immune system. Immunol Today 1980;11:170–174.

Klimek V, Mogilnicka E: The influence of mianserin and danitracen on the disappearance of noradrenaline in the rat brain. Pol J Pharmacol Pharmac 1978;30:255–261.

Kobayashi RM, Palkovits M, Kizer JS, Jacobowitz DM, Kopin LJ: Selective alterations of catecholamines and tyrosine hydroxylase activity in the hypothalamus following acute and chronic stress; in Usdin E, Kvetnansky R, Kopin IJ (eds): Catecholamines and Stress. Oxford, Pergamon Press, 1975, pp 29–38.

Konarska M, Stewart RE, McCarty R: Habituation of sympathetic adrenal medullary responses following exposure to chronic intermittent stress. Physiol Behav 1989;46:255–261.

Koyama T, Meltzer HY: A biochemical and neuroendocrine study of the serotonergic system in depression; in Hyppius H (ed): New Results in Depression Research. Berlin, Springer, 1986, pp 169–188.

Kraemer GW, McKinney WT: Interactions of pharmacological agents which alter biogenic amine metabolism and depression: An analysis of contributing factor within a primate model of depression. J Affect Dis 1979;1:33–39.

Kvetnansky R, Mitro A, Palkovitz M, Brownstein M: Catecholamines in individual hypothalamic nuclei in stressed rats; in Usdin E, Kvetnansky R, Kopin IJ (ed): Catecholamines and Stress. New York, Pergamon Press, 1976, p 29.

Kvetnansky R, Weiss VK, Thoa NB, Kopin IJ: Effects of chronic guanethidine treatment and adrenal medullectomy on plasma levels of catecholamines and corticosterone in forcibly immobilized rats. J Pharmacol Exp Ther 1979; 209:287–291.

Lake CR, Picker D, Ziegler MG, Slipper S, Slater S, Murphy DL: High plasma norepinephrine levels in patients with major affective disorders. Am J Psychiatry 1982;139:1315–1321.

Lake CR, Ziegler MG, Kopin IJ: Use of plasma norepinephrine for evaluation of sympathetic neuronal function in man. Life Sci 1976;18: 1315–1321.

LaPierre YD: Pharmacological therapy of dysthymia. Acta Psychiatr Scand 1994;89(suppl 383):4248.

Larson PT, Hjemdahl PJ, Olsson G, Egberg N, Hornstra G: Altered platelet function during mental stress and adrenaline infusion in humans: Evidence for an increased aggregability in vivo as measured by filtragometry. Clin Sci 1989;76:369–376.

Lechin AE, Jara H, Cabrera A, Villa S, Jimenez V, Guerrero H, van der Dijs B, Lechin F: Plasma neurotransmitters profile in reactive hypoglycemia. Proceedings of the III Interamerican Congress of Clinical Pharmacology and Therapeutics. Arch Ven Farm Terap 1988a;7(suppl 1):abstr 111.

Lechin AE, Jara H, Rada I, Villa S, Cabrera A, Jimenez V, van der Dijs B, Lechin F: Plasma neurotransmitters profile in irritable bowel syndrome (lBS): Diarrheic patients. Proceedings of the III Interamerican Congress of Clinical Pharmacology and Therapeutics. Arch Ven Farm Terap 1988b;7(suppl 1):abstr 88.

Lechin AE, Villa S, Jara H, Cabrera A, Jimenez V, van der Dijs B, Lechin F: Plasma neurotransmitters profile in bronchial asthma. Proceedings of the III Interamerican Congress of Clinical Pharmacology and Therapeutics. Arch Ven Farm Terap 1988c;7(suppl 1):abstr 10.

Lechin AE, Varon J, van der Dijs B, Lechin F: Plasma catecholamines and indoleamines during attacks and remission on severe bronchial asthma: Possible role of stress. Am J Respir Crit Care Med 1994a;149:A778.

Lechin AE, Varon J, van der Dijs B, Lechin F: Plasma neurotransmitters, blood pressure and heart rate during rest and exercise. Am J Respir Crit Care Med 1994b;149:A482.

Lechin F: Central and plasma 5HT, vagal tone and airways. Trends Pharmacol Sci 2000;21:425.

Lechin F, van der Dijs B: A new treatment for headache: Pathophysiologic considerations. Headache 1977;16:318–321.

Lechin F, van der Dijs B: Physiological, clinical and therapeutical basis of a new hypothesis for headache. Headache 1980;20:77–83.

Lechin F, van der Dijs B: Intestinal pharmacomanometry and glucose tolerance: Evidence for two antagonistic dopaminergic mechanisms in the human. Biol Psychiatry 1981a;16:969–986.

Lechin F, van der Dijs B: Colon motility and psychological traits in irritable bowel syndrome. Dig Dis Sci 1981b;26:474–475.

Lechin F, van der Dijs B: Noradrenergic or dopaminergic activity in chronic schizophrenia? Br J Psychiatry 1981c;139:472.

Lechin F, van der Dijs B: Clonidine therapy for psychosis and tardive dyskinesia. Am J Psychiatry 1981d;38:390.

Lechin F, van der Dijs B: Intestinal pharmacomanometry as a guide to psychopharmacological therapy; in Velazco M (ed): Clinical Pharmacology and Therapeutics. International Congress Series No 604. Amsterdam, Excerpta Medica, 1982, pp 166–173.

Lechin F, van der Dijs B: Slow wave sleep (SWS), REM sleep (REMS) and depression. Res Commun Psychol Psychiatr Behav 1984;9:227–262.

Lechin F, van der Dijs B: Serotonin and pulmonary vasoconstriction. J Appl Physiol 2002;92: 1363–1364.

Lechin F, van der Dijs B, Bentolila A, Peña F: The spastic colon syndrome: Pathophysiological considerations. J Clin Pharmacol 1977a;17: 431–440.

Lechin F, van der Dijs B, Bentolila A, Peña F: Antidiarrheal effects of dihydroergotamine. J Clin Pharmacol 1977b;17:339–349.

Lechin F, van der Dijs B, Lechin E. Peña F, Bentolila A: The noradrenergic and dopaminergic blockades: A new treatment for headache. Headache 1978;18:69–74.

Lechin F, van der Dijs B, Lechin E: The Autonomic Nervous System: Physiological Basis of Psychosomatic Therapy. Barcelona, Editorial Cientifico-Medica, 1979a, chap VIII, pp 119–149.

Lechin F, van der Dijs B, Lechin E: The Autonomic Nervous System: Physiological Basis of Psychosomatic Therapy. Barcelona, Editorial Cientifico-Medica, 1979b, chap V, pp 65–72.

Lechin F, Gomez F, van der Dijs B, Lechin E: Distal colon motility in schizophrenic patients. J Clin Pharmacol 1980a;20:459–465.

Lechin F, van der Dijs B, Gomez F, Valls JM, Acosta E, Arocha L: Pharmacomanometric studies of colonic motility as a guide to the chemotherapy of schizophrenia. J Clin Pharmacol 1980b; 20:664–671.

Lechin F, van der Dijs B, Gomez F, Acosta E, Arocha L: On the use of clonidine and thioproperazine in a woman with Gilles de La Tourette's disease. Biol Psychiatry 1982a;17:103–108.

Lechin F, van der Dijs B, Gomez F, Acosta E, Arocha L: Comparison between the effects of d-amphetamine and fenfluramine on distal colon motility in non-psychotic patients. Res Commun Psychol Psychiatr Behav 1982b;7:411–430.

Lechin F, van der Dijs B, Gomez F, Arocha L, Acosta E: Effects of d-amphetamine, clonidine and clonazepam on distal colon motility in non-psychotic patients. Res Commun Psychol Psychiatr Behav 1982c;7:385–410.

Lechin F, van der Dijs B, Insausti CL, Gomez F: Treatment of ulcerative colitis with thioproperazine. J Clin Gastroenterol 1982d;4:445–449.

Lechin F, van der Dijs B, Acosta E, Gomez F, Lechin E, Arocha L: Distal colon motility and clinical parameters in depression. J Affect Dis 1983a;5:19–26.

Lechin F, van der Dijs B, Gomez F, Arocha L, Acosta E, Lechin E: Distal colon motility as a predictor of antidepressant response to fenfluramine, imipramine and clomipramine. J Affect Dis 1983b;5:27–35.

Lechin F, van der Dijs B, Gomez F, Lechin E, Oramas O, Villa S: Positive symptoms of acute psychosis: Dopaminergic or noradrenergic overactivity? Res Commun Psychol Psychiatr Behav 1983c;8:23–54.

Lechin F, van der Dijs B, Insausti CL, Gomez F. Villa S, Lechin AE, Arocha L, Oramas O: Treatment of ulcerative colitis with clonidine. J Clin Pharmacol 1985a;25:219–226.

Lechin F, van der Dijs B, Jackubowicz D, Camero RE, Villa S, Arocha L, Lechin AE: Effects of clonidine on blood pressure, noradrenaline, cortisol, growth hormone, and prolactin plasma levels in high and low intestinal tone depressed patients. Neuroendocrinology 1985b; 41:156–162.

Lechin F, van der Dijs B, Jackubowicz D, Camero RE, Villa S, Lechin E, Gomez F: Effects of clonidine on blood pressure, noradrenaline, cortisol, growth hormone, and prolactin plasma levels in high and low intestinal tone subjects. Neuroendocrinology 1985c;40:253–261.

Lechin F, van der Dijs B, Azocar J, Amat J, Vitelli-Florez G, Martinez C, Lechin-Baez S, Jimenez V, Cabrera A, Cardenas M, Villa S: Stress, immunology and cancer: Effect of psychoactive drugs. Arch Ven Farmac Terap 1987a;6:28–43.

Lechin F, van der Dijs B, Jackubowicz D, Camero RE, Lechin S, Villa S, Reinfeld B, Lechin ME: Role of stress in the exacerbation of chronic illness: Effects of clonidine administration on blood pressure and plasma norepinephrine, cortisol, growth hormone and prolactin concentrations. Psychoneuroendocrinology 1987b; 12:117–129.

Lechin F, van der Dijs B, Amat J, Lechin AE, Cabrera A, Lechin ME, Gomez F, Arocha L, Jimenez V: Definite and sustained improvement with pimozide of two patients with severe trigeminal neuralgia: Some neurochemical, neurophysiological and neuroendocrinological findings. J Med 1988a;19:243–256.

Lechin F, van der Dijs B, Azocar J, Vitelli-Florez G, Lechin S, Villa S, Jara H, Cabrera A: Neurochemical and immunological profiles of three clinical stages in 50 advanced cancer patients. Proceedings of the III Interamerican Congress of Clinical Pharmacology and Therapeutics. Arch Ven Farm Terap 1988b;7(suppl 1):abstr 39.

Lechin F, van der Dijs B, Gomez F, Villa S, Cabrera A, Jimenez V, Guerrero H, Lechin AE: Plasma neurotransmitters profile in depressive syndromes. Proceedings of the III Interamerican Congress of Clinical Pharmacology and Therapeutics and the XII Latinamerican Congress of Pharmacology. Arch Ven Farm Terap 1988c;7(suppl 1): abstr 7.

Lechin F, van der Dijs B, Villa S, Jara H, Rada I, Lechin ME, Jimenez V, Gomez F: Plasma neurotransmitters profile in chronic illness. Proceedings of the III Interamerican Congress of Clinical Pharmacology and Therapeutics. Arch Ven Farm Terap 1988d;7(suppl 1):abstr 38.

Lechin F, van der Dijs B, Amat J, Lechin ME: Central neuronal pathways involved in depressive syndrome: Experimental findings; in Lechin F, van der Dijs B (eds): Neurochemistry and Clinical Disorders: Circuitry of Some Psychiatric and Psychosomatic Syndromes. Boca Raton, CRC Press, 1989a, pp 6–89.

Lechin F, van der Dijs B, Gomez F, Lechin E, Acosta E, Arocha L: Biological markers in the assessment of central autonomic nervous functioning: An approach to the diagnosis of some psychiatric and psychosomatic syndromes; in Lechin F, van der Dijs B (eds): Neurochemistry and Clinical Disorders: Circuitry of Some Psychiatric and Psychosomatic Syndromes. Boca Raton, CRC Press, 1989b, pp 151–226.

Lechin F, van der Dijs B, Lechin ME, Amat J, Lechin AE, Cabrera A, Gomez F, Acosta E, Arocha L, Villa S, Jimenez V: Pimozide therapy for trigeminal neuralgia. Arch Neurol 1989c;46:960–963.

Lechin F, van der Dijs B, Lechin S, Vitelli-Florez G, Lechin ME, Cabrera A: Neurochemical, hormonal and immunological views of stress: Clinical and therapeutic implications in Crohn's disease and cancer; in Velazco M (ed): Recent Advances in Pharmacology and Therapeutics. International Congress Series 839. Amsterdam, Excerpta Medica, 1989d, pp 57–70.

Lechin F, van der Dijs B, Rada I, Jara H, Lechin AE, Cabrera A, Lechin ME, Jimenez V, Gomez F, Villa S, Acosta E, Arocha L: Plasma neurotransmitters and cortisol in duodenal ulcer patients: Role of stress. Dig Dis Sci 1990a;35:1313–1319.

Lechin F, van der Dijs B, Vitelli-Florez G, Lechin-Baez S, Azocar J, Cabrera A, Lechin AE, Jara H, Lechin ME, Gomez F, Arocha L: Psychoneuroendocrinological and immunological parameters in cancer patients: Involvement of stress and depression. Psychoneuroendocrinology 1990b;15:435–451.

Lechin F, van der Dijs B, Lechin AE, Lechin ME, Coll-Garcia- E, Jara H, Cabrera A, Jimenez V, Gomez F, Tovar D, Rada I, Arocha L: Doxepin therapy for postprandial symptomatic hypoglycemic patients: Neurochemical, hormonal and metabolic disturbances. Clin Sci 1991;80:373–384.

Lechin F, van der Dijs B, Lechin ME, Baez S, Jara H, Lechin A, Orozco B, Rada I, Cabrera A, Jimenez V, Leon G: Effects of an oral glucose load on plasmaneurotransmitters in humans: Involvement of REM sleep? Neuropsychobiology 1992a;26:4–11.

Lechin F, van der Dijs B, Lechin ME, Jara H, Lechin AE, Cabrera A, Rada I, Orozco B, Jimenez V, Valderrama T: Dramatic improvement with clonidine of acute pancreatitis showing raised catecholamines and cortisol plasma levels: Case report of five patients. J Med 1992b;23:339–351.

Lechin F, van der Dijs B, Lechin ME, Jara H, Lechin A, Baez S, Orozco B, Rada I, Cabrera A, Arocha L, Jimenez V, Leon G: Plasma neurotransmitters throughout oral glucose tolerance test in non-depressed essential hypertension patients. Clin Exp Hypertens 1993;15:209–240.

Lechin F, van der Dijs B, Baez-Lechin S, Lechin AE, Orozco B, Lechin ME, Rada I, Jara H, Gomez F, Cabrera A, Jimenez V, Arocha L, Leon G: Two types of irritable bowel syndrome: Pathophysiologic and pharmacological considerations. Arch Ven Farmacol Terap 1994a;12:105–114.

Lechin F, van der Dijs B, Lechin AE, Orozco B, Lechin ME, Baez S, Rada I, Leon G, Acosta E: Plasma neurotransmitters and cortisol in chronic illness: Role of stress. J Med 1994b;25:181–192.

Lechin F, van der Dijs B, Vitelli-Florez G, Lechin-Baez S, Lechin ME, Lechin AE, Orozco B, Rada I, Leon G, Jimenez V: Peripheral blood immunological parameters in long-term benzodiazepine users. Neuropharmacology 1994c;17:63–72.

Lechin F, van der Dijs B, Orozco B, Lechin AE, Baez S, Lechin ME, Rada I, Acosta E, Arocha L, Jimenez V, Leon G, Garcia Z: Plasma neurotransmitters, blood pressure and heart rate during supine-resting, orthostasis and moderate exercise in dysthymic depressed patients. Biol Psychiatry 1995a;37:884–891.

Lechin F, van der Dijs B, Orozco B, Lechin ME, Baez S, Lechin AE, Rada I, Acosta E, Arocha L, Jimenez V, Leon G, Garcia Z: Plasma neurotransmitters, blood pressure, and heart rate during supine-resting, orthostasis, and moderate exercise conditions in major depressed patients. Biol Psychiatry 1995b;38:166–173.

Lechin F, van der Dijs B, Lechin AE, Orozco B, Lechin ME, Baez-Lechin S, Rada I, Leon G, Garcia Z, Jimenez V: Plasma neurotransmitters, blood pressure and heart rate during supine-resting, orthostasis and moderate exercise stress test in healthy humans before and after the parasympathetic blockade with atropine. Res Commun Biol Psychol Psychiat 1996a;21:55–72.

Lechin F, van der Dijs B, Orozco B, Lechin AE, Baez S, Lechin ME, Benaim M, Acosta E, Arocha L, Jimenez V, Leon G, Garcia Z: Plasma neurotransmitters, blood pressure and heart rate during supine-resting, orthostasis, and moderate exercise in severely ill patients: A model of failing to cope with stress. Psychother Psychosom 1996b;65:129–136.

Lechin F, van der Dijs B, Orozco B, Lechin ME, Lechin AE: Increased levels of free-serotonin in plasma of symptomatic asthmatic patients. Ann Allergy Asthma Immunol 1996c;77:245–253.

Lechin F, van der Dijs B, Orozco B, Jara H, Rada I, Lechin ME, Lechin AE: Neuropharmacological treatment of bronchial asthma with an antidepressant drug: tianeptine. A double-blind crossover placebo-controlled study. Clin Pharmacol Ther 1998a;64:223–232.

Lechin F, van der Dijs B, Lechin A, Orozco B, Lechin ME, Lechin AE: The serotonin uptake-enhancing drug tianeptine suppresses asthmatic symptoms in children: A double-blind crossover placebo-controlled study. J Clin Pharmacol 1998b;38:918–925.

Lechin ME, Jara H, Villa S, Gomez F, Cabrera A, Guerrero H, van der Dijs B, Lechin F: Plasma neurotransmitters profile in somatoform disorders. Proceedings of the III Interamerican Congress of Clinical Pharmacology and Therapeutics. Arch Ven Farm Terap 1988a;7(suppl 1): abstr 2.

Lechin ME, Jara H, Rada I, Villa S, Cabrera A, Jimenez V, van der Dijs B, Lechin F: Plasma neurotransmitters profile in irritable bowel syndrome (IBS): Spastic colon. Proceedings of the III Interamerican Congress of Clinical Pharmacology and Therapeutics. Arch Ven Farm Terap 1988b;7(suppl 1):abstr 87.

Lechin ME, Jara H, Villa S, Gomez F, Jimenez V, Cabrera A, van der Dijs B, Lechin F: Plasma neurotransmitters profile in tension headache. Proceedings of the III Interamerican Congress of Clinical Pharmacology and Therapeutics. Arch Ven Farm Terap 1988c;7(suppl 1): abstr 1.

Lechin ME, Villa S, Rada I, Jara H, Cabrera A, Jimenez V, van der Dijs B, Lechin F: Plasma neurotransmitters profile in reflux esophagitis. Proceedings of the III Interamerican Congress of Clinical Pharmacology and Therapeutics. Arch Ven Farm Terap 1988d;7(suppl 1):abstr 85.

Lechin S, Vitelli G, Martinez C, Fernandez M, Cabrera A, van der Dijs B, Azocar J, Lechin F: Plasma neurotransmitters, lymphocyte subpopulations and natural killer cell activity in terminal cancer patients. Proceedings of the III Interamerican Congress of Clinical Pharmacology and Therapeutics. Arch Ven Farm Terap 1988;7(suppl 1):abstr 37.

Leonard BE, Kafoe W: A comparison of acute and chronic effects of four antidepressant drugs on the turnover of serotonin, dopamine and noradrenaline in the rat brain. Biochem Pharmacol 1976;25:1939–1942.

Levine SP, Towell BL, Suarez AM, Knieriem LK, Harris MM, George JN: Platelet activation and secretion associated with emotional stress. Circulation 1985;71:1129–1134.

Liang-Fu T: 5-Hydroxytryptamine uptake inhibitors block induced 5HT release. Br J Pharmacol 1979;66:185–190.

Lucki Y, Frazer A: Performance and extinction of lever press behavior following chronic administration of desipramine to rats. Psychopharmacology 1985;85:253–259.

Maes M, Lambrechts J, Suy E, van der Vorst C, Bosmans E: Absolute number and percentage of circulating natural killer, non-MHC-restricted T cytotoxic, and phagocytic cells in unipolar depression. Biol Psychiatry 1994;29:157–163.

Maes M, Meltzer H, Jacobs J, Suy E, Calabrese J, Minner B, Raus J: Autoimmunity in depression: Increased antiphospholipid autoantibodies. Acta Psychiatr Scand 1993;87:160–166.

Maier SF: Learned helplessness and animal models of depression. Prog Neuropsychopharmacol Biol Psychiatry 1984;8:435–446.

Maj J: Pharmacological spectrum of some new antidepressants; in Dumond C (ed): Advances in Pharmacology and Therapeutics. New York, Pergamon Press, 1978, pp 161–170.

Matussek N, Ackenheil M, Hippius H, Muller F, Chroeder HT, Schultes H, Wasilewski B: Effect of clonidine on growth hormone release in psychiatric patients and controls. Psychiatry Res 1980;2:25–36.

McWilliam JR, Meldrum BS: Noradrenergic regulation of growth hormone in the baboon. Endocrinology 1983;112:254–259.

Meltzer HY, Lowy MT: The serotonin hypothesis of depression; in Meltzer HY (ed): Psychopharmacology: The Third Generation of Progress. New York, Raven Press, 1987, pp 513–526.

Mormede P, Dantzer R, Michaud B, Kelley KW, Le Moal M: Influence of stressor predictability and behavioral control on lymphocyte reactivity, antibody responses and neuroendocrine activation in rats. Physiol Behav 1988;43:577–583.

Morris JB, Beck AT: The efficacy of antidepressant drugs. Arch Gen Psychiatry 1974;30:667–674.

Murphy DL, Campbell Y, Costa JL: Current status of indoleamine hypothesis of the affective disorders; in Lipton MA, DiMascio A, Kiliam KF (eds): Psychopharmacology: A generation of Progress. New York, Raven Press, 1978, pp 1235–1248.

Nagayama H, Hingtgen JN, Aprison MH: Postsynaptic action by four antidepressive drugs in an animal model of depression. Pharmacol Biochem Behav 1981;15:650–655.

Natelson BH, Creighton D, McCarty R, Tapp WN, Pitman D, Ottenweller JE: Adrenal hormonal indices of stress in laboratory rats. Physiol Behav 1987;39:117–125.

Natelson BH, Ottenweller JE, Cook JA, Pitman D, McCarty R, Tapp WN: Effect of stressor intensity on habituation of the adrenocortical stress response. Physiol Behav 1988;43:41–48.

Nielsen M, Braestrup C: Chronic treatment with desipramine caused a sustained decrease of 3,4-dihydroxyphenylglycol-sulfate and total 3-methoxy-4-hydroxyphenylglycol in rat brain. Arch Pharmacol 1977;300:87–92.

Nybaeck HV, Walters JR, Aghajanian GK: Tricyclic antidepressants: Effects on the firing rate of brain noradrenergic neurons. Eur J Pharmacol 1975;32:302–312.

Ogren SO, Fuxe K, Archer T, Johansson G, Holm AC: behavioral and biochemical studies on the effects of acute and chronic administration of antidepressant drugs on central serotonergic receptor mechanisms; in Langer S, Takahashi R, Segawa T, Briley M (eds): New Vistas in Depression. New York, Pergamon Press, 1982, pp 171–178.

Ogren SO, Fuxe K, Agnati LF, Gustafsson JA, Johnson G, Holm AC: Reevaluation of the indoleamine hypothesis of depression: Evidence for a reduction of functional activity of central 5HT systems by antidepressant drugs. J Neural Transm 1979;46:85–103.

Ottenweller JR, Natelson BH, Pitman DL, Drastal SD: Adrenocortical and behavioral responses to repeated stressors: Toward an animal model of chronic stress and stress-related mental illness. Biol Psychiatry 1989;26:829–841.

Pavlidis N, Chirigos M: Stress-induced impairment of macrophage tumoricidal function. Psychosom Med 1980;42:47–54.

Paykel ES: Monoamine oxidase inhibitors: When should they be used? In Hawton K, Cowen P (eds): Dilemma and Difficulties in the Management of Psychiatric Patients. Oxford, Oxford University Press, 1990, pp 17–30.

Petty F, Sherman AD: Learned helplessness induction decreases in vivo cortical serotonin release. Pharmacol Biochem Behav 1983;18:649–650.

Porsolt RD, Anton G, Blavet N, Jalfre M: 'Behavioral despair' in rats: A new model sensitive to antidepressant treatments. Eur J Pharmacol 1978;47:379–391.

Przegalinski E, Kordecka-Magiera A, Mogilnicka E, Maj J: Chronic treatment with some atypical antidepressant increases the brain level of 3-methoxy-4-hydroxyphenylglycol (MHPG) in rats. Psychopharmacology 1981;74:187–190.

Pujol JF, Keane P, McRae A, Lewis BD, Renaud B: Biochemical evidence for serotonergic control of the locus coeruleus; in Garattini S, Pujol JF, Samanin R (eds): Interactions between Putative Neurotransmitters in the Brain. New York, Raven Press, 1978, pp 401–410.

Quitkin FM, Harrison WM, Stewart JW, McGrath PJ, Tricamo E, Ocepek-Welikson K, Rabkin JG, Wager SG, Nunes E, Klein DF: Response to phenelzine and imipramine in placebo responders with atypical depression. Arch Gen Psychiatry 1991;48:319–323.

Raiteri M, Angellini F, Bertollini A: Comparative study of the effects of mianserine, a tetracyclic antidepressant, and of imipramine on uptake and release of neurotransmitters in synaptosomas. J Pharm Pharmacol 1976;28:483–488.

Rimon R, Jaaskelainen J, Kaatinen P: Meclobamide versus imipramine in depressed outpatients: A double-blind multicentre study. Int Clin Psychopharmacol 1993;1:141–148.

Rodriguez-Echandia EL, Broitman ST, Foscolo MR: Effect of the chronic ingestion of clorimipramine on the whole board response to acute stresses in male rats. Pharmacol Biochem Behav 1987;26:207–210.

Roffman M, Kling MK, Cassens G, Orsulak PJ, Reigle TG, Schildkraut JJ: The effects of acute and chronic administration of tricyclic antidepressants of MHPG-SO$_4$ in rat brain. Commun Psychopharmacol 1977;1:195–206.

Rosenbaum AH, Schatzberg AF, Maruta T, Orsulak PJ, Cole JO, Grab EL, Schildkraut JJ: MHPG as a predictor of antidepressant response to imipramine and maprotyline. Am J Psychiatry 1980;137:1090–1097.

Roth KA, Mefford IM, Barchas JD: Epinephrine, norepinephrine, dopamine, and serotonin: Differential effects of acute and chronic stress on regional brain amines. Brain Res 1982;239:417–424.

Roy A, Pickar D, Linnoila M, Potter WZ: Plasma norepinephrine in affective disorders: Relationship to melancholia. Arch Gen Psychiatry 1985;42:1181–1185.

Rubin RT, Poland RE, Hays SE: Psychoneuroendocrine research in endogenous depression: A review; in Obiols J, Bailus C, Gonzalez-Monclus E, Pujol J (eds): Biological Psychiatry Today. Amsterdam, Elsevier, 1979, pp 684–688.

Sachser N: Short-term responses of plasma norepinephrine, epinephrine, glucocorticoid and testosterone titers to social and non-social stressors in male guinea pigs of different social status. Physiol Behav 1987;39:11–20.

Schatzberg AF: Classification of depressive disorders; in Cole JO, Schatzberg AF, Frazier SH (eds): Depression, Biology, Psychodynamics and Treatment. New York, Plenum Press, 1978, pp 13–40.

Schildkraut JJ, Orsulak PJ, Gudeman JE: Recent studies of the role of catecholamines in the pathophysiology and classification of depressive disorders; in Schildkraut JJ, Orsulak PJ (eds): Neuroregulators and Psychiatric Disorders. New York, Oxford Press, 1977, pp 122–128.

Scuvee-Moreau JJ, Dresse AL: Effect of various antidepressant drugs on the spontaneous firing rate of locus coeruleus and raphe dorsalis neurons of the rat. Eur J Pharmacol 1979;57:219–225.

Segal M: Serotonergic innervation of the locus coeruleus from the dorsal raphe and its action on responses to noxious stimuli. J Physiol 1979;286:401–415.

Sherman AD, Petty F: Neurochemical basis of the action of antidepressants on learned helplessness. Behav Neural Biol 1980;30:119–134.

Siever LJ, Risch SC, Murphy DL: Central cholinergic-adrenergic imbalance in the regulation of affective state. Psychiatr Res 1981;4:108–114.

Siever LJ, Uhde TW: New studies and perspectives on the noradrenergic receptor system in depression: Effects of the alpha-adrenergic agonist clonidine. Biol Psychiatry 1984;19:131–156.

Siever LJ, Uhde TW, Silberman EK, Jimerson DG, Aloi JA, Post RM, Murphy DL: Growth hormone response to clonidine as a probe of noradrenergic receptor responsiveness in affective disorder patients and controls. Psychiatr Res 1982;6:171–183.

Sourkes TL: Neurotransmitters and central regulation of adrenal functions. Biol Psychiatry 1985;20:182–191.

Steplewski Z, Vogel WH, Ekya H, Poropatich C, McDonald-Smith J: Effects of restraint stress on inoculated tumor growth and immune response in rats. Cancer Res 1985;45:5128–5133.

Stoddard SL, Bergdall VK, Towsend DW, Levin BE: Plasma catecholamines associated with hypothalamically-elicited defense behavior. Physiol Behav 1986;36:867–673.

Sugrue MF: Changes in rat brain monoamine turnover following chronic antidepressant administration. Life Sci 1980;26:423–429.

Sulser F, Mobley PL: Regulation of central noradrenergic receptor function: new vistas on the mode of action of antidepressant treatments; in Usdin E, Bunney WB, Davis JM (eds): Neuroreceptors: Basic Clinical Aspects. New York, Wiley, 1981, pp 55–63.

Swenson RM, Vogel WH: Plasma catecholamine and corticosterone as well as brain catecholamine changes during coping in rats exposed to stressful foot-shock. Pharmacol Biochem Behav 1983;18:689–693.

Tanaka M, Ida Y, Tsuda A, Tsujimaru S, Shirao Y, Oguchi M: Metenkephalin, injected during the early phase of stress, attenuates stress-induced increases in noradrenaline release in rat brain regions. Pharmacol Biochem Behav 1989;32: 791–795.

Targum SD: Persistent neuroendocrine disregulation in major depressive disorder: a marker for early relapse. Biol Psychiatry 1984;19:305–318.

Tecoma ES, Huey LY: Psychic distress and the immune response. Life Sci 1985;36:1799–1812.

Thierry AM, Tassin JP, Blanc G, Glowinski J: Selective activation of the mesocortical dopaminergic system by stress. Nature 1976;263: 242–244.

Tissari AH, Argiolas A, Fadda F, Serra G, Gessa GL: Foot-shock stress accelerates non-striatal dopamine synthesis without activating tyrosine hydroxylase. Arch Pharmacol 1979;308:155–157.

Tonnesen E, Huttel MS, Christensen NJ, Schmitz O: Natural killer cell activity in patients undergoing upper abdominal surgery: Relationship to the endocrine stress response. Acta Anaesthesiol Scand 1984;28:654–660.

van der Dijs B, Lechin AE, Villa S, Gomez F, Cabrera A, Jimenez V, Guerrero H, Lechin F: Plasma neurotransmitters profile in cluster headache. Proceedings of the III Interamerican Congress of Clinical Pharmacology and Therapeutics. Arch Ven Farm Terap 1988a;7(suppl 1):abstr 3.

van der Dijs B, Lechin S, Vitelli G, Cabrera A, Fernandez M, Martinez C, Azocar J, Lechin F: Plasma neurotransmitters, lymphocyte subpopulations and natural killer cell activity in progressive cancer patients. Proceedings of the III Interamerican Congress of Clinical Pharmacology and Therapeutics. Arch Ven Farm Terap 1988b;7(suppl 1):abstr 35.

van der Dijs B, Lechin S, Vitelli G, Cabrera A, Fernandez M, Martinez C, Azocar J, Lechin F: Plasma neurotransmitters, lymphocyte subpopulations and killer cell activity in short-term symptomless cancer patients. Proceedings of the III Interamerican Congress of Clinical Pharmacology and Therapeutics. Arch Ven Farm Terap 1988;7(suppl 1):abstr 34.

Vesifeld IL, Vasilijiev VN, Luicheva RF: Relationship of catecholamines, histamine and serotonin in men under different kinds of stress; in Usdin E, Kvetnansky R, Kopin IJ (eds): Catecholamines and Stress. Oxford, Pergamon Press, 1976, pp 527–534.

Vetulani J, Antkiewicz-Michaluk L, Rokosz-Pelc A: Chronic administration of antidepressant drugs increased the density of cortical (^{3}H)-prazosin binding site in the rat. Brain Res 1984; 310:360–362.

Vitelli G, Lechin S, Cabrera A, Fernandez M, Azocar J, van der Dijs B, Lechin, F: Plasma neurotransmitters, lymphocyte subpopulations and natural killer cell activity in long-term symptomless cancer patients. Proceedings of the III Interamerican Congress of Clinical Pharmacology and Therapeutics. Arch Ven Farm Terap 1988;7(suppl 1):abstr 36.

Vogel GW: A review of REM sleep deprivation. Arch Gen Psychiatry 1975;32:749–761.

Von Zerssen D, Berger M, Doerr P: Neuroendocrine dysfunction in subtypes of depression; in Shah NS, Donald AG (eds): Psychoneuroendocrine Dysfunction in Psychiatric and Neurological Illness: Influence of Psychopharmacological Agents. New York, Plenum Press, 1984.

Weiss JM, Goodman PA, Losito PG, Corrigan S, Charry JM, Bailey WH: Behavioral depression produced by an uncontrollable stressor: Relationship to norepinephrine, dopamine and serotonin levels in various regions of rat brain. Brain Res Rev 1981;3:167–205.

Weisse CS, Pato CN, McAllister CG, Liuman R, Breier A, Paul SM, Baum A: Differential effects of controllable and uncontrollable acute stress on lymphocyte proliferation and leukocyte percentages in humans. Brain Behav Immunity 1990;4:339–351.

Weizman R, Laor N, Podliszewski E, Notti I, Djaldeui M, Bessler H: Cytokine production in major depressed patients before and after clomipramine treatment. Biol Psychiatry 1994;35: 42–47.

Wolfe BB, Harden TK, Sporn JR, Molinoff PB: Presynaptic modulation of beta adrenergic receptors in rat cerebral cortex after treatment with antidepressants. J Pharmacol Exp Ther 1978;207:446–457.

Wyatt RJ, Portnoy B, Kupfer DJ: Resting plasma catecholamine concentrations in patients with depression and anxiety. Arch Gen Psychiatry 1971;24:65–70.

Yoshimatsu H, Oomura Y, Katafuchi T, Niijim A, Sato A: Lesions of the ventromedial hypothalamic nucleus enhance sympatho-adrenal function. Brain Res 1985;339:390–392.

Young JB, Rosa RM, Landsberg L: Dissociation of sympathetic nervous system and adrenal medullary responses. Am J Physiol 1984;247: E35–E40.

Ziegler MG, Lake CR, Wood JH: Relationship between norepinephrine in blood and cerebrospinal fluid in the presence of a blood cerebrospinal fluid barrier for NE. J Neurochem 1977; 28:677–679.

Zimmerman M, Coryell W, Pfohl B: The categorical and dimensional models of endogenous depression. J Affect Dis 1985;9:181–186.

References for Chapter 6

Artigas F, Sarrias MJ, Martínez E, Gelpí E, Alvarez E, Udina C: Increased plasma free serotonin but unchanged platelet serotonin in bipolar patients treated chronically with lithium. Psychopharmacology 1989;99:328–332.

Bowden CHL, Calabrese JR, McElroy SL, Rhodes LJ, Keck PE, Cookson J, Anderson J, Bolden-Watson C, Ascher J, Monaghan E, Zhou J: The efficacy of lamotrigine in rapid cycling and non-rapid cycling patients with bipolar disorder. Biol Psychiatry 1999;45:953–958.

Chouinard G, Young SN, Annable L: Antimanic effect of clonazepam. Biol Psychiatry 1983;18: 451–456.

Evins AE, Tisdale T: Olanzapine-induced obsessive-compulsive disorder. Am J Psychiatry 1999;156:5.

Hotta I, Yamawaki S, Segawa T: Long-term lithium treatment causes serotonin receptor down-regulation via serotonergic presynapses in rat brain. Neuropsychobiology 1986;16:19–26.

Khan S, Haddad P, Montague L, Summerton C: Systemic lupus erythematosus presenting as mania. Act Psychiatr Scand 2000;101:406–408.

Koek RJ, Yerevanian BI, Tachiki KH, Smith JC, Alcock J, Kopelowicz A: Hemispheric asymmetry in depression and mania a longitudinal QEEG study in bipolar disorder. J Affect Dis 1999;53:109–122.

Lechin F, Gómez F, Acosta E, Arocha L, van der Dijs B: Treatment of manic syndrome patients with dopaminergic antagonists. Arch Ven Farm Clin Terap 1982;1:150.

Lechin F, van der Dijs B, Gómez F, Valls JM, Acosta E, Arocha L: Pharmacomanometric studies of colonic motility as a guide to the chemotherapy of schizophrenia. J Clin Pharmacol 1980; 20:664–671.

Lechin F, van der Dijs B: Antimanic effect of clonazepam. Biol Psychiatry 1983;18:1511.

Lechin F, van der Dijs B: Noradrenergic or dopaminergic activity in chronic schizophrenia? Br J Psychiatry 1981;139:472.

Perugi G, Akiskal HS, Ramacciotti S, Nassini S, Toni C, Milanfranchi A, Musetti L: Depressive comorbidity of panic, social phobic, and obsessive-compulsive disorders re-examined: Is there a-bipolar II connection? J Psychiat Res 1999;33:53–61.

Sharp T, Bramwell SR, Lambert P, Grahame-Smith DG: Effect of short-and long-term administration of lithium on the release of endogenous 5-HT in the hippocampus of the rat in vivo and in vitro. Neuropharmacology 1991; 30:977–984

Shouse MN, Bier M, Langer J, Alcalde O, Richkind M, Szymusiak R: The α2-agonist clonidine suppresses seizures, whereas the α$_2$-antagonist idazoxan promotes seizures: A microinfusion study in amygdala-kindled kittens. Brain Res 1994;648:352–356.

Stoop R, Epiney S, Meier E, Pralong E: Modulation of epileptiform discharges in the rat limbic system in vitro by noradrenergic agents. Neurosci Lett 2000;287:5–8.

Tohen M, Sanger TM, McElroy SL, Tollefson GD, Chengappa KNR, Daniel DG, Petty F, Centorrino F, Wang R, Grundy SL, Greaney MG, Jacobs TG, David SR, Toma V, The Olanzapine HGEH study Group: Olanzapine versus placebo in the treatment of acute mania. Am J Psychiatry 1999;156:702–709.

Tsai SY, Chen KP, Yang YY, Chen CC, Lee JC, Singh VK, Leu SJC: Activation of indices of cell-mediated immunity in bipolar mania. Biol Psychiatry 1999;45:989–994.

Van Zijderveld GA, Veltman DJ, van Dyck R, van Doornen LJP: Epinephrine-induced panic attacks and hyperventilation. J Psychiatr Res 1999;33:73–78.

Velayudhan A, Sunitha TA, Balachander S, Reddy JYC, Khanna S: A study of platelet serotonin receptor in mania. Biol Psychiatry 1999;45: 1059–1062.

Wilkinson DJ, Thompson JM, Lambert GW, Jennings GL, Schwarz RG, Jefferys D, Turner AG, Esler MD: Sympathetic activity in patients with panic disorder at rest, under laboratory mental stress, and during panic attacks. Arch Gen Psychiatry 1998;55:511–520.

References for Chapter 7

Abi-Dargham A, Gil R, Krystal J, Baldwin RM, Seibyl JP, Bowers M, Van Dyck CH, Charney DS, Innis RB, Laruelle M: Increased striatal dopamine transmission in schizophrenia: Confirmation in a second cohort. Am J Psychiatry 1998;155:761–767.

Ågmo A, Belzung C, Rodriguez C: A rat model of distractibility: Effects of drugs modifying dopaminergic, noradrenergic and GABAergic neurotransmission. J Neural Transm 1997;104: 11–29.

Anand A, Charney DS, Oren DA, Berman RM, Hu XS, Cappiello A, Krystal JH: Attenuation of the neuropsychiatric effects of ketamine with lamotrigine. Arch Gen Psychiatry 2000;57: 270–276.

Anderson GM, Freedman DX, Cohen DJ: Whole blood serotonin in autistic and normal subjects. J Child Psychol Psychiatry 1987;28:885–900.

Asberg M, Nordstrom P, Traskman-Bendz L: Cerebrospinal fluid studies in suicide, an overview. Ann NY Acad Sci 1986;487:243–255.

Assaf SY, Miller JJ: The role of a raphe serotonin system in the control of septal unit activity and hippocampal desynchronization. Neuroscience 1978;3:539–550.

Brown CS, Kent TA, Bryant SG, Gevedon RM, Campbell JL, Felthous A, Barratt ES, Rose RM: Blood platelet uptake of serotonin in episodic aggression. Psychiatry Res 1989;27:5–12.

Brown GL, Ebert MH, Goyer PF, Jimerson DC, Klein WJ, Bunney WEJ: Aggression, suicide and serotonin: Relationship to CSF amine metabolites. Am J Psychiatry 1982;139:741–746.

Brown GL, Goodwin FK, Bunney WEJ: Human aggression and suicide: Their relationship to neuropsychiatric diagnoses and serotonin metabolism. Adv Biochem Psychopharmacol 1982;34:287–307.

Carboni E, Rolando M, Silvagni A, Di Chiara G: Increase of dialysate dopamine in the bed nucleus of stria terminalis by clozapine and related neuroleptics. Neuropsychopharmacology 2000;22:140–147.

Carlsson A, Waters N, Carlsson ML: Neurotransmitter interactions in schizophrenia-therapeutic implications. Biol Psychiatry 1999;46:1388–1395.

Cases O, Seif I, Grimsby J, Gaspar P, Chen K, Pournin S, Muller U, Aguet M, Babinet C, Shih JC: Aggressive behavior and altered amounts of brain serotonin and norepinephrine in mice lacking MAOA. Science 1995;268:1763–1766.

Chamberlain B, Ervin FR, Pihl RO, Young SN: The effect of raising or lowering tryptophan levels on aggression in vervet monkeys. Pharmacol Biochem Behav 1987;28:503–510.

Coccaro EF, Siever LJ, Klar HM, Maurer G, Cochrane K, Cooper TB, Mohs RC, Davis KL: Serotonergic studies in patients with affective and personality disorders: Correlates with suicidal and impulsive aggressive behavior. Arch Gen Psychiatry 1989;46:587–599.

Coccaro EF, Silverman JM, Klar HK, Horvath TB, Siever LJ: Familial correlates of reduced central serotonergic system function in patients with personality disorders. Arch Gen Psychiatry 1994;51:318–324.

Coccaro EF: Central serotonin and impulsive aggression. Br J Psychiatry 1989;155:52–62.

Cochran E, Robins E, Grote S: Regional serotonin levels in brain: A comparison of depressive suicides and alcoholic suicides with controls. Biol Psychiatry 1976;11:283–294.

Cook EH, Arora RC, Anderson GM, Berry-Kravis EM, Yan SY, Yeoh HC, Sklena PJ, Charak DA, Leventhal BL: Platelet serotonin studies in hyperserotonemic relatives of children with autistic disorder. Life Sci 1993;52:2005–2015.

Cook EH, Leventhal BL, Freedman DX: Serotonin and measured intelligence. J Autism Dev Disord 1988;18:553–559.

Cook EH, Stein MA, Ellison T, Unis AS, Leventhal BL: Attention deficit hyperactivity disorder and whole blood serotonin levels: Effects of comorbidity. Psychiatry Res 1995;57:13–20.

Duncan GE, Miyamoto S, Leipzig JN, Lieberman JA: Comparison of the effects of clozapine, risperidone, and olanzapine on ketamine-induced alterations in regional brain metabolism. J Pharmacol Exp Ther 2000;293:8–14.

Ellenbroek B, Cools AR: The neurodevelopment hypothesis of schizopharenia: Clinical evidence and animal models. Neurosci Res Commun 1998;22:127–132.

Faraone SV, Bierderman J, Spencer T, Wilens T, Seidman LJ, Mick E, Doyle AE: Attention-deficit/hyperactivity disorder in adults: An overview. Biol Psychiatry 2000;48:9–20.

Fernstrom JD, Wurtman RJ: Brain serotonin content: Physiological dependence on plasma tryptophan levels. Science 1971;173:149–152.

Galinowski A, Poirier MF, Aymard N, Leyris A, Beauverie P, Bourdel MC, Loo H: Evolution of plasma homovanillic acid (HVA) in chronic schizophrenic patients treated with haloperidol. Acta Psychiatr Scand 1998;97:458–466.

Gessa GL, Devoto P, Diana M, Flore G, Melis M, Pistis M: Dissociation of haloperidol, clozapine, and olanzapine effects on electrical activity of mesocortical dopamine neurons and dopamine release in the prefrontal cortex. Neuropsychopharmacology 2000;22:642–649.

Hanna G, Yuwiler A, Cantwell DP: Whole blood serotonin in juvenile obsessive-compulsive disorder. Biol Psychiatry 1991;29:738–744.

Hirata-Hibi M, Higashi S, Tachibana T, Watanabe N: Stimulated lymphocytes in schizophrenia. Arch Gen Psychiatry 1982;39:82–87.

Ichikawa J, Kuroki T, Dai J, Meltzer HY: Effect of antipsychotic drugs on extracellular serotonin levels in rat medial prefrontal cortex and nucleus accumbens. Eur J Pharmacol 1998;351: 163–171.

Jäkälä P, Riekkinen M, Sirviö J, Koivisto E, Kejonen K, Vanhanen M, Riekkinen P: Guanfacine, but not clonidine, improves planning and working memory performance in humans. Neuropsychopharmacology 1999;20:460–470.

Jakovljevic M, Mück-Šeler D, Pivac M, Ljubicic D, Bujas M, Dodig G: Seasonal influence on platelet 5-HT levels in patients with recurrent major depression and schizophrenia. Biol Psychiatry 1997;41:1028–1034.

Jones H, Curtis VA, Wright P, Lucey JV: Neuroendocrine evidence that clozapine's serotonergic antagonism is relevant to its efficacy in treating hallucinations and other positive schizophrenic symptoms. Am J Psychiatry 1998;155:838–840.

Kaneko M, Honda K, Kanno T, Horikoshi R, Manome T, Watanabe A, Kumashiro H: Plasma free 3-methoxy-4-hydroxyphenylglycol in acute schizophrenics before and after treatment. Neuropsychobiology 1992;25:126–129.

Keshavan MS, Reynolds CF, Montrose D, Miewald J, Downs C, Sabo EM: Sleep and suicidality in psychotic patients. Acta Psychiatr Scand 1994;89:122–125.

Kremer HPH, Goekoop JG, Van Kempen GMJ: Clinical use of the determination of serotonin in whole blood. J Clin Psychopharmacol 1990;10:83–87.

Kruesi MJP, Rapoport JL, Hamburger S, Hibbs E, Potter WZ, Lenane M: CSF monoamine metabolites, aggression, and impulsivity in disruptive behavior disorders of children and adolescents. Arch Gen Psychiatry 1990;47:419–426.

Lechin F, van der Dijs B, Amat J, Lechin ME: Central neuronal pathways involved in psychotic syndromes; in Lechin F, van der Dijs B (eds): Neurochemistry and Clinical Disorders: Circuitry of Some Psychiatric and Psychosomatic Syndromes. Boca Raton, CRC Press, 1989, pp 91–120.

Lechin F, van der Dijs B, Gómez F, Lechin E, Oramas O, Villas S: Positive symptoms of acute psychosis: Dopaminergic or noradrenergic overactivity? Res Commun Psychol Psychiatr Behav 1983;8:23.

Lechin F, van der Dijs B, Gómez F, Lechin E: Distal colon motility in schizophrenic patients. J Clin Pharmacol 1980;20:459–464.

Lechin F, van der Dijs B, Gómez F, Oramas O, Lechin E: On the use of clonidine and levodopa in minimal brain dysfunction syndrome. Arch Ven Farm Clin Terap 1982;1:159.

Lechin F, van der Dijs B, Gómez F, Valls JM, Acosta E, Arocha L: Pharmacomanometric studies of colonic motility as a guide to the chemotherapy of schizophrenia. J Clin Pharmacol 1980;20:664–671.

Lechin F, van der Dijs B: Clonidine therapy for psychosis and tardive dyskinesia. Am J Psychiatry 1981;138:390.

Lechin F, van der Dijs B: Noradrenergic or dopaminergic activity in chronic schizophrenia? Br J Psychiatry 1981;139:472.

Linnoila M, Virkkunen M, Scheinin M, Nuutila A, Rimon R, Goodwin FK: Low CSF 5HIAA concentration differentiates impulsive from nonimpulsive violent behavior. Life Sci 1983;33:2609–2614.

Mann JJ, McBride A, Anderson GM, Mieczkowski TA: Platelet and whole blood serotonin content in depressed inpatients: Correlations with acute and life-time psychopathology. Biol Psychiatry 1992;32:243–257.

Moffitt TE, Brammer GL, Caspi A, Fawcett JP, Raleigh M, Yuwiler A, Silva P: Whole blood serotonin relates to violence in an epidemiological study. Biol Psychiatry 1998;43:446–457.

Müller N, Ackenheil M, Hofschuster E, Mempel W, Eckstein R: Cellular immunity in schizophrenic patients before and during neuroleptic treatment. Psychiatry Res 1991;37:147–160.

Murphy DL, Campbell IC, Costa JL: The brain serotonergic system in the effective disorders. Prog Neuropsychopharmacol 1978;2:1–31.

Pliszka SR, Graham AR, Rogeness MD, Renner P, Sherman J, Broussard T: Plasma neurochemistry in juvenile offenders. J Am Acad Child Adolesc Psychiatry 1988;27:588–594.

Post RM, Rubinow DR, Uhde TW, Ballenger JC, Linnoila M: Dopaminergic effects of carbamazepine. Arch Gen Psychiatry 1986;43:392–396.

Printz DJ, Strauss DH, Goetz R, Sadiq S, Malaspina D, Krolewski J, Gorman JM: Elevation of CD5+B lymphocytes in schizophrenia. Biol Psychiatry 1999;46:110–118.

Pucilowski O, Kostowski W: Aggressive behavior and the central serotonergic systems. Behav Brain Res 1983;9:33–48.

Ritvo ER, Yuwiler A, Geller E, Plotkin S, Mason A, Saeger K: Maturational changes in blood serotonin levels and platelet counts. Biochem Med 1971;5:90–96.

Ritvo ER, Yuwiler A, Geller E: Increased blood serotonin and platelets in early infantile autism. Arch Gen Psychiatry 1970;25:566–572.

Rothermundt M, Arolt V, Weitzsch C, Eckhoff D, Kirchner H: Immunological dysfunction in schizophrenia: A systematic approach. Neuropsychobiology 1998;37:186–193.

Roy A, Adinoff B, Linnoila M: Acting out hostility in normal volunteers: Negative correlation with levels of 5HIAA in cerebrospinal fluid. Psychiatry Res 1988;24:187–194.

Sarrias MJ, Cabre P, Martinez E, Artigas F: Relationship between serotonergic measures in blood and cerebrospinal fluid simultaneously obtained in humans. J Neurochem 1990;54:783–786.

Scheepers FE, Gispen de Wied CC, Hulshoff HE, Van de Flier W, Van der Linden JA, Kahn RS: The effect of clozapine on caudate nucleus volume in schizophrenic patients previously treated with typical antpsychotics. Neuropsychopharmacology 2001;24:47–54.

Siefert WE, Foxx JL, Butler IJ: Age effect on dopamine and serotonin metabolite levels in CSF. Ann Neurol 1980;8:38–42.

Tamminga CA, Gotts MD; Thaker GK, Alphs LD, Foster NL: Dopamine agonist treatment of schizophrenia with N-propyl-norapomorphine. Arch Gen Psychiatry 1986;43:398–402.

Tassin JP: NE/DA interactios in prefrontal cortex and their possible roles as neuromodulators in schizophrenia. J Neural Transm 1992;36 (suppl):135–62.

Wirz-Justice A, Lichtsteiner M, Freer H: Diurnal and seasonal variations in human platelet serotonin in man. J Neural Transm (GenSect) 1977;41:7–15.

Youngren KD, Inglis FM, Pivirotto PJ, Jedema HP, Bradberry CW, Goldman-Rakic PS, Roth RH, Moghaddam B: Clozapine preferentially increases dopamine release in the rhesus monkey prefrontal cortex compared with the caudate nucleus. Neuropsychopharmacology 1999;20:403–412.

Yuwiler A, Brammer GL, Morley JE, Raleigh MU, Flannert JW, Gelle E: Short-term and repetitive administration of oral tryptophan in normal man. Arch Gen Psychiatry 1981;38:619–626.

References for Chapter 8

Abelson JL, Curtis GC, Cameron OG: Hypothalamic-pituitary-adrenal axis activity in panic disorder: effects of alprazolam on 24 h secretion of adrenocorticotropin and cortisol. J Psychiatr Res 1996;30:79–93.

Biber B, Alkin T: Panic disorder subtypes: Differential responses to CO_2 challenge. Am J Psychiatry 1999;156:739–744.

Bystritsky A, Leuchter AF, Vapnik T: EEG abnormalities in nonmedicated panic disorder. J Nerv Mental Dis 1999;187:113–114.

Caillard V, Rouillon F, Viel JF, Markabi S, The French University Antidepressant Group: Comparative effects of low and high doses of clomipramine and placebo in panic disorders: A double-blind controlled study. Acta Psychiatr Scand 1999;99:51–58.

Coplan JD, Lydiard RB: Brain circuits in panic disorder. Biol Psychiatry 1998;44:1264–1276.

Davis M: Are different parts of the extended amygdala involved in fear versus anxiety? Biol Psychiatry 1998;44:1239–1247.

De Beurs E, van Balkom AJLM, Van Dyck R, Lange A: Long-term outcome of pharmacological and psychological treatment for panic disorder with agoraphobia: A 2-year naturalistic follow-up. Acta Psychiatr Scand 1999;99:59–67.

Friedman BH, Thayer JF, Borkovec TD, Tyrrell RA, Johnson BH, Columbo R: Autonomic characteristics of nonclinical panic and blood phobia. Biol Psychiatry 1993;34:298–310.

Goodard AW, Sholomskas DE, Walton KE, Augeri FM, Charney DS, Heninger GR, Goodman WK, Price LH: Effects of tryptophan depletion in panic disorder. Biol Psychiatry 1994;36:775–777.

Gurguis GNM, Antai-Otong D, Vo SP, Blakeley JE, Orsulak PJ, Petty F, Rush J: Adrenergic receptor function in panic disorder. I. Platelet α_2-receptors: Gi protein coupling, effects of imipramine, and relationship to treatment outcome. Neuropsychopharmacology 1999;20:162–170.

Hyman SE: Brain neurocircuitry of anxiety and fear: implications for clinical research and practice (editorial). Biol Psychiatry 1998;44:1201–1203.

Jäkälä P, Sirviö J, Riekkinen M, Koivisto E, Kejonen K, Vanhanen M, Riekkinen P: Guanfacine and clonidine, alpha₂-agonists, improve paired associates learning but not delayed matching to sample, in humans. Neuropsychopharmacology 1999;20:119–130.

Koyama S, Kubo CH, Rhee JS, Akaike N: Presynaptic serotonergic inhibition of GABAergic synaptic transmission in mechanically dissociated rat basolateral amygdala neurons. J Physiol 1999;518:525–538.

Lechin F, van der Dijs B, Amat J, Lechin S: Central neuronal pathways involved in anxiety behavior: experimental findings; in Lechin F, van der Dijs B (eds): Neurochemistry and Clinical Disorders: Circuitry of Some Psychiatric and Psychosomatic Syndromes. Boca Raton, CRC Press, 1989, pp 49–64.

Lechin F, van der Dijs B, Jara H, Orozco B, Baez S, Jahn E, Benaim M, Lechin E, Lechin ME, Jimenez V, Lechin AE: Plasma neurotransmitter profiles of anxiety, phobia and panic disorder patients: Acute and chronic effects of buspirone. Res Commun Biol Psychol Psychiatry 1997;22:95–110.

Leyton M, Bélanger C, Martial J, Beaulieu S, Corin E, Pecknold J, Kin NY, Meaney M, Thavundayil J, Larue S, Nair V: Cardiovascular, neuroendocrine, and monoaminergic responses to psychological stressors: possible differences between remitted panic disorder patients and healthy controls. Biol Psychiatry 1996;40:353–360.

Lydiard RB, Steiner M, Burnham D, Gergel I: Efficacy studies of paroxetine in panic disorder. Psychopharmacol Bull 1998;34:175–182

Meltzer HY, Flemming R, Robertson A: The effect of buspirone on prolactin and growth hormone in man. Arch Gen Psychiatry 1983;40:1099–1104.

Mongeau R, Marsden CHA: Effect of imipramine treatments on the 5-HT$_{1A}$-receptor-mediated inhibition of panic-like behaviours in rats. Psychopharmacology 1997;131:321–328.

Papp LA, Martinez J, Gorman JM: Arterial epinephrine levels in panic disorder. Psychiatr Res 1998;25:111–112.

Slaap BR, van Vliet IM, Westenberg HGM, Den Boer JA: MHPG and heart rate as correlates of nonresponse to drug therapy in panic disorder patients. Psychopharmacology 1996;127:353–358.

Stein MB, Delaney SM, Chartier MJ, Kroft CD, Hazen AL: [³H]paroxetine binding to platelets of patients with social phobia: Comparison to patients with panic disorder and healthy volunteers. Biol Psychiatry 1995;37:224–228.

Villacres EC, Hollifield M, Katon WJ, Wilkinson CHW, Veith RC: Sympathetic nervous system activity in panic disorder. Psychiatr Res 1987;21:313–321.

Worthington III JJ, Pollack MH, Otto MW, McLean RY, Moroz G, Rosenbaum JF: Long-term experience with clonazepam in patients with a primary diagnosis of panic disorder. Psychopharmacol Bull 1998;34:199–205.

Zacharko RM, Koszycki D, Mendella PD, Bradwejn J: Behavioral, neurochemical, anatomical and electrophysiological correlates of panic disorder: Multiple transmitter interaction and neuropeptide colocalization. Prog Neurobiol 1995;47:371–423.

References for Chapter 9

Abraham WT, Hensen J, Schrier RW: Elevated plasma noradrenaline concentrations in patients with low-output cardiac failure: Dependence on increased noradrenaline secretion rates. Clin Sci 1990;79:429–435.

Adachi M, Oda N, Kokubu F, Minoguchi K: IL-10 induces a Th2 cell tolerance in allergic asthma. Int Arch Allergy Immunol 1999;118:391–394.

Allen DB, Julius JR, Breen TJ, Attie KM: Treatment of glucocorticoid-induced growth suppression with growth hormone. J Clin Endocrinol Metab 1998;83:2824–2829.

Alstergren P, Kopp S: Pain and synovial fluid concentration of serotonin in arthritic temporomandibular joints. Pain 1997;72:137–143.

Amat J, Torres A, Lechin F: Differential effect of footshock stress on humoral and cellular responses of the cat. Life Sci 1993;53:315–322.

Anderson E, Lee G: The polycystic ovarian (PCO) condition: Apoptosis and epithelialization of the ovarian antral follicles are aspects of cystogenesis in the dehydroepiandrosterone (DHEA)-treated rat model. Tissue Cell 1997;29:171–189.

Anderson G, Jenkinson EJ: Thymus organ cultures and T-cell receptor repertoire development. Immunology 2000;100:405–410.

Antel JP, Owens T: Immune regulation and CNS autoimmune disease. J Neuroimmunol 1999;100:181–189.

Aspinall R, Andrew D: Thymic involution in aging. J Clin Immunol 2000;20:250–262.

Ballieux RE: Bidirectional communication between the brain and the immune system. Eur J Clin Invest 1992;22:6–9.

Barbarino A, Corsello SM, Casa SD, Tofani A, Sciuto R, Rota CA, Bollanti L, Barini A: Corticotropin-releasing hormone inhibition of growth hormone-releasing hormone-induced growth hormone release in man. J Clin Endocrinol Metab 1990;71:1368–1374.

Barili P, Bronzetti E, Felici L, Ferrante F, Ricci A, Zaccheo D, Amenta F: Age-dependent changes in the expression of dopamine receptor subtypes in human peripheral blood lymphocytes. J Neuroimmunol 1996;71:45–50.

Bauer J, Herrmann F: Interleukin-6 in clinical medicine. Ann Haematol 1991;62:203–210.

Behbehani MM, Da Costa-Gomez TM: Properties of a projection pathway from the medial preoptic nucleus to the midbrain periaqueductal gray of the rat and its role in the regulation of cardiovascular function. Brain Res 1996;740:141–150.

Bellinghausen I, Brand U, Enk AH, Knop J, Saloga J: Signals involved in the early TH1/TH2 polarization of an immune response depending on the type of antigen. J Allergy Clin Immunol 1999;103:298–306.

Benarroch EE, Balda MS, Finkielman S, Nahmod VE: Neurogenic hypertension after depletion of norepinephrine in anterior hypothalamus induced by 6-hydroxydopamine administration into the ventral pons: Role of serotonin. Neuropharmacology 1983;22:29–34.

Bergquist J, Tarkowski A, Ewing A, Ekman R: Catecholaminergic suppression of immunocompetent cells. Immunol Today 1998;19:562–567.

Berridge MJ: Lymphocyte activation in health and disease. Crit Rev Immunol 1997;17:155–178.

Blalock JE, Bost KL, Smith EM: Neuroendocrine peptide hormones and their receptors in the immune system-production, processing and action. J Neuroimmunol 1985;10:31–40.

Blalock JE: A molecular basis for bidirectional communication between the immune and neuroendocrine systems. Am Physiol Soc 1989;69:1–32.

Bondy B, de Jonge S, Pander S, Primbs J, Ackenheil M: Identification of dopamine D4 receptor mRNA in circulating human lymphocytes using nested polymerase chain reaction. J Neuroimmunol 1996;71:139–144.

Brown GM, Seggie J: Effects of antidepressants on entrainment of circadian rhythms. Prog Neuropsychopharmacol Biol Psychiatry 1988;12: 299–306.

Brown MR, Fisher LA: Glucocorticoid suppression of the sympathetic nervous system and adrenal medulla. Life Sci 1986;39:1003–1012.

Caggiula AR, McAllister CG, Matthews KA, Berga SL, Owens JF, Miller AL: Psychological stress and immunological responsiveness in normally cycling, follicular-stage women. J Neuroimmunol 1995;59:103–111.

Carlson SL, Fox S, Abell KM: Catecholamine modulation of lymphocyte homing to lymphoid tissues. Brain Behav Immunity 1997;11:307–320.

Cash E, Charreire J, Rott O: B-cell activation by superstimulatory influenza virus hemagglutinin: A pathogenesis for autoimmunity? Immunol Rev 1996;152:67–88.

Cerwenka A, Carter LL, Reome JB, Swain SL, Dutton RW: In vivo persistence of CD8 polarized T cell subsets producing type 1 or type 2 cytokines. J Immunol 1998;161:97–105.

Chikanza IC, Panayi GS: Hypothalamic-pituitary mediated modulation of immune function: prolactin as a neuroimmune peptide. Br J Rheumatol 1991;30:203–207.

Chirkov YY: Chirkov LP, Horowitz JD: Suppressed anti-aggregating and cGMP-elevating effects of sodium nitroprusside in platelets from patients with stable angina pectoris. Arch Pharmacol 1996;354:520–525.

Christ AD, Stevens AC, Koeppen H, Walsh S, Omata F, Devergne O, Birkenbach M, Blumberg RS: An interleukin 12-related cytokine is up-regulated in ulcerative colitis but not in Crohn's disease. Gastroenterology 1998;115: 307–313.

Christophers E: The immunopathology of psoriasis. Int Arch Allergy Immunol 1996;110:199–206.

Conti LH, Youngblood KL, Printz MP, Foote SL: Locus coeruleus electrophysiological activity and responsivity to corticotropin-releasing factor in inbred hypertensive and normotensive rats. Brain Res 1997;774:27–34.

Correa SG, Riera CM, Spiess J, Bianco ID: Modulation of the inflammatory response by corticotropin-releasing factor. Eur J Pharmacol 1997; 319:85–90.

Crocker IC, Church MK, Newton S, Townley RG: Glucocorticoids inhibit proliferation and interleukin-4 and interleukin-5 secretion by aeroallergen-specific T-helper type 2 cell lines. Ann Allergy Asthma Immunol 1998;80:509–16.

Cross AH, Lyons JA, San M, Keeling RM, Ku G, Racke MK: T-cells are the main cell type expressing B7-1 and B7-2 in the central nervous system during acute, relapsing and chronic experimental autoimmune encephalomyelitis. Eur J Immunol 1999;29:3140–3147.

D'Ambrosio D, Iellem A, Colantonio L, Clissi B, Pardi R, Sinigaglia F: Localization of Th-cell subsets in inflammation: Differential thresholds for extravasation of Th1 and Th2 cells. Immunol Today 2000;21:183–186.

Dahle CH, Vrethem M, Ernerudh J: T lymphocyte subset abnormalities in peripheral blood from patients with the Guillain-Barré syndrome. J Neuroimmunol 1994;53:219–225.

Dampney RAL: The subretrofacial vasomotor nucleus: Anatomical, chemical and pharmacological properties and role in cardiovascular regulation. Prog Neurobiol 1994;42:197–227.

Davila DR, Brief S, Simon J, Hammer RE, Brinster RL, Kelley KW: Role of growth hormone in regulating T-dependent immune events in aged, nude, and transgenic rodents. J Neurosci Res 1987;18:108–116.

De Simoni MG: Two-way communication pathways between the brain and the immune system. Neurosci Res Commun 1997;21:163–172.

Disshon KA, Dluzen DE: Estrogen reduces acute striatal dopamine responses in vivo to the neurotoxin MPP+ in female, but not male rats. Brain Res 2000;868:95–104.

Douek DC, Koup RA: Evidence for thymic function in the elderly. Vaccine 2000;18:1638–1641.

Downing JEG, Miyan JA: Neural immunoregulation: Emerging roles for nerves in immune homeostasis and disease. Immunol Today 2000;21:281–289.

Drugarin D, Negru S, Koreck A, Zosin I, Cristea C: The pattern of a Th1 cytokine in autoimmune thyroiditis. Immunol Lett 2000;71:73–77.

Durelli L, Ferrero B, Oggero A, Verdun E, Bongioanni MR, Gentile E, Isoardo GL, Ricci A, Rota E, Bergamasco B, Durazzo M, Saracco G, Biava MA, Brossa PC, Giorda L, Pagni R, Aimo G: Autoimmune events during interferon beta-1b treatment for multiple sclerosis. J Neurol Sci 1999;162:74–83.

Egwuagu ChE, Sztein J, Mahdi RM, Li W, Chao-Chan Ch, Smith JA, Charukamnoetkanok P, Chepelinsky AB: IFN-β increases the severity and accelerates the onset of experimental autoimmune uveitis in transgenic rats. J Immunol 1999;162:510–517.

Eisenberg R: Mechanisms of systemic autoimmunity in murine models of SLE. Immunol Res 1998;17:41–47.

Elenkov IJ, Vizi ES: Presynaptic modulation of release of noradrenaline from the sympathetic nerve terminals in the rat spleen. Neuropharmacology 1991;30:1319–1324.

Evans DL, Leserman J, Pedersen CA, Golden RN, Lewis MH, Folds JA, Ozer H: Immune correlates of stress and depression. Psychopharmacol Bull 1989;25:319–328.

Fecho K, Maslonek KA, Dykstra LA, Lysle DT: Alterations of immune status induced by the sympathetic nervous system: Immunomodulatory effects of DMPP alone and in combination with morphine. Brain Behav Immunity 1993;7: 253–270.

Feifel D, Vaccarino FJ: Growth hormone-regulatory peptides (GHRH and somatostatin) and feeding: A model for the integration of central and peripheral function. Neurosci Behav Rev 1994;18:421–433.

Fioroni L, Fava M, Genazzani AD, Facchinetti F, Genazzani R: Life events impact in patients with secondary amenorrhoea. J Psychosom Res 1994;38:617–622.

Flatmark T: Catecholamine biosynthesis and physiological regulation in neuroendocrine cells. Act Physiol Scand 2000;168:1–17.

Forrester AJ, Sullivan V, Simmons A, Blacklaws BA, Smith GL, Nash AA, Minson AC: Induction of protective immunity with antibody to herpes simplex virus type 1 glycoprotein H (gH) and analysis of the immune response to GH expressed in recombinant vaccinia virus. J Gen Virol 1991;72:369–375.

Frank MG, Hendricks SE, Johnson DR, Wieseler JL, Burke WJ: Antidepressants augment natural killer cell activity: In vivo and in vitro. Neuropsychobiology 1999;39:18–24.

Fuchs BA, Campbell KS, Munson AE: Norepinephrine and serotonin content of the murine spleen: Its relationship to lymphocyte β-adrenergic receptor density and the humoral immune response in vivo and in vitro. Cell Immunol 1988;117:339–351.

Fujimura T, Yamanashi R, Masuzawa M, Fujita Y, Katsuoka K, Nishiyama S, Mitsuyama M, Nomoto K: Conversion of the CD4+ T cell profile from Th2- dominant type to Th1-dominant type after varicella-zoster virus infection in atopic dermatitis. J Allergy Clin Immunol 1997;100:274–282.

Fukui Y, Sudo N, Yu XN, Nukina H, Sogawa H, Kubo Ch: The restraint stress-induced reduction in lymphocyte cell number in lymphoid organs correlates with the suppression of in vivo antibody production. J Neuroimmunol 1997;79:211–217.

Fuxe K, Andersson K, Eneroth P, Siegel RA, Agnati LF: Immobilization stress-induced changes in discrete hypothalamic catecholamine levels and turnover, their modulation by nicotine and relationship to neuroendocrine function. Acta Physiol Scand 1983;117:421–426.

Galdiero M, De Martino L, Marcatili A, Nuzzo I, Vitiello M, Cipollaro De L'ero G: Th1 and Th2 cell involvement in immune response to Salmonella typhimurium porins. Immunology 1998;94:5–13.

Gauthier P: Pressor responses and adrenomedullary catecholamine release during brain stimulation in the rat. Can J Physiol Pharmacol 1981; 59:485–492.

Ghigo E, Arvat E, Valente F, Nicolasi M, Boffano GM, Procopio M, Bellone J, Maccario M, Mazza E, Camanni F: Arginine reinstates the somatotrope responsiveness to intermittent growth hormone-releasing hormone administration in normal adults. Neuroendocrinology 1991;54: 291–294.

Gilbey MP, Coote JH, Fleetwood-Walker S, Peterson DF: The influence of the paraventriculospinal pathway, and oxytocin and vasopressin on sympathetic neurones. Brain Res 1982;251: 283–290.

Gill HS, Altmann K, Cross ML, Husband AJ: Induction of T helper 1- and T helper 2-type immune responses during haemonchus contortus infection in sheep. Immunology 2000;99: 458–463.

Ginaldi L, De Martinis M, D'Ostilio A, Marini L, Loreto MF, Corsi MP, Quaglino D: The immune system in the elderly. Immunol Res 1999;20:101–108.

Giustina A, Doga M, Bodini C, Girelli A, Legati F, Bossoni S, Romanelli G: Acute effects of cortisone acetate on growth hormone response to growth hormone-releasing hormone in normal adult subjects. Acta Endocrinol (Copenh) 1990;122:206–210.

Goedegebuure PS, Eberlein TJ: The role of CD4+ tumor-infiltrating lymphocytes in human solid tumors. Immunol Res 1995;14:119–131.

Grignaschi G, Invernizzi RW, Fanelli E, Fracasso C, Caccia S, Samanin R: Citalopram-induced hypophagia is enhanced by blockade of 5-HT$_{1A}$ receptors: role of 5-HT$_{2c}$ receptors. Br J Pharmacol 1998;124:1781–1787.

Gross JA: TNF-R homologues in autoimmune disease. Immunol Today 2000;404:995–999.

Halse AK, Wahren-Herlenius M, Jonsson R: Ro/SS-A- and La/ss-B-reactive B lymphocytes in peripheral blood of patients with Sjögren's syndrome. Clin Exp Immunol 1999;115:208–213.

Halse A, Harley JB, Kroneld U, Jonsson R: Ro/SS-A-reactive B lymphocytes in salivary glands and peripheral blood of patients with Sjögren's syndrome. Clin Exp Immunol 1999;115:203–207.

Harling-Berg CHJ, Park JT, Knopf PM: Role of the cervical lymphatics in the Th2-type hierarchy of CNS immune regulation. J Neuroimmunol 1999;101:111–127.

Herbert TB, Cohen S: Stress and immunity in humans: A meta-analytic review. Psychosom Med 1993;55:364–379.

Holtman JR, Dick TE, Berger AJ: Serotonin-mediated excitacion of recurrent laryngeal and phrenic motoneurons evoked by stimulation of the raphe obscurus. Brain Res 1987;417:12–20.

Homey B, Dieu-Nosjean MC, Wiesenborn A, Massacrier C, Pin JJ, Oldham E, Catron D, Buchanan ME, Müller A, de Waal Malefyt R, Deng G, Orozco R, Ruzicka T, Lehmann P, Lebecque S, Caux CH, Zlotnik A: Up-regulation of macrophage inflammatory protein-3/CCL20 and CC chemokine receptor 6 in psoriasis. J Immunol 2000;164:6621–6632.

Houzen H, Hattori Y, Kanno M, Kikuchi S, Tashiro K, Motomura M, Nakao Y, Nakamura T: Functional evaluation of inhibition of autonomic transmitter release by autoantibody from Lambert-Eaton myasthenic syndrome. Ann Neurol 1998;43:677–680.

Huang FP, Niedbala W, Wei XQ, Xu D, Feng GJ, Robinson JH, Lam Ch, Liew FY: Nitric oxide regulates Th1 cell development through the inhibition of IL-12 synthesis by macrophages. Eur J Immunol 1998;28:4062–4070.

Jackson JC, Walker RF, Brooks WH, Roszman TL: Specific uptake of serotonin by murine macrophages. Life Sci 1988;42:1641–1650.

Jafarian-Tehrani M, Sternberg EM: Animal models of neuroimmune interactions in inflammatory diseases. J Neuroimmunol 1999;100:13–20.

Jayachandran M, Panneerselvam C: Cellular immune responses to vitamin C supplementation in ageing humans assessed by the in vitro leucocyte migration inhibition test. Med Sci Res 1998;26:227–230.

Jendreyko N, Uttenreuther-Fischer MM, Lerch H, Gaedicke G, Fischer P: Genetic origin of IgG antibodies cloned by phage display and anti-idiotypic panning from three patients with autoimmune thrombocytopenia. Eur J Immunol 1998;28:4236–4247.

Kanda N, Tsuchida T, Tamaki K: Testosterone inhibits immunoglobulin production by human peripheral blood mononuclear cells. Clin Exp Immunol 1996;106:410–415.

Kappel M, Poulsen TD, Galbo H, Pedersen BK: Influence of minor increases in plasma catecholamines on natural killer cell activity. Horm Res 1998;49:22–26.

Karalis K, Muglia LJ, Bae D, Hilderbrand H, Majzoub JA: CRH and the immune system. J Neuroimmunol 1997;72:131–136.

Kawahara Y, Kawahara H, Westerink BHC: Comparison of effects of hypotension and handling stress on the release of noradrenaline and dopamine in the locus coeruleus and medial prefrontal cortex of the rat. Arch Pharmacol 1999; 360:42–49.

Kaye WH, Ebert MH, Gwirtsman HE, Weiss SR: Differences in brain serotonergic metabolism between nonbulimic and bulimic patients with anorexia nervosa. Am J Psychiatry 1984;141: 1598–1684.

Kelley KW: Growth hormone, lymphocytes and macrophages. Biochem Pharmacol 1989;38: 705–713.

Kemeny DM: CD8+ T cells in atopic disease. Curr Opin Immunol 1998;10:628–633.

Kerttula TO, Collin P, Mäki M, Hurme M: Normal T-helper 1/T-helper 2 balance in peripheral blood of coeliac disease patients. Scand J Immunol 1999;49:197–202.

Khorram O, Vu L, Yen SSC: Activation of immune function by dehydro-epiandrosterone (DHEA) in age-advanced men. J Ger Soc Am 1997;52: 1–7.

Kjeldsen SE, Rostrup M, Gjesdal K, Eide I: The epinephrine-blood platelet connection with special reference to essential hypertension. Am Heart J 1991;122:330–336.

Kleemann R, Scott FW, Wörz-Pagenstert U, Ratnayake WMN, Kolb H: Impact of dietary fat on Th1/Th2 cytokine gene expression in the pancreas and gut of diabetes-prone BB rats. J Autoimmun 1998;11:97–103.

Kohama T, Terada S, Suzuki N, Inoue M: Effects of dehydroepiandrosterone and other sex steroid hormones on mammary carcinogenesis by direct injection of 7,12-dimethylbenz(a) anthracene (DMBA) in hyperprolactinemic female rats. Breast Cancer Res Treat 1997;43:105–115.

Kohm AP, Sanders VM: Suppression of antigen-specific Th2 cell-dependent IgM and IgG1 production following norepinephrine depletion in vivo. J Immunol 1999;162:5299–5308.

Köller H, Siebler M, Hartung HP: Immunologically induced electrophysiological dysfunction: Implications for inflammatory diseases of the CNS and PNS. Prog Neurobiol 1997;52:1–26.

Korte SM, Van Duin S, Bouws GAH, Koolhaas JM, Bohus B: Involvement of hypothalamic serotonin in activation of the sympathoadrenomedullary system and hypothalamo-pituitary-adrenocortical axis in male wistar rats. Eur J Pharmacol 1991;197:225–228.

Kraemer WJ, Patton JF, Knuttgen HG, Hannan ChJ, Kettler T, Gordon SE, Dziados JE, Fry AC, Frykman PN, Harman EA: Effects of high-intensity cycle exercise on sympathoadrenal-medullary response patterns. J Appl Physiol 1991;70:8–14.

Kubera M, Kenis G, Bosmans E, Scharpé S, Maes M: Effects of serotonin and serotonergic agonists and antagonists on the production of interferon-γ and interleukin-10. Neuropsychopharmacology 2000;23:89–98.

Kuis W, de Jong-de Vos van Steenwijk CCE, Sinnema G, Kavelaars A, Prakken B, Helders PJM, Heijnen CJ: The autonomic nervous system and the immune system in juvenile rheumatoid arthritis. Brain Behav Immunity 1996;10:387–398.

Kwok RP, Juorio AV: Facilitating effect of insulin on brain 5-hydroxytryptamine metabolism. Neuroendocrinology 1987;45:267–273.

Laguzzi R, Talman WT, Reis DJ: Serotonergic mechanisms in the nucleus tractus solitarius may regulate blood pressure and behaviour in the rat. Clin Sci 1982;63:323–326.

Lanzi R, Tannenbaum GS: Time-dependent reduction and potentiation of growth hormone (GH) responsiveness to GH-releasing factor induced by exogenous GH: Role for somatostatin. Endocrinology 1992;130:1822–1828.

Laue L, Peck GL, Loriaux DL, Gallucci W, Chrousos GP: Adrenal androgen secretion in postadolescent acne: Increased adrenocortical function without hypersensitivity to adrenocorticotropin. J Clin Endocrinol Metab 1991;73:380–384.

Lauw FN, Ten-Hove T, Dekkers PEP, de Jonge E, van Deventer SJH, van der Poll T: Reduced Th1, but not Th2, cytokine production by lymphocytes after in vivo exposure of healthy subjects to endotoxin. Infect Immunity 2000;68: 1014–1018.

Lechin F, van der Dijs B, Jakubowicz D, Camero RE, Villa S, Arocha L, Lechin A: Effects of clonidine on blood pressure, noradrenaline, cortisol, growth hormone, and prolactin plasma levels in high and low intestinal tone depressed patients. Neuroendocrinology 1985;41:156–162.

Lechin F, van der Dijs B, Jakubowicz D, Camero RE, Villa S, Lechin E, Gómez F: Effects of clonidine on blood pressure, noradrenaline, cortisol, growth hormone and prolactin plasma levels in low and high intestinal tone subjects. Neuroendocrinology 1985;40:253–261.

Lechin F, van der Dijs B, Jakubowicz D, Camero RE, Lechin S, Villa S, Reinfeld B, Lechin ME: Role of stress in the exacerbation of chronic illness: Effects of clonidine administration on blood pressure, nor-epinephrine, cortisol, growth hormone and prolactin plasma levels. Psychoneuroendocrinology 1987;12:117–129.

Lechin F, van der Dijs B, Vitelli G, Lechin-Baez S, Azócar J, Cabrera A, Lechin A, Jara H, Lechin M, Gómez F, Arocha L: Psychoneuroendocrinological and immunological parameters in cancer patients: Involvement of stress and depression. Psychoneuroendocrinology 1990;15:435–451.

Lechin F, van der Dijs B, Lechin AE, Orozco B, Lechin ME, Báez S, Rada I, León G, Acosta E: Plasma neurotransmitters and cortisol in chronic illness: Role of stress. J Med 1994;25:181–192.

Lechin F, van der Dijs B, Vitelli-Flores G, Báez S, Lechin ME, Lechin AE, Orozco B, Rada I, León G, Jiménez V: Peripheral blood immunological parameters in long-term benzodiazepine users. Clin Neuropharmacol 1994;17:63–72.

Lechin F, van der Dijs B, Benaim M: Benzodiazepines: Tolerability in elderly patients (review). Psychother Psychosom 1996;65:171–182.

Lechin F, van der Dijs B, Lechin M: Plasma neurotransmitters and functional illness (review). Psychother Psychosom 1996;65:293–318.

Lechin F, van der Dijs B, Jara H, Baez S, Orozco B, Jahn E, Lechin ME, Jimenez V, Lechin AE: Successful neuropharmacological treatment of myasthenia gravis: Report of eight cases. Res Commun Biol Psychol Psychiatry 1997;22:81–94.

Lechin F, van der Dijs B, Pardey-Maldonado B, Jahn E, Jiménez V, Orozco B, Baez S, Lechin ME: Enhancement of noradrenergic neural transmission: An effective therapy of myasthenia gravis. Report of 52 consecutive patients. J Med 2000;31:333–362.

Lechner O, Hu Y, Jafarian-Tehrani M, Dietrich H, Schwarz S, Herold M, Haour F, Wick G: Disturbed immunoendocrine communication via the hypothalamo-pituitary-adrenal axis in murine lupus. Brain Behav Immunity 1996;10:337–350.

LeMay LG, Vander AJ, Kluger MJ: The effects of psychological stress on plasma interleukin-6 activity in rats. Physiol Behav 1990;47:957–961.

Li L, Gotta S, Mauviel A, Varga J: L-Tryptophan induces expression of collagenase gene in human fibroblasts: Demonstration of enhanced AP-1 binding and AP-1 binding site-driven promoter activity. Cell Mol Biol Res 1995;41:361–368.

Lindsey BG, Arata A, Morris KF, Hernandez YM, Shannon R: Medullary raphe neurones and baroreceptor modulation of the respiratory motor pattern in the cat. J Physiol 1998;512:863–882.

Lio D, Balistreri CR, Candore G, D'Anna C, Di Lorenzo G, Gervasi F, Listi F, Scola L, Caruso C: In vitro treatment with interleukin-2 normalizes type.1 cytokine production by lymphocytes from elderly. Immunopharmacol Immunotoxicol 2000;22:195–203.

Liu Y, Wolfe SA: Haloperidol and spiperone potentiate murine splenic B cell proliferation. Immunopharmacology 1996;34:147–259.

Livnat S, Felten SY, Carlson SL, Bellinger DL, Felten D: Involvement of peripheral and central catecholamine systems in neural-immune interactions. J Neuroimmunol 1985;10:5–30.

Lonati A, Licenziati S, Canaris AD, Fiorentini S, Pasolini G, Marcelli M, Seidenary S, Caruso A, De Panfilis G: Reduced production of both Th1 and Tc1 lymphocyte subsets in atopic dermatitis. Clin Exp Immunol 1999;115:1–5.

Madden KS, Moynihan JA, Brenner GJ, Felten SY, Felten DL, Livnat S: Sympathetic nervous system modulation of the immune system. III. Alterations in T and B cell proliferation and differentiation in vitro following chemical sympathectomy. J Neuroimmunol 1994;49:77–87.

Majori M, Corradi M, Caminati A, Cacciani G, Bertacco S, Pesci A: Predominant TH1 cytokine pattern in peripheral blood from subjects with chronic obstructive pulmonary disease. J Allergy Clin Immunol 1999;103:458–462.

Matera L, Mori M, Geuna M, Buttiglieri S, Palestro G: Prolactin in autoimmunity and antitumor defence. J Neuroimmunol 2000;109:47–55.

Mathé G, Florentin I, Bruley-Rosset M: Restoration of aging reduced immunity is possible with immunomodulators and is applicable to cancer treatment and prevention. Biomed Pharmacol 1997;51:193–199.

Matheson GK, Gage D, White G, Dixon V, Gipson D: A comparison of the effect of busperone and diazepam on plasma corticosterone levels in rat. Neuropharmacology 1988;27:823–830.

Mazzarella G, Bianco A, Catena E, De Palma R, Abbate GF: Th1/Th2 lymphocyte polarization in asthma. Allergy 2000;55:6–9.

McEwen BS, Biron ChA, Brunson KW, Bulloch K, Chambers WH, Dhabhar FS, Goldfarb RH Kitson RP, Miller AH, Spencer RL, Weiss JM: The role of adrenocorticoids as modulators of immune function in health and disease: Neural, endocrine and immune interactions. Brain Res Rev 1997;23:79–133.

McIntosh R, Watson P, Weetman A: Somatic hypermutation in autoimmune thyroid disease. Immunol Rev 1998;162:219–231.

Mellor AL, Munn DH: Tryptophan catabolism and T-cell tolerance: Immunosuppression by starvation? Rev Immunol Today 1999;20:469–473.

Melvin WS, Boros Lg, Muscarella P, Brandes JL, Johnson JA, Fisher WE, Schirmer WJ, Ellison EC: Dehydroepiandrosterone-sulfate inhibits pancreatic carcinoma cell proliferation in vitro in vivo. Surgery 1997;121:392–397.

Mendlovic S, Mozes E, Eilat E, Doron A, Lereya J, Zakuth V, Spirer Z: Immune activation in non-treated suicidal major depression. Immunol Lett 1999;67:105–108.

Merahi N, Orer HS, Laguzzi R: 5-HT2 receptors in the nucleus tractus solitarius: Characterisation and role in cardiovascular regulation in the rat. Brain Res 1992;575:74–78.

Metz DP, Bottomly K: Function and regulation of memory CD4 T cells. Immunol Res 1999;19:127–141.

Miller RA: Effect of aging on T lymphocyte activation. Vaccine 2000;18:1654–1660.

Mills CD, Kincaid K, Alt JM, Heilman MJ, Hill AM: M-1/M-2 macrophages and the Th1/Th2 paradigm. J Immunol 2000;164:6166–6173.

Mills PJ, Berry ChC, Dimsdale JE, Ziegler MG, Nelesen RA, Kennedy BP: Lymphocyte subset redistribution in response to acute experimental stress: effects of gender, ethnicity, hypertension, and the sympathetic nervous system. Brain Behav Immunity 1995;9:61–69.

Modlin R, Rickinson A: Immunity to infection. Current Opinion Immunol 2000;12:387–389.

Monteleone P, Catapano F, Fabrazzo M, Tortorella A, Maj M: Decreased blood levels of tumor necrosis factor-alpha in patients with obsessive-compulsive disorder. Neuropsychobiology 1998;37:182–185.

Morton ChL, Potter PM: Rhabdomyosarcoma – specific expression of the herpes simplex virus thymidine kinase gene confers sensitivity to ganciclovir. J Pharmacol Exp Ther 1998;286:1066–1073.

Moseley P: Stress proteins and the immune response. Immunopharmacology 2000;48:299–302.

Mouthon L, Lacroix-Desmazes S, Kazatchkine MD: Analysis of self-reactive antibody repertoires in normal pregnancy. J Autoimmunity 1998;11:279–286.

Mulligan K, Grunfeld C, Hellerstein MK, Neese RA, Schambelan M: Anabolic effects of recombinant human growth hormone in patients with wasting associated with human immunodeficiency virus infection. J Clin Endocrinol Metab 1993;77:956–962.

Murphy WJ, Longo DL: Growth hormone as an immunomodulating therapeutic agent. Immunol Today 2000;21:211–212.

Muth ER, Koch KL, Stern RM: Significance of autonomic nervous system activity in functional dyspepsia. Dig Dis Sci 2000;45:854–863.

Nakamura H, Seto T, Nagase H, Yoshida M, Dan S, Ogino K: Inhibitory effect of pregnancy on stress-induced immunosuppression through corticotropin releasing hormone (CRH) and dopaminergic systems. J Neuroimmunol 1997;75:1–8.

Nicholson LB, Kuchroo VK: Manipulation of the Th1/Th2 balance in autoimmune disease. Curr Opin Immunol 1996;8:837–842.

Nimmagadda SR, Spahn JD, Nelson HS, Jenkins J, Szefler SJ, Leung DYM: Fluticasone propionate results in improved glucocorticoid receptor binding affinity and reduced oral glucocorticoid requirements in severe asthma. Ann Allergy Asthma Immunol 1998;81:35–40.

Nisticò G: Communications among central nervous system, neuroendocrine and immune systems: Interleukin-2. Prog Neurobiol 1993;40:463–475.

Odeh M: New insights into the pathogenesis and treatment of rheumatoid arthritis. Clin Immunol Immunopathol 1997;83:103–116.

Ohashi Y, Tanaka A, Kakinoki Y, Ohno Y, Sakamoto H, Kato A, Masamoto T, Washio Y, Nakai Y: Serum level of soluble interleukin-2 receptor in patients with seasonal allergic rhinitis. Scand J Immunol 1997;45:315–321.

Ostenson RC, Lum LG: In vitro differences in lymphocyte subpopulation reactivity in lung cancer patients: Purified protein derivative-specific suppressor T lymphocytes in patients who have received bacillus Calmette-Guerin. Clin Immunol Immunopathol 1984;30:233–240.

Ostrowski K, Hermann C, Bangash A, Schjerling P, Nis Nielsen J, Pedersen KB: A trauma-like elevation of plasma cytokines in humans in response to treadmill running. J Physiol 1998; 513:889–894.

Pan W, Zadina JE, Harlan RE, Weber JT, Banks WA, Kastin AJ: Tumor necrosis factor-α: A neuromodulator in the CNS. Neurosci Behav Rev 1997;21:603–613.

Patel JN, Eisenhofer G, Coppack SW, Miles JM: Norepinephrine spillover in forearm and subcutaneous adipose tissue before and after eating. J Clin Endocrinol Metab 1999;84:2815–2819.

Perine P, Wadhwa M, Buttarello M, Meager A, Facchinetti A, Thorpe R, Biasi G, Gallo P: Effect of IFNγ and anti-IFNγ antibodies on NK cells in multiple sclerosis patients. J Neuroimmunol 2000;105:91–95.

Perini P, Devinsky O, Hauser P, Gallucci WT, Theodore WH, Chrousos GP, Gold PW, Kling MA: Effects of carbamazepine on pituitary-adrenal function in healthy volunteers. J Clin Endocrinol Metab 1992;74:406–412.

Pers JO, Jamin Ch, Le Corre R, Lydyard PM, Youinou P: Ligation of CD5 on resting B cells, but not on resting T cells, results in apoptosis. Eur J Immunol 1998;28:4170–4176.

Petersen KG, Zeisel HJ, Kerp L: The immune response to GHRH, relationship to conformation. Horm Metab Res 1989;21:427–430.

Piccinni MP, Scaletti C, Maggi E, Romagnani S: Role of hormone-controlled Th1-and Th2-type cytokines in successful pregnancy. J Neuroimmunol 2000;109:30–33.

Pierce PA, Xie GX, Peroutka SJ, Green PG, Levine JD: 5-Hydroxytryptamine-induced synovial plasma extravasation is mediated via 5-hydroxytryptamine$_{2A}$ receptors on sympathetic efferent terminals. J Pharmacol Exp Ther 1995;275:502–508.

Porges SW: Cardiac vagal tone: A physiological index of stress. Neurosci Biobehav Rev 1995; 19:225–233.

Prasad AS, Fitzgerald JT, Bao B, Beck FWJ, Chandrasekar PH: Duration of symptoms and plasma cytokine levels in patients with the commom cold treated with zinc acetate. Ann Intern Med 2000;133:245–252.

Raber J, Sorg O, Horn TFW, Yu N, Koob GF, Campbell IL, Bloom FE: Inflammatory cytokines: Putative regulators of neuronal and neuro-endocrine function. Brain Res Rev 1998;26:320–328.

Rapaport R, Oleske J, Ahdieh H, Skuza K, Holland BK, Passannante MR, Denny T: Effects of human growth hormone on immune functions: In vitro studies on cells of normal and growth hormone-deficient children. Life Sci 1987;41:2319–2324.

Ricci A, Bronzetti E, Felici L, Tayebati SK, Amenta F: Dopamine D4 receptor in human peripheral blood lymphocytes: A radioligand binding assay study. Neurosci Lett 1997;229:130–134.

Ricci A, Bronzetti E, Magnini F, Tayebati SK, Zaccheo D, Amenta F: Dopamine D1-like receptor subtypes in human peripheral blood lymphocytes. J Neurosci 1999;96:234–240.

Richard ChA, Stremel RW: Involvement of the raphe in the respiratory effects of gigantocellular area activation. Brain Res Bull 1990;25:19–23.

Rinner I, Schauenstein K, Mangge H, Porta S, Kvetnansky R: Opposite effects of mild and severe stress on in vitro activation of rat peripheral blood lymphocytes. Brain Behav Immunity 1992;6:130–140.

Romagnani S: Th1 and Th2 in human diseases. Clin Immunol Immunopathol 1996;80:225–235.

Roszman TL, Brooks WH: Neural modulation of immune function. J Neuroimmunol 1985;10:59–69.

Sacerdote P, Bianchi M, Panerai AE: In vivo and in vitro clomipramine treatment decreases the migration of macrophages in the rat. Eur J Pharmacol 1997;319:287–290.

Schlesinger I, Rabinowitz R, Brenner T, Abramsky O, Schlesinger M: Changes in lymphocyte subsets in myasthenia gravis: Correlation with level of antibodies to acetylcholine receptor and age of patient. Neurology 1992;42:321–357.

Schmidt HH, Neumeister P, Kainer F, Karpf EF, Linkesch W, Sill H: Treatment of essential thrombocythemia during pregnancy: Antiabortive effect of interferon-α? Ann Hematol 1998; 77:291–292.

Schultz DR, Arnold PI, Jy W, Valant PA, Gruber J, Ahn YS, Mao FW, Mao WW, Horstman LL: Anti-CD36 autoantibodies in thrombotic thrombocytopenic purpura and other thrombotic disorders: Identification of an 85 kD form of CD36 as a target antigen. Br J Haematol 1998;103:849–857.

Schwarz MJ, Späth M, Müller-Bardorff H, Pongratz DE, Bondy B, Ackenheil M: Relationship of substance P, 5-hydroxyindole acetic acid and tryptophan in serum of fibromyalgia patients. Neurosci Lett 1999;259:196–198.

Scolding NJ, Zajicek JP, Wood N, Compston DAS: The pathogenesis of demyelinating disease. Prog Neurobiol 1994;43:143–173.

Shanks N, Francis D, Zalcman S, Meaney MJ, Anisman H: Alterations in central catecholamines associated with immune responding in adult and aged mice. Brain Res 1994;666:77–87.

Shimoda K, Yamada N, Ohi K, Tsujimoto T, Takahashi K, Takahashi S: Chronic administration of tricyclic antidepressants suppresses hypothalamo-pituitary-adrenocortical activity in male rats. Psychoneuroendocrinology 1988; 13:431–440.

Shomali ME: The use of anti-aging hormones. Melatonin, growth hormone, testosterone, and dehydroepiandrosterone: Consumer enthusiasm for unproven therapies. Med J 1997;46:181–186.

Shukitt-Hale B, Stillman MJ, Lieberman HR: Tyrosine administration prevents hypoxia-induced decrements in learning and memory. Physiol Behav 1996;59:867–871.

Sigmundsdottir H, Sigurgeirsson B, Troye-Blomberg M, Good MF, Valdimarsson H, Jonsdottir I: Circulating T cells of patients with active psoriasis respond to streptococcal M-peptides sharing sequences with human epidermal keratins. Scand J Immunol 1997;45:688–697.

Sigola LB, Zinyama RB: Adrenaline inhibits macrophage nitric oxide production through α1 and α2 adrenergic receptors. Immunology 2000;100:359–363.

Skok J, Poudrier J, Gray D: Dendritic cell-derived IL-12 promotes B cell induction of Th2 differentiation: A feedback regulation of Th1 development. J Immunol 1999;163:4284–4291.

Smit AB, Van Kesteren RE, Li KW, Van Mínnen J, Spijker S, Van Heerikhuizen H, Geraerts WPM: Towards understanding the role of insulin in the brain: Lessons from insulin-related signaling systems in the invertebrate brain. Prog Neurobiol 1998;54:35–54.

Smith EM, Cadet P, Stefano GB, Opp MR, Hughes TK: IL-10 as a mediator in the HPA axis and brain. J Neuroimmunol 1999;100:140–148.

Soper WY, Melzack R: Stimulation-produced analgesia: Evidence for somatotopic organization in the midbrain. Brain Res 1982;251:301–311.

Sortino MA, Aleppo G, Scapagnini U, Canonico PL: Different responses of gonadotropin-releasing hormone (GnRH) release to glutamate receptor agonists during aging. Brain Res Bull 1996;41:359–362.

Sporton SCE, Shepheard SL, Jordan D, Ramage AG: Microinjection of 5-HT$_{1A}$ agonists into the dorsal motor vagal nucleus produce a bradycardia in the atenolol-pretreated anaesthetized rat. Br J Pharmacol 1991;104:466–470.

Stein RC, Dalgleish AG: Immunomodulatory agents: The cytokines. Eur J Cancer 1994;30:400–404.

Storms WW, Theen Ch: Clinical adverse effects of inhaled corticosteroids: Results of a questionnaire survey of asthma specialists. Ann Allergy Asthma Immunol 1998;80:391–394.

Straub RH, Miller LE, Schölmerich J, Zietz B: Cytokines and hormones as possible links between endocrinosenescence and immunosenescence. J Neuroimmunol 2000;109:10–15.

Suarez GA, Giannini C, Bosch EP, Barohn RJ, Wodak J, Ebeling P, Anderson R, McKeever PE, Bromberg MB, Dyck PJ: Immune brachial plexus neuropathy: Suggestive evidence for an inflammatory-immune pathogenesis. Neurology 1996;46:559–561.

Sugahara M, Shiraishi H: Dopamine D$_1$ and D$_2$ receptor agents and their interaction influence the synaptic density of the rat prefrontal cortex. Neurosci Lett 1999;259:141–144.

Tamada K: T-cell costimulation in a new light. Immunol Today 2000;6:283–289.

Tang Y, Shankar R, Gamelli R, Jones S: Dynamic norepinephrine alterations in bone marrow: Evidence of functional innervation. J Neuroimmunol 1999;96:182–189.

Tews DS, Goebel HH: Cytokine expression profile in idiopathic inflammatory myopathies. J Neuropathol Exp Neurol 1996;55:342–347.

Thompson TL, Moss RL: Estrogen regulation of dopamine release in the nucleus accumbens: Genomic-and nongenomic-mediated effects. J Neurochem 1994;62:1750–1756.

Thompson TL, Moss RL: Modulation of mesolimbic dopaminergic activity over the rat estrous cycle. Neurosci Lett 1997;229:145–148.

Thyaga-Rajan S, Madden KS, Stevens SY, Felten DL: Effects of L-deprenyl treatment on noradrenergic innervation and immune reactivity in lymphoid organs of young F344 rats. J Neuroimmunol 1999;96:57–65.

Tourbah A, Clapin A, Gout O, Fontaine B, Liblau R, Batteux F, Stiévenart JL, Weill B, Lubetzki C, Lyion-Caen O: Systemic autoimmune features and multiple sclerosis. Arch Neurol 1998; 55:517–521.

Tsukamoto K, Sved AF, Ito S, Komatsu K, Kanmatsuse K: Enhanced serotonin-mediated responses in the nucleus tractus solitarius of spontaneously hypertensive rats. Brain Res 2000;863:1–8.

Tsunoda S, Kawano M, Koni I, Kasahara Y, Yachie A, Miyawaki T, Seki H: Diminished expression of CD59 on activated CD8+ T cells undergoing apoptosis in systemic lupus erythematosus and Sjögren's syndrome. Scand J Immunol 2000;51:293–299.

Umetsu DT, DeKruyff RH: Updates on cells and cytokines. TH1 and TH2 CD4+ cells in human allergic diseases. J Allergy Clin Immunol 1997; 100:1–6.

Van Giersbergen PL, Palkovits M, De Jong W: Involvement of neurotransmitters in the nucleus tractus solitarii in cardiovascular regulation. Physiol Rev 1992;72:789–817.

Vile JM, Strange PG: D2-like dopamine receptors are not detectable on human peripheral blood lymphocytes. Biol Psychiatry 1996;40:881–885.

Walker RF, Codd EE: Neuroimmunomodulatory interactions of norepinephrine and serotonin. J Neuroimmunol 1985;10:41–58.

Watanabe N, Maeda M, Okamoto T, Sasaki H, Tsuji N, Akiyama S, Kobayashi D, Sato T, Yamauchi N, Niitsu Y: Tumor necrosis factor and interferon-β augment anticolon antibody-dependent cellular cytotoxicity in ulcerative colitis. Immunopharmacol Immunotoxicol 1996;18:15–26.

Watanabe T, Kawada T, Kurosawa M, Sato A, Iwai K: Adrenal sympathetic efferent nerve and catecholamine secretion excitation caused by capsaicin in rats. Am J Physiol 1988;255:E23–E27.

Wehrenberg WB, Janowski BA, Piering AW, Culler F, Jones KL: Glucocorticoids: Potent inhibitors and stimulators of growth hormone secretion. Endocrinology 1990;126:3200–3203.

Weksler ME, Szabo P: The effect of age on the B-cell repertoire. J Clin Immunol 2000;20:240–249.

Widner B, Weiss G, Fuchs D: Tryptophan degradation to control T-cell responsiveness. Comment Immunol Today 2000;21:250–252.

Willette RN, Punnen S, Krieger AJ, Sapru HN: Interdependence of rostral and caudal ventrolateral medullary areas in the control of blood pressure. Brain Res 1984;321:169–174.

Yang QS, Jobe PC, Dailey JW: Noradrenergic mechanisms for the anticonvulsant effects of desipramine and yohimbine in genetically epilepsy-prone rats: studies with microdialysis. Brain Res 1993;610:24–31.

Yang Z, Coote JH: Influence of the hypothalamic paraventricular nucleus on cardiovascular neurones in the rostral ventrolateral medulla of the rat. J Physiol 1998;513:521–530.

Yau JC, Germond C, Gluck S, Cripps Ch, Verma S, Burns BF, Koski TM, Lister DC, Goss GD: Mitoxantrone, prednimustine, and vincristine for elderly patients with aggressive non-Hodgkin's lymphoma. Am J Hematol 1998;59:156–160.

Yin D: Stress-related immunosuppression and opioid-dependent Fas expression. Immunol Today 2000;191:1423–1428.

Yong VW, Chabot S, Stuve O, Williams G: Interferon beta in the treatment of multiple sclerosis: Mechanisms of action. Neurobiol 1996;51: 682–689.

Zamir N, Skofitsch G, Jacobowitz DM: Distribution of immunoreactive melanin-concentrating hormone in the central nervous system of the rat. Brain Res 1986;373:241–245.

Zhang D, Kishihara K, Wang B, Mizobe K, Kubo CH, Nomoto K: Restraint stress-induced immunosuppression by inhibiting leukocyte migration and Th1 cytokine expression during the intraperitoneal infection of Listeria monocytogenes. J Neuroimmunol 1998;92:139–151.

Zuñiga E, Motran C, Montes CL, Diaz FL, Bocco JL, Gruppi A: Trypanosoma cruzi-induced immunosuppression: B cells undergo spontaneous apoptosis and lipopolysaccharide (LPS) arrests their proliferation during acute infection. Clin Exp Immunol 2000;119:507–515.

References for Chapter 10

Agrewala JN, Wilkinson RJ: Differential regulation of Th1 and Th2 cells by p91–110 and p21–40 peptides of the 16-kD α-crystallin antigen of Mycobacterium tuberculosis. Clin Exp Immunol 1998;114:392–397.

Aharoni R, Teitelbaum D, Sela M, Arnon R: Bystander suppression of experimental autoimmune encephalomyelitis by T cell lines and clones of the Th2 type induced by copolymer 1. J Neuroimmunol 1998;91:135–146.

Amital H, Swissa M, Bar-Dayan Y, Buskila D, Shoenfeld Y: New therapeutic avenues in autoimmunity. Res Immunol 1996;147:361–376.

Benschop RJ, Schedlowski M, Wienecke H, Jacobs R, Schmidt RE: Adrenergic control of natural killer cell circulation and adhesion. Brain Behav Immunity 1997;11:321–332.

Blom B, Res PCM, Spits H: T cell precursors in man and mice. Clin Rev Immunol 1998;18: 371–388.

Brady LS: Stress, antidepressant drugs, and the locus coeruleus. Brain Res Bull 1994;35:545–556.

Bright JJ, Du C, Coon M, Sriman S, Klaus SJ: Prevention of experimental allergic encephalomyelitis via inhibition of IL-12 signaling and IL-12-mediated Th1 differentiation: An effect of the novel anti-inflammatory drug lisofylline. J Immunol 1998;161:7015–7022.

Carpenter S: Inclusion body myositis: A review. J Neuropathol Exp Neurol 1996;55(11):1105–1114.

Cope AP: Regulation of autoimmunity by proinflammatory cytokines. Curr Opin Immunol 1998;10:669–676.

Dedhia V, Goluszko E, Wu B, Deng C, Christadoss P: The effect of B cell deficiency on the immune response to acetylcholine receptor and the development of experimental autoimmune myasthenia gravis. Clin Immunol Immunopathol 1998;87:266–275.

Demissie S, Rogers CF, Hiramoto NS, Ghanta VK, Hiramoto RN: Are coline a muscarinic cholinergic agent conditions central pathways that modulate natural killer cell activity? J Neuroimmunol 1995;59:57–63.

Di Renzo M, Rubegni P, De Aloe G, Paulesu L, Pasqui AL, Andreassi L, Auteri A: Extracorporeal photochemotherapy restores Th1/Th2 imbalance in patients with early stage cutaneous T-cell lymphoma. Immunology 1997;92: 99–103.

Dieleman LA, Palmen MJ, Akol H, Bloemena E, Peña AS, Meuwissen SGM, Van Rees EP: Chronic experimental colitis induced by dextran sulphate sodium (DSS) is characterized by Th1 and Th2 cytokines. Clin Exp Immunol 1998;114:385–391.

Drugarin D, Negru S, Koreck A, Zosin I, Cristea C: The pattern of a TH1 cytokine in autoimmune thyroiditis. Immunol Lett 2000;71:73–77.

Funakoshi K, Kadota T, Atobe Y, Nakano M, Goris RC, Kishida R: Serotonin-immunoreactive axons in the cell column of sympathetic preganglionic neurons in the spinal cord of the filefish *Stephanolepis cirrhifer*. Neurosci Lett 2000;280:115–118.

Gollob JA, Murphy EA, Mahajan S, Schnipper CP, Ritz J, Frank DA: Altered interleukin-12 responsiveness in Th1 and Th2 cells is associated with the differential activation of STAT5 and STAT1. Blood 1998;91:1341–1354.

Graeff FG, Viana MB, Mora PO: Dual role of 5-HT in defense and anxiety. Neurosci Biobehav Rev 1997;21:791–799.

Haas DA, George SR: Single or repeated mild stress increases synthesis and release of hypothalamic corticotropin-releasing factor. Brain Res 1988; 461:230–237.

Haddad A, Bienvenu J, Miossec P: Increased production of a Th2 cytokine profile by activated whole blood cells from rheumatoid arthritis patients. J Clin Immunol 1998;18:399–406.

Hakonarson H, Maskeri N, Carter C, Grunstein MM: Regulation of TH1-and TH2-type cytokine expression and action in atopic asthmatic sensitized airway smooth muscle. J Clin Invest 1999;103:1077–1087.

Harold KL, Schlinkert RT, Mann DK, Reeder CB, Noel P, Fitch TR, Braich TA, Camoriano JK: Long-term results of laparoscopic splenectomy for immune thrombocytopenic purpura. Mayo Clin Proc 1999;74:37–39.

Homey B, Dieu-Nosjean MC, Wiesenborn A, Massacrier C, Pin JJ, Oldham E, Catron D, Buchanan ME, Müller A, de Waal MR, Deng G, Orozco R, Ruzicka T, Lehmann P, Lebecque S, Caux CH, Zlotnik A: Up-regulation of macrophage inflammatory protein-3α /CCL20 and CC chemokine receptor 6 in psoriasis. J Immunol 2000;164:6621–6632.

Homo-Delarche F, Dardenne M: The neuroendocrine-immune axis. Semin Immunopathol 1993;14:221–238.

Jendreyko N, Uttenreuther-Fischer MM, Lerch H, Gaedicke G, Fischer P: Genetic origin of IgG antibodies cloned by phage display and antiidiotypic panning from three patients with autoimmune thrombocytopenia. Eur J Immunol 1998;28:4236–4247.

Kalinkovich A, Weisman Z, Greenberg Z, Nahmias J, Eitan S, Stein M, Bentwich Z: Decreased CD4 and increased CD8 counts with T cell activation is associated with chronic helminth infection. Clin Exp Immunol 1998;114: 414–421.

Kaufmann S, Jones KL, Wehrenberg WB, Culler FL: Inhibition by prednisone of growth hormone (GH) response to GH-releasing hormone in normal men. J Clin Endocrinol Metab 1988; 67:1258–1262.

Kemeny DM: CD8+ T cells in atopic disease. Curr Opin Immunol 1998;10:628–633.

Kemp EH, Gawkrodger DJ, Watson PF, Weetman AP: Autoantibodies to human melanocyte-specific protein Pmel17 in the sera of vitiligo patients: a sensitive and quantitative radioimmunoassay (RIA). Clin Exp Immunol 1998; 114:333–338.

Khan S, Haddad P, Montague L, Summerton C: Systemic lupus erythematosus presenting as mania. Acta Psychiatr Scand 2000;101:406–408.

Kuwabara S, Asahina M, Koga M, Mori M, Yuki N, Hattori T: Two patterns of clinical recovery in Guillain-Barré syndrome with IgG anti-GM1 antibody. Neurology 1998;51:1656–1660.

Laaris N, Le Poul E, Hamon M, Lanfumey L: Stress-induced alterations of somatodendritic 5-HT1A autoreceptor sensitivity in the rat dorsal raphe nucleus-in vitro electrophysiological evidence. Fundam Clin Pharmacol 1997;11: 206–214.

Laugero KD, Moberg GP: Summation of behavioral and immunological stress: Metabolic consequences to the growing mouse. Am J Physiol Endocrinol Metab 2000;279:44–49.

Maecker H, Desai A, Dash R, Rivier J, Vale W, Sapolsky R: Astressin, a novel and potent CRF antagonist, is neuroprotective in the hippocampus when administered after a seizure. Brain Res 1997;744:166–170.

Mason D, Powrie F: Control of immune pathology by regulatory T cells. Curr Opin Immunol 1998;10:649–655.

Melero J, Tarragó D, Núñez-Roldán A, Sánchez B: Human polyreactive IgM monoclonal antibodies with blocking activity against self-reactive IgG. Scand J Immunol 1997;45:393–400.

Menon JN, Bretscher PA: Parasite dose determines the Th1/Th2 nature of the response to Leishmania major independently of infection route and strain of host or parasite. Eur J Immunol 1998;28:4020–4028.

Mouthon L, Lacroix-Desmazes S, Kazatchkine MD: Analysis of self-reactive antibody repertoires in normal pregnancy. J Autoimmun 1998;11:279–286.

Murray JS: How the MHC selects Th1/Th2 immunity. Immunol Today 1998;19:157–163.

Nagumo H, Agematsu K, Shinozaki K, Hokibara S, Ito S, Takamoto M, Nikaido T, Yasui K, Uehara Y, Yachie A, Komiyama A: CD27/CD70 interaction augments IgE secretion by promoting the differentiation of memory B cells into plasma cells. J Immunol 1998;161:6496–6502.

Nakamura H, Seto T, Nagase H, Yoshida M, Dan S, Ogino K: Inhibitory effect of pregnancy on stress-induced immunosuppression through corticotropin releasing hormone (CRH) and dopaminergic systems. J Neuroimmunol 1997; 75:1–8.

Nicholson LB, Kuchroo VK: Manipulation of the Th1/Th2 balance in autoimmune disease. Curr Opinion Immunol 1996;8:837–842.

Ohta Y, Yamane M, Sohda T, Makino H: Tak-603 selectively suppresses Th1-type cytokine production and inhibits the progression of adjuvant arthritis. Immunology 1997;92:75–83.

Pers JO, Jamin Ch, Le Corre R, Lydyard PM, Youinou P: Ligation of CD5 on resting B cells, but not on resting T cells, results in apoptosis. Eur J Immunol 1998;28:4170–4176.

Pohl-Koppe A, Burchett SK, Thiele EA, Hafler DA: Myelin basic protein reactive Th2 T cells are found in acute disseminated encephalomyelitis. J Neuroimmunol 1998;91:19–27.

Prinz JC: Psoriasis vulgaris, streptococci and the immune system: A riddle to be solved soon? Scand J Immunol 1997;45:583–586.

Puertas A, Frias J, Ruiz E, Ortega E: Effect of CRF injected into the median eminence on GH secretion in female rats under different steroid status. Neurochem Res 1996;21:897–901.

Schmidt HH, Neumeister P, Kainer F, Karpf EF, Linkesch W, Sill H: Treatment of essential thrombocythemia during pregnancy: Antiabortive effect of interferon-α? Ann Hematol 1998; 77:291–292.

Schreiber S, Nikolaus S, Hampe J, Hämling J, Koop I, Groessner B, Lochs H, Schraedler A: Tumour necrosis factor α and interleukin 1β in relapse of Crohn's disease. Lancet 1999;353: 459–461.

Schultz DR, Arnold PI, Jy W, Valant PA, Gruber J, Ahn YS, Mao FW, Mao WW, Horstman LL: Anti-CD36 autoantibodies in thrombotic thrombocytopenic purpura and other thrombotic disorders: Identification of an 85 kD form of CD36 as a target antigen. Br J Haematol 1998;103:849–857.

Setijoso E, Robberecht W, van Eycken P, Roskams T, Tack J, Van Steenbergen W: Myasthenia gravis: Another autoimmune disease associated with hepatitis C virus infection. Dig Dis Sci 1999;44:186–189.

Teller WM: Recent progress in research on the central regulation of growth hormone secretion. Monatsschr Kinderheilkd 1977;125:812–817.

Thyaga-Rajan S, Madden KS, Kalvass JC, Dimitrova SS, Felten SY, Felten DL: L-Deprenyl-induced increase in IL-2 and NK cell activity accompanies restoration of noradrenergic nerve fibers in the spleens of old F344 rats. J Neuroimmunol 1998;92:9–21.

Von Boehmer H, Rajewsky K: Lymphocyte development commitment, selection and switching. Curr Opin Immunol 2000;12:141–143.

Wang ZY, Okita DK, Howard JF, Conti-Fine BM: CD4+ T cell repertoire on the α-subunit of muscle acetylcholine receptor in myasthenia gravis. J Neuroimmunol 1998;91:33–42.

Windhagen A, Anderson DE, Carrizosa A, Balashov K, Weiner HL, Hafler DA: Cytokine secretion of myelin basic protein reactive T cells in patients with multiple sclerosis. J Neuroimmunol 1998;91:1–9.

Zhang GX, Yu LY, Shi FD, Xiao BG, Björk J, Hedlund G, Link H: Linomide suppresses both Th1 and Th2 cytokines in experimental autoimmune myasthenia gravis. J Neuroimmunol 1997;73:175–182.

Zorrilla EP, McKay JR, Luborsky L, Schmidt K: Relation of stressors and depressive symptoms to clinical progression of viral illness. Am J Psychiatry 1996;153:626–635.

Barnard CJ, Behnke JM, Gage AR, Brown H, Smithurst PR: Modulation of behaviour and testosterone concentration in immunodepressed male laboratory mice *(Mus musculus).* Physiol Behav 1997;61:907–917.

Bonneau RH, Brehm MA, Kern AM: The impact of psychological stress on the efficacy of anti-viral adoptive immunotherapy in an immunocompromised host. J Neuroimmunol 1997;78:19–33.

Charles PC, Weber KS, Cipriani B, Brosnan CF: Cytokine, chemokine and chemokine receptor mRNA expression in different strains of normal mice: Implications for establishment of a Th1/Th2 bias. J Neuroimmunol 1999;100:64–73.

Cohen S, Doyle WJ, Skoner DP: Psychological stress, cytokine production, and severity of upper respiratory illness. Psychosom Med 1999;61:175–180.

Correa SG, Rodriguez-Galán MC, Rivero V, Riera CM: Chronic varied stress modulates experimental autoimmune encephalomyelitis in Wistar rats. Brain Behav Immunity 1998;12:134–148.

Cunnick JE, Lysle DT, Kucinski BJ, Rabin BS: Evidence that shock-induced immune suppression is mediated by adrenal hormones and peripheral β adrenergic receptors. Biochem Behav 1990;36:645–651.

Dantzer R, Kelley KW: Stress and Immunity: An integrated view of relationships between the brain and the immune system. Life Sci 1989;44:1995–2008.

De Souza E: Neuroendocrine effects of benzodiazepines. J Psychiatr Res 1990;24(suppl 2):111–119.

Diamant M, Wied D: Autonomic and behavioral effects of centrally administered corticotropin-releasing factor in rats. Endocrinology 1991;129:446–454.

Dotti C, Taleisnik S: Beta-adrenergic receptors in the premammillary nucleus mediate the inhibition of LH release evoked by locus coeruleus stimulation. Neuroendocrinology 1984;38:6–11.

Fotoulaki M, Nousia-Arvanitakis S, Augoustidou-Savvopoulou P, Kanakoudi-Tsakalides F, Zaramboukas T, Vlachonikolis J: Clinical application of immunological markers as monitoring tests in celiac disease. Dig Dis Sci 1999;44:2133–2138.

Friedman Y, Bacchus R, Raymond R, Joffe RT, Nobrega JN: Acute stress increases thyroid hormone levels in rat brain. Biol Psychiatry 1999;45:234–237.

Gagro A , Gordon J: The interplay between T helper subset cytokines and IL-12 in directing human B lymphocyte differentiation. Eur J Immunol 1999;29:3369–3379.

Griffin AC, Lo WD, Wolny AC, Whitacre CC: Suppression of experimental autoimmune encephalomyelitis by restraint stress: Sex differences. J Neuroimmunol 1993;44:103–116.

Gupta S: Molecular steps of cell suicide: An insight into immune senescence. J Clin Immunol 2000;20:229–239.

Hahn YS, Kim Y, Jo SO, Han HS: Reduced frequencies of peripheral interferon-γ- producing CD4+ and CD4– cells during acute Kawasaki disease. Int Arch Allergy Immunol 2000;122:293–298.

Hernández F, Blanquer A, Linares M, López A, Tarín F, Cerveró A: Autoimmune thrombocytopenia associated with hepatitis C virus infection. Acta Haematol 1998;99:217–220.

Hinrichsen H, Fölsch U, Kirch W: Modulation of the immune response to stress in patients with systemic lupus erythematosus: Review of recent studies. Eur J Clin Invest 1992;22(suppl 1):21–25.

Hohagen F, Timmer J, Weyerbrock A, Fritsch-Montero R, Ganter U, Krieger S, Berger M, Bauer J: Cytokine production during sleep and wakefulness and its relationship to cortisol in healthy humans. Neuropsychobiology 1993;28:9–16.

Ihan A, Tepes B, Gubina M: Diminished TH1-type cytokine production in gastric mucosa T-lymphocytes after *H. pylori* eradication in duodenal ulcer patients. Eur J Physiol 2000;440 (suppl 5):89–90.

Kocjan T, Wraber B, Repnik , Hojker S: Changes in Th1/Th2 cytokine balance in Graves' disease. Eur J Physiol 2000;440(suppl 1):94–95.

Košnik M, Wraber B: Shift from th2 to th1 response in immunotheraphy with venoms. Eur J Physiol 2000;440(suppl 1):R71-R72.

Kovalovsky D, Refojo D, Holsboer F, Arzt E: Molecular mechanisms and Th1/Th2 pathways in corticosteroid regulation of cytokine production. J Neuroimmunol 2000;109:23–29.

Kulkarni A, Jan-Ravi T, Brodmerkel GJ, Agrawal RM: Inflammatory myositis in association with inflammatory bowel disease. Dig Dis Sci 1997;42:1142–1145.

Larsson PT, Hjemdahl P, Olsson G, Egberg N, Hornstra G: Altered platelet function during mental stress and adrenaline infusion in humans: Evidence for an increased aggregability in vivo as measured by filtragometry. Clin Sci 1989;76:369–376.

Lechin F, van der Dijs B, Insausti CL, Gomez F: Treatment of ulcerative colitis with thioproperazine. J Clin Gastroenterol 1982d;4:445–449.

Lechin F, van der Dijs B, Acosta E, Gomez F, Lechin E, Arocha L: Distal colon motility and clinical parameters in depression. J Affect Dis 1983a;5:19–26.

Lechin F, van der Dijs B, Gomez F, Arocha L, Acosta E, Lechin E: Distal colon motility as a predictor of antidepressant response to fenfluramine, imipramine and clomipramine. J Affect Dis 1983b;5:27–35.

Lechin F, van der Dijs B, Gomez F, Lechin E, Oramas O, Villa S: Positive symptoms of acute psychosis: Dopaminergic or noradrenergic overactivity? Res Commun Psychol Psychiatr Behav 1983c;8:23–54.

Lechin F, van der Dijs B, Insausti CL, Gomez F, Villa S, Lechin AE, Arocha L, Oramas O: Treatment of ulcerative colitis with clonidine. J Clin Pharmacol 1985a;25:219–226.

Lechin F, van der Dijs B, Jackubowicz D, Camero RE, Villa S, Arocha L, Lechin AE: Effects of clonidine on blood pressure, noradrenaline, cortisol, growth hormone, and prolactin plasma levels in high and low intestinal tone depressed patients. Neuroendocrinology 1985b;41:156–162.

Lechin F, van der Dijs B, Jackubowicz D, Camero RE, Villa S, Lechin E, Gomez F: Effects of clonidine on blood pressure, noradrenaline, cortisol, growth hormone, and prolactin plasma levels in high and low intestinal tone subjects. Neuroendocrinology 1985c;40:253–261.

Lechin F, van der Dijs B, Azocar J, Amat J, Vitelli-Florez G, Martinez C, Lechin-Baez S, Jimenez V, Cabrera A, Cardenas M, Villa S: Stress, immunology and cancer: Effect of psychoactive drugs. Arch Ven Farmac Terap 1987a;6:28–41.

Lechin F, van der Dijs B, Jackubowicz D, Camero RE, Lechin S, Villa S, Reinfeld B, Lechin ME: Role of stress in the exacerbation of chronic illness: Effects of clonidine administration on blood pressure and plasma norepinephrine, cortisol, growth hormone and prolactin concentrations. Psychoneuroendocrinology 1987b;12:117–129.

Lechin F, van der Dijs B, Azocar J, Vitelli-Florez G, Lechin S, Villa S, Jara H, Cabrera A: Neurochemical and immunological profiles of three clinical stages in 50 advanced cancer patients. Proceedings of the III Interamerican Congress of Clinical Pharmacology and Therapeutics. Arch Ven Farm Terap 1988b;7(suppl 1):abstr 39.

Lechin F, van der Dijs B, Gomez F, Villa S, Cabrera A, Jimenez V, Guerrero H, Lechin AE: Plasma neurotransmitters profile in depressive syndromes. Proceedings of the III Interamerican Congress of Clinical Pharmacology and Therapeutics and the XII Latinamerican Congress of Pharmacology. Arch Ven Farm Terap 1988c;7(suppl 1):abstr 7.

Lechin F, van der Dijs B, Villa S, Jara H, Rada I, Lechin ME, Jimenez V, Gomez F: Plasma neurotransmitters profile in chronic illness. Proceedings of the III Interamerican Congress of Clinical Pharmacology and Therapeutics. Arch Ven Farm Terap 1988d;7(suppl 1):abstr 38.

Lechin F, van der Dijs B, Amat J, Lechin ME: Central neuronal pathways involved in depressive syndrome: Experimental findings; in Lechin F, van der Dijs B (eds): Neurochemistry and Clinical Disorders: Circuitry of Some Psychiatric and Psychosomatic Syndromes. Boca Raton, CRC Press, 1989a, pp 6–89.

Lechin F, van der Dijs B, Gomez F, Lechin E, Acosta E, Arocha L: Biological markers in the assessment of central autonomic nervous functioning: An approach to the diagnosis of some psychiatric and psychosomatic syndromes; in Lechin F, van der Dijs B (eds): Neurochemistry and Clinical Disorders: Circuitry of Some Psychiatric and Psychosomatic Syndromes. Boca Raton, CRC Press, 1989b, pp 151–226.

Lechin F, van der Dijs B, Lechin S, Vitelli-Florez G, Lechin ME, Cabrera A: Neurochemical, hormonal and immunological views of stress: Clinical and therapeutic implications in Crohn's disease and cancer; in Velazco M (ed): Recent Advances in Pharmacology and Therapeutics. International Congress Series 839. Amsterdam, Excerpta Medica, 1989d, pp 57–70.

Lechin F, van der Dijs B, Rada I, Jara H, Lechin AE, Cabrera A, Lechin ME, Jimenez V, Gomez F, Villa S, Acosta E, Arocha L: Plasma neurotransmitters and cortisol in duodenal ulcer patients: Role of stress. Dig Dis Sci 1990a;35:1313–1319.

Lechin F, van der Dijs B, Vitelli-Florez G, Lechin-Baez S, Azocar J, Cabrera A, Lechin AE, Jara H, Lechin ME, Gomez F, Arocha L: Psychoneuroendocrinological and immunological parameters in cancer patients: Involvement of stress and depression. Psychoneuroendocrinology 1990b;15:435–451.

Lechin F, van der Dijs B, Lechin ME, Jara H, Lechin AE, Cabrera A, Rada I, Orozco B, Jimenez V, Valderrama T: Dramatic improvement with clonidine of acute pancreatitis showing raised catecholamines and cortisol plasma levels: Case report of five patients. J Med 1992b;23:339–351.

Lechin F, van der Dijs B, Lechin ME, Jara H, Lechin A, Baez S, Orozco B, Rada I, Cabrera A, Arocha L, Jimenez V, Leon G: Plasma neurotransmitters throughout oral glucose tolerance test in non-depressed essential hypertension patients. Clin Exp Hypertens 1993;15:209–240.

Lechin F, van der Dijs B, Baez-Lechin S, Lechin AE, Orozco B, Lechin ME, Rada I, Jara H, Gomez F, Cabrera A, Jimenez V, Arocha L, Leon G: Two types of irritable bowel syndrome: Pathophysiologic and pharmacological considerations. Arch Ven Farmacol Terap 1994a;12:105–114.

Lechin F, van der Dijs B, Lechin AE, Orozco B, Lechin ME, Baez S, Rada I, Leon G, Acosta E: Plasma neurotransmitters and cortisol in chronic illness: Role of stress. J Med 1994b;25:181–192.

Lechin F, van der Dijs B, Vitelli-Florez G, Lechin-Baez S, Lechin ME, Lechin AE, Orozco B, Rada I, Leon G, Jimenez V: Peripheral blood immunological parameters in long-term benzodiazepine users. Neuropharmacology 1994c;17:63–72.

Lechin F, van der Dijs B, Orozco B, Lechin AE, Baez S, Lechin ME, Rada I, Acosta E, Arocha L, Jimenez V, Leon G, Garcia Z: Plasma neurotransmitters, blood pressure and heart rate during supine-resting, orthostasis and moderate exercise in dysthymic depressed patients. Biol Psychiatry 1995a;37:884–891.

Lechin F, van der Dijs B, Orozco B, Lechin ME, Baez S, Lechin AE, Rada I, Acosta E, Arocha L, Jimenez V, Leon G, Garcia Z: Plasma neurotransmitters, blood pressure, and heart rate during supine-resting, orthostasis, and moderate exercise conditions in major depressed patients. Biol Psychiatry 1995b;38:166–173.

Lechin F, van der Dijs B, Lechin AE, Orozco B, Lechin ME, Baez-Lechin S, Rada I, Leon G, Garcia Z, Jimenez V: Plasma neurotransmitters, blood pressure and heart rate during supine-resting, orthostasis and moderate exercise stress test in healthy humans before and after the parasympathetic blockade with atropine. Res Commun Biol Psychol Psychiatry 1996a; 21:55–72.

Lechin F, van der Dijs B, Orozco B, Lechin AE, Baez S, Lechin ME, Benaim M, Acosta E, Arocha L, Jimenez V, Leon G, Garcia Z: Plasma neurotransmitters, blood pressure and heart rate during supine-resting, orthostasis, and moderate exercise in severely ill patients: A model of failing to cope with stress. Psychother Psychosom 1996b;65:129–136.

Lechin F, van der Dijs B, Orozco B, Lechin ME, Lechin AE: Increased levels of free-serotonin in plasma of symptomatic asthmatic patients. Ann Allergy Asthma Immunol 1996c;77:245–253.

Lechin F, van der Dijs B, Lechin ME: Plasma neurotransmiters and functional illness. Psychother Psychosom 1996d;65:293–318.

Lechin F, van der Dijs B, Benaim M: Benzodiazepines: Tolerability in elderly patients. Psychother Psychosom 1996e;65:171–182.

Lechin F, van der Dijs B, Orozco B, Jara H, Rada I, Lechin ME, Lechin AE: Neuropharmacological treatment of bronchial asthma with an antidepressant drug: tianeptine: a double-blind cross-over placebo-controlled study. Clin Pharmacol Ther 1998a;64:223–232.

Lechin F, van der Dijs B, Lechin A, Orozco B, Lechin ME, Lechin AE: The serotonin uptake-enhancing drug tianeptine suppresses asthmatic symptoms in children: A double-blind cross-over placebo-controlled study. J Clin Pharmacol 1998b;38:918–925.

Lechin ME, Jara H, Villa S, Gomez F, Cabrera A, Guerrero H, van der Dijs B, Lechin F: Plasma neurotransmitters profile in somatoform disorders. Proceedings of the III Interamerican Congress of Clinical Pharmacology and Therapeutics. Arch Ven Farm Terap 1988a;7(suppl 1):abstr 2.

Lechin ME, Jara H, Rada I, Villa S, Cabrera A, Jimenez V, van der Dijs B, Lechin F: Plasma neurotransmitters profile in irritable bowel syndrome (IBS): Spastic colon. Proceedings of the III Interamerican Congress of Clinical Pharmacology and Therapeutics. Arch Ven Farm Terap 1988b;7(suppl 1):abstr 87.

Lechin S, Vitelli G, Martinez C, Fernandez M, Cabrera A, van der Dijs B, Azocar J, Lechin F: Plasma neurotransmitters, lymphocyte subpopulations and natural killer cell activity in terminal cancer patients. Proceedings of the III Interamerican Congress of Clinical Pharmacology and Therapeutics. Arch Ven Farm Terap 1988;7(suppl 1):abstr 37.

Maes M, Van Bockstaele DR, Van Gastel A, Song C, Schotte CH, Neels H, DeMeester I, Scharpe S, Janca A: The effects of psychological stress on leukocyte subset distribution in humans: Evidence of immune activation. Neuropsychobiology 1999;39:1–9.

Martínez V, Rivier J, Wang L , Taché Y: Central injection of a new corticotropin-releasing factor (CRF) antagonist, astressin, blocks CRF- and stress-related alterations of gastric and colonic motor function. J Pharmacol Exp Ther 1997;280:754–760.

Mizobe K, Kishihara K, El-Naggar RE, Madkour GA, Kubo CH, Nomoto K: Restraint stress-induced elevation of endogenous glucocorticoid suppresses migration of granulocytes and macrophages to an inflammatory locus. J Neuroimmunol 1997;73:81–89.

Morley JE, Raleigh MJ, Brammer GL, Yuwiler A, Geller E, Flannery J, Hershman JM: Serotonergic and catecholaminergic influence on thyroid function in the vervet monkey. Eur J Pharmacol 1980;67:283–288.

Nagata T, Kiriike N, Tobitani W, Kawarada Y, Matsunaga H, Yamagami S: Lymphocyte subset, lymphocyte proliferative response, and soluble interleukin-2 receptor in anorexic patients. Biol Psychiatry 1999;45:471–474.

Ostrowski K, Hermann C, Bangash A, Schjerling P, Nielsen JN, Pedersen BK: A trauma-like elevation of plasma cytokines in humans in response to treadmill running. J Physiol 1998;513:889–894.

Pedersen BK, Kappel M, Klokker M, Nielsen HB, Secher NH: The immune system during exposure to extreme physiologic conditions. Int J Sports Med 1994;15(suppl 3):116–121.

Platzer C, Döcke WD, Volk HD, Prösch S: Catecholamines trigger IL-10 release in acute systemic stress reaction by direct stimulation of its promoter/enhancer activity in monocytic cells. J Neuroimmunol 2000;105:31–38.

Pradalier A, Launay JM: Immunological aspects of migraine. Biomed Pharmacother 1996;50:64–70.

Shanks N, Renton C, Zalcman S, Anisman H: Influence of change from grouped to individual housing on a T-cell-dependent immune response in mice: Antagonism by diazepam. Pharmacol Biochem Bebav 1994;47:497–502.

Stefanski V, Engler H: Social stress, dominance and blood cellular immunity. J Neuroimmunol 1999;94:144–152.

Suzuki K, Totsuka M, Nakaji S, Yamada M, Kudoh S, Liu Q, Sugawara K, Yamaya K, Sato K: Endurance exercise causes interaction among stress hormones, cytokines, neutrophil dynamics, and muscle damage. J Appl Physiol 1999; 87:1360–1367.

Wakelkamp IM, Gerding MN, Van Der Meer JW, Prummel MF, Wiersinga WM: Both Th1- and Th2-derived cytokines in serum are elevated in Graves' ophthalmopathy. Clin Exp Immunol 2000;121:453–457.

Yehuda R, Meyer JS: A role for serotonin in the hypothalamic-pituitary-adrenal response to insulin stress. Neuroendocrinology 1984;38:25–32.

Zaccone P, Hutchings P, Nicoletti F, Penna G, Adorini L, Cooke A: The involvement of IL-12 in murine experimentally induced autoimmune thyroid disease. Eur J Immunol 1999;29:1933–1942.

References for Chapter 12

Cazzola M, Matera MG: 5-HT modifiers as a potential treatment of asthma. Trends in Pharmacol Sci 2000;21:13–16.

Dupont LJ, Pype JL,Dernedts MG, De Leyn P, Denefhe G, Verleden GM: The effects of 5-HT on cholinergic contraction in human airways in vitro. Eur Respir J 1999;14:642–649.

Hervé P, Launay JM, Scrobohaci ML, Brenot F, Simonneau G, Petitpretz P, Poubeau P, Cerrina J, Duroux P, Drouet L: Increased plasma serotonin in primary pulmonary hypertension. Am J Med 1995;99:249–254.

Lechin AE, Varon J, van der Dijs B, Lechin F: Plasma catecholamines and indoleamines during attacks and remission on severe bronchial asthma: possible role of stress. Am J Respir Crit Care Med 1994;149:A778.

Lechin F: Central and plasma 5HT, vagal tone and airways. Trends in Pharmacol Sci 2000;21: 425.

Lechin F: Asthma, asthma medication and autonomic nervous system dysfunction. Clin Physiol 2001;6:723.

Lechin F, van der Dijs B, Lechin AE: Severe asthma and plasma serotonin. Allergy 2002;57: 258–259.

Lechin F, van der Dijs B: Serotonin and pulmonary vasoconstriction. J Appl Physiol 2002;92: 1363–1364.

Lechin F, van der Dijs B, Orozco B, Lechin ME, Lechin AE: Increased levels of free-serotonin in plasma of symptomatic asthmatic patients. Ann Allergy Asthma Immunol 1996;77:245–253.

Lechin F, van der Dijs B, Orozco B, Jara H, Rada I, Lechin ME, Lechin AE: Neuropharmacological treatment of bronchial asthma with an antidepressant drug: tianeptine. A double-blind crossover placebo-controlled study. Clin Pharmacol Ther 1998a;64:223–232.

Lechin F, van der Dijs B, Lechin A, Orozco B, Lechin ME, Lechin AE: The serotonin uptake-enhancing drug tianeptine suppresses asthmatic symptoms in children. A double-blind crossover placebo-controlled study. J Clin Pharmacol 1998b;38:918–925.

Subject Index